Neurology

AN ILLUSTRATED COLOUR TEXT

Commissioning Editor: Michael Parkinson
Development Editor: Lulu Stader
Project Manager: Frances Affleck
Design Direction: Erik Bigland
Illustration Manager: Bruce Hogarth

Neurology

SECOND EDITION

AN ILLUSTRATED COLOUR TEXT

Geraint Fuller MA MD FRCP
Consultant Neurologist,
Gloucestershire Royal Hospital,
Gloucester, UK

Mark Manford MD MRCP
Consultant Neurologist,
Bedford Hospital,
Bedford, UK
Addenbrooke's Hospital
Cambridge, UK

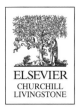

ELSEVIER
CHURCHILL
LIVINGSTONE

EDINBURGH   LONDON   NEW YORK   OXFORD   PHILADELPHIA   ST LOUIS   SYDNEY   TORONTO   2006

ELSEVIER
CHURCHILL
LIVINGSTONE

© Harcourt Publishers Limited 2000
© 2006, Elsevier Limited. All rights reserved.

First edition 2000
Second edition 2006

ISBN 0441-0071-3

British Library Cataloguing in Publication Data
A catalogue record for this book is available from the British Library

Library of Congress Cataloging in Publication Data
A catalog record for this book is available from the Library of Congress

your source for books, journals and multimedia in the health sciences
www.elsevierhealth.com

Working together to grow libraries in developing countries

www.elsevier.com | www.bookaid.org | www.sabre.org

ELSEVIER   BOOK AID International   Sabre Foundation

The publisher's policy is to use **paper manufactured from sustainable forests**

Printed in China

Preface

Neurology has a reputation for being one of the more difficult medical specialities. Medical students in the United Kingdom usually have only brief neurology firm attachments and infrequently work in neurology departments after qualification. And yet neurological problems are very common, accounting for 10% of general practice consultations and 20% of acute medical admissions. How can medical students and junior doctors get to grips with a difficult subject that is met with in everyday practice?

This book aims to provide a framework on which to build the clinical skills to cope with most common neurological problems. The first section describes the basic principles, the second section provides an approach to history taking and examination, the third describes current methods of neurological investigation, the fourth outlines an approach to common presenting problems and the fifth section provides information about different neurological diseases. The final section provides some clinical cases for you to practise on.

The format aims to be 'more magazine than textbook' in its approach, dividing the subject into 'bite-sized' chunks. A book this size clearly cannot be exhaustive; there are whole books written about subjects mentioned in passing in a single sentence. But hopefully this introductory text will form the basis of a sound approach to the diagnosis and management of most patients with neurological problems.

Gloucester and Bedford   G.F.
2005   M.M.

Acknowledgements

We are grateful to all those who have helped with this project. In particular we would like to thank the medical illustration department at Gloucestershire Royal Hospital for their help in producing the images. We are indebted to Dr Liz Brown, Dr Shelly Renowden, Professor Seth Love, Mrs Barbara Harney, Vashti Bond and Peter Murphy for providing some of the illustrations for this book. We are also grateful for the help and patience of our editor, Lulu Stader.

Contents

Organization of the nervous system

The practice of clinical neurology depends on an appreciation of the structure and function of the nervous system. However, a detailed knowledge of neuroanatomy is not essential. This section will outline some of the important neuroanatomy needed for clinical neurology. Some areas, for example the anatomy of the visual system, will be described in the relevant section.

The levels of the nervous system

The nervous system is very complicated, in terms of both its structure and its physiology. Fortunately, when things go wrong they can be categorized on the basis of a relatively simple scheme of neuroanatomy. The nervous system can be thought of as having different levels (Fig. 1). The distribution and type of the clinical problem will often point to the affected level. For example, a patient who is confused must have a disturbance affecting the cerebral hemispheres. There are some situations when the level cannot immediately be determined: for example, a patient with foot drop could have a problem in the peripheral nerve, nerve root, spinal cord or cerebral hemisphere. Terminology used to describe disturbances at different levels is given in Box 1.

The central nervous system

The cerebral hemispheres

The cerebral hemispheres contain the apparatus of higher function. The dominant hemisphere (left in right-handed people) controls speech and the non-dominant hemisphere provides more spatial awareness. Different lobes undertake different functions (Fig. 2).

- frontal – motor control of the opposite side of the body, insight and control of emotions, and, in the dominant hemisphere, output of speech
- temporal – memory and emotions and dominant hemisphere, comprehension of speech

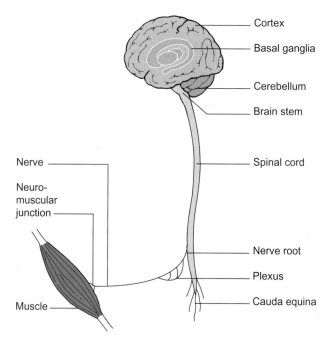

Fig. 1 **Levels of the nervous system.**

Labels: Cortex, Basal ganglia, Cerebellum, Brain stem, Spinal cord, Nerve root, Plexus, Cauda equina, Nerve, Neuro-muscular junction, Muscle

---

> ## Box 1
>
> **Terminology**
> Abnormalities in the different levels of the nervous system can be referred to according to different terms. One commonly used system is described here. The suffix -opathy can be replaced by -itis if there is thought to be an inflammatory basis to the disturbance.
>
> - **Encephalopathy**: abnormality of the brain (may be refined by terms such as focal, diffuse, metabolic or toxic).
> - **Myelopathy**: abnormality of the spinal cord.
> - **Radiculopathy**: abnormality of a single nerve root.
> - **Polyradiculopathy**: abnormality of many nerve roots.
> - **Plexopathy**: abnormality of a plexus (brachial or lumbar).
> - **Polyneuropathy or neuropathy**: abnormality of many nerves.
> - **Mononeuropathy**: abnormality of single named nerve.
> - **Mononeuritis multiplex**: an abnormality of multiple named nerves.
> - **Myopathy**: abnormality of muscle (myositis or polymyositis – inflammation of muscle).
> - **Meningitis**: inflammation of the meninges.
>
> These terms can be combined with one another or other qualifiers to produce descriptions such as focal encephalopathy, or meningoencephalomyelitis (inflammation of the meninges, brain and spinal cord).

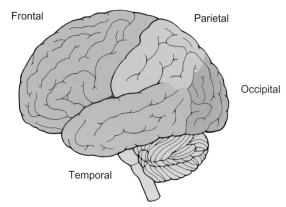

Fig. 2 **Lobes of the brain.**

Labels: Frontal, Parietal, Occipital, Temporal

- parietal – sensation of the opposite side of the body and appreciation of space, especially in the non-dominant hemisphere
- occipital – appreciation of vision.

The basal ganglia

The basal ganglia are interconnected deep nuclei including the putamen, caudate, globus pallidum and substantia nigra with complicated interrelations. They are involved in the integration of motor and sensory inputs. For the most part, detailed appreciation of their anatomy is not essential because when things go wrong they produce clinical syndromes such as Parkinson's disease.

Cerebellum

The cerebellum coordinates movement and is important in the control of balance and posture. The cerebellar

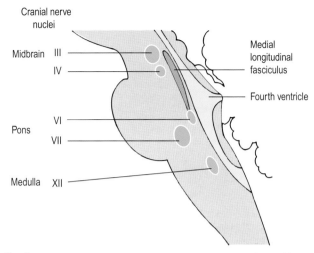

Fig. 3 **Level of cranial nerve nuclei in the brain stem, indicated by Roman numerals.**

hemispheres control coordination on the same side of the body. The central cerebellar structures are important in gait and sitting balance.

Brain stem
The brain stem contains nuclei, including the reticular formation, which maintains consciousness, and those for the cranial nerves (3–12), and the large white matter tracts running from the spinal cord to more central structures and vice versa. The descending motor tract, the corticospinal tract, mostly crosses over (decussates) in the pyramids in the medulla. The ascending dorsal column crosses in the medulla. The most useful nuclei for localization are the 3rd, 4th, 6th, 7th and 12th (Fig. 3). The fact that these tracts cross in the brain stem is helpful in localization of any lesion. A brain stem lesion can produce a cranial nerve lesion on one side and limb signs on the other side (for example, a left-sided facial sensory loss and a right-sided sensory loss in the arm and leg in the lateral medullary syndrome).

The spinal cord
The spinal cord contains the sensory and motor tracts and within it are the anterior horn cells, the cell bodies of the motor neurones that run through the ventral root. These motor fibres in the ventral root join the dorsal root and leave the spinal canal. The sensory cell bodies lie outside the spinal cord, though within the spinal canal, in the dorsal root ganglion. The organization of the internal structure is helpful for localizing lesions and is described on pages 80–81.

The spinal cord is organized segmentally. This means that the nerves that arise in one segment innervate particular muscle groups (myotomes) and provide sensation for particular areas of skin (dermatomes). The dermatomes and myotomes are summarized on pages 23–25, 27 and 83. The spinal cord segments are referred to by the level at which the nerve root leaves the spinal canal. In the cervical spine these are numbered so that the root leaves the spinal canal above the vertebral body, except C8, which goes out below the 7th cervical vertebra and above the 1st thoracic vertebra. In the thoracic (T1 to T12), lumbar (L1 to L5) and sacral (S1 to S5) spine the segment goes out below the respective vertebra. However, the segments are not adjacent to the vertebral body as the spinal cord stops growing before the spinal column. This difference is most marked in the lumbar spine. In adults, the spinal cord ends (segmental level S5) at the level of the L1 vertebra.

The peripheral nervous system
The *nerve roots* leave the spinal canal through their exit foramina. In the lumbar spine the nerve roots from the lower end of the spinal cord form the *cauda equina* before leaving the lumbosacral spinal canal.

The roots combine in the cervical and lumbosacral regions to form the *brachial plexus* and *lumbosacral plexus*. The detailed anatomy of this area is occasionally useful, but most neurologists would refer to diagrams in these situations.

The brachial and lumbosacral plexuses then divide into named nerves. Lesions of nerve roots and named nerves produce a characteristic distribution of motor and sensory loss.

Stimulation of the motor nerves will then lead to the release of acetylcholine at the neuromuscular junction, which binds to acetylcholine receptors, leading to muscle contraction.

Motor levels
In addition to considering these anatomical levels, clinicians group patterns of muscle weakness together as follows:

- upper motor neurone, including the corticospinal system from the cortex up to the synapse with the anterior horn cell
- lower motor neurone, which includes the anterior horn cell within the spinal cord and its axon extending to the neuromuscular junction
- neuromuscular junction
- muscle weakness.

These are the major divisions in the motor system and most motor deficits can be classified on clinical grounds.

Autonomic nervous system
The autonomic nervous system controls the automatic aspects of the nervous system. It is classified into two divisions:

- *sympathetic 'alarm' system*, which arises from the spinal segments T1 to L2
- *parasympathetic 'holiday' system*, which arises from the brain stem (associated with cranial nerves 3, 7 and 9) and the spinal segments S2–4.

This is considered further on pages 114–115.

Other levels of the nervous system
Not all types of neurological disorder fall into the system described above. One of the most difficult areas in clinical neurology is the diagnosis and management of patients with symptoms or signs that are not organically determined. These can be manifestations of overt psychiatric problems (e.g. the weakness and lethargy of a patient with depression) or they can be the sole manifestation of the psychiatric illness (e.g. a patient with a non-organic weakness or with non-epileptic seizures). These are discussed in pages 116–119.

> *Organization of the nervous system*
>
> - It is useful to think of the organization of the nervous system in terms of different levels.
> - The cerebral hemispheres control the opposite side of the body.
> - Language is found in the dominant hemisphere.
> - The spinal cord is organized segmentally.

Neurological thinking

How does an experienced clinical neurologist come to a clinical diagnosis? Considering how this is done helps to appreciate the knowledge and skills that are needed and to understand how they are applied.

The process of diagnosis involves:

■ *Background knowledge* of neurological symptoms and signs, the clinical features of neurological syndromes and diseases, neuroanatomy and an appreciation of the incidence of different neurological syndromes.
■ *The techniques* of taking a neurological history and conducting a neurological examination. The techniques that are used will depend on the patient's problem and different approaches will be used in different clinical settings.
■ A method of *synthesizing* this information: 'neurological thinking' (Fig. 1).

The background knowledge of the different neurological conditions is dealt with mainly in section 5 of this book. The techniques of history taking and examination are described in section 2, and their application in particular situations in section 4. The process of synthesis of information is best acquired with clinical experience and is learnt from teaching at the bedside or by watching a neurologist in outpatients. However, it is easier to learn if you understand what is involved in the process.

Making a neurological diagnosis

There are two ways of making a neurological diagnosis clinically.

'Wiring diagram analysis' or anatomical localization

This method tends to be emphasized in teaching because it involves deduction of the site of a lesion from knowledge of neuroanatomy and of the neuropathological process from the history, e.g. the recognition that a combined trigeminal, facial and auditory nerve lesion is sited at the cerebellopontine angle. This is useful, and having seen one constellation of signs, the pattern is recognized the next time.

This process is led by the history but is primarily a synthesis of findings on clinical examination. In trying to make sense of the physical signs, one should think about which level of the nervous system is being affected (p. 2). The onset and progression of the anatomically determined symptoms reflect the underlying pathology; this information is taken from the history, and is discussed further on pages 8–9.

Pattern recognition or syndromic diagnosis

This is the only method in many neurological diagnoses where the site of the lesion cannot be deduced

neuroanatomically, e.g. migraine, Parkinson's disease, myotonic dystrophy and some forms of epilepsy. In addition, once experienced, pattern recognition can be used to work out the site of lesions, for example recognition of the clinical picture of Brown–Séquard syndrome (Fig. 2), which is due to a lesion of one half of the spinal cord, rather than working out the localization from first principles (see p. 80 for more on Brown–Séquard syndrome).

Different levels of diagnosis

It is important to understand that neurological diagnoses can be made with different degrees of sophistication (Fig. 3; Table 1). For example, it can be deduced that a right-handed patient with a slowly progressive right-sided hemiparesis and aphasia has a left hemisphere lesion (anatomical diagnosis) and that it is likely to be a space-occupying lesion because of the slow onset (clinical diagnosis). A brain scan demonstrates a mass that is thought to be an intrinsic brain tumour (radiological diagnosis), and biopsy and neuropathological examination finds an astrocytoma (pathological diagnosis).

Following a clinical examination there may well not be a definitive diagnosis, but there should be a working diagnosis, usually with a differential diagnosis. This could be a

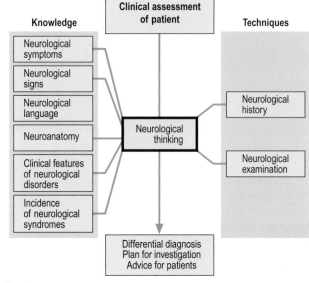

Fig. 1 **Neurological thinking.**

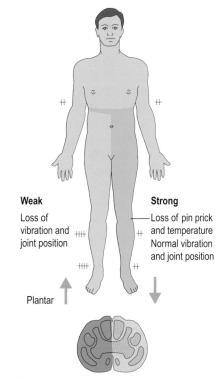

Fig. 2 **Brown–Séquard syndrome: a right-sided T8 lesion.**

definitive syndromic diagnosis (e.g. migraine with aura, clinically definite multiple sclerosis), a syndromic diagnosis requiring further investigation (e.g. motor neurone disease), an anatomical diagnosis (e.g. myopathy), a description of the clinical problem (e.g. single seizure or left sixth nerve palsy) or simply a description of the symptom (e.g. blackout ?cause).

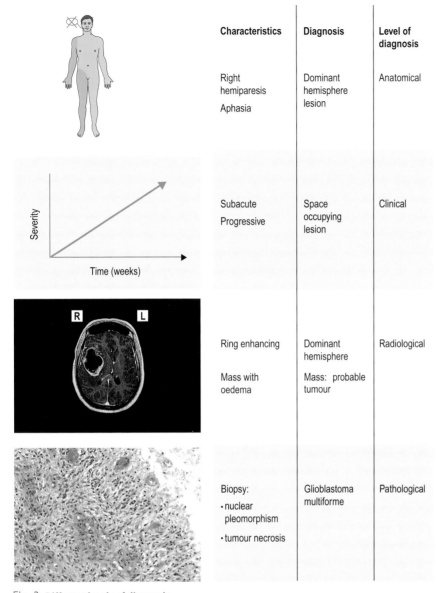

Characteristics	Diagnosis	Level of diagnosis
Right hemiparesis Aphasia	Dominant hemisphere lesion	Anatomical
Subacute Progressive	Space occupying lesion	Clinical
Ring enhancing Mass with oedema	Dominant hemisphere Mass: probable tumour	Radiological
Biopsy: • nuclear pleomorphism • tumour necrosis	Glioblastoma multiforme	Pathological

Fig. 3 **Different levels of diagnosis.**

Table 1 **Different types of diagnosis**	
■ Anatomical	■ Aetiological
■ Syndromic	■ Pathological
■ Radiological	■ Genetic

Common and important disorders

In considering any clinical problem it is useful to think about the common disorders, as these occur most commonly. However, in most clinical situations there are rare but important disorders that need to be considered much more often than their incidence merits, for example:

■ Wilson's disease is a rare abnormality of copper metabolism that can present with Parkinsonism. Drug therapy to prevent further accumulation of copper is the specific treatment. This is rare but needs to be considered in younger patients with movement disorders.

■ Migraine and tension headache are common. Temporal arteritis, subarachnoid haemorrhage and meningitis are rarer, but are life-threatening and require specific treatments and therefore need to be considered frequently despite occurring rarely.

Throughout this book, estimates of the incidence of the conditions discussed will be given. This is important information in reaching a diagnosis. The example often given to illustrate this is in the identification of a small bird outside a window. It is much more likely to be a sparrow than a canary. However, this is not a good illustration as canaries are bright yellow and if it was bright yellow it probably is a canary. A better example is a bird of prey circling above; it is a buzzard, but what type? A bird book tells you there are three European

buzzards (the common buzzard, rough-legged buzzard and the honey buzzard) that differ in minor ways *but also* that the common buzzard is common, whereas the rough-legged and honey buzzards are rare visitors to the UK. It is almost certainly a common buzzard, but one should watch out for the differences in wing length and width that distinguish these other buzzards.

Investigation

The next stage is planning the investigation. This depends on the condition concerned. Investigations are used in four ways:

■ To confirm the diagnosis, e.g. finding a positive anti-acetylcholine receptor antibody confirms the diagnosis of myasthenia gravis.

■ To support the diagnosis, e.g. finding periventricular white matter changes on magnetic resonance imaging supports the clinical diagnosis of multiple sclerosis.

■ To exclude alternative diagnoses, e.g. an erythrocyte sedimentation rate test in a patient with late-onset headaches to exclude the diagnosis of temporal arteritis. Investigations are undertaken for alternative diagnoses if they are common, or if rarer and responsive to specific treatment.

■ To look for the cause of the neurological problem, e.g. seeking risk factors for atherosclerosis and evidence of carotid stenosis in a patient following a small anterior circulation stroke (pp. 70–71).

In undertaking these investigations it is important to be aware of the sensitivity (how often does the test find true positives?) and specificity (reflecting false priorities) of the different investigations in different clinical settings. Accurate clinical assessment enables the best use of investigations.

Neurological thinking

■ Clinical assessment involves the *synthesis* of information obtained using *clinical skills*, history taking and neurological examination, combined with *background knowledge* about neurological disease.

■ Diagnoses can be made at different levels, for example syndromic, radiological or pathological.

■ Common disorders are important because they are common. For different clinical problems there are a few rare but important conditions to consider.

Pathological processes in neurology

It is useful to appreciate the ways in which the nervous system malfunctions. This is important clinically because the time course of any pathological process is described by the patient in the history. It also provides a framework for understanding different types of disease, particularly rarer diseases that you might not otherwise know about.

Broadly, pathological processes can be divided into (Fig. 1):

- **S**ystemic – abnormalities in the nervous system secondary to systemic disease
- **I**ntrinsic – arising within the nervous system
- **V**ascular – resulting from disturbances in the blood supply to the nervous system
- **E**xtrinsic – affecting the nervous system from outside.

Hint: remember this as SIVE. There is some overlap between these categories.

Systemic

These changes are usually due to metabolic, toxic, nutritional, immunological or endocrine disorders (Table 1).

Metabolic

The function of the nervous system requires appropriate systemic homeostasis. If disrupted, this commonly produces a metabolic encephalopathy, with confusion or coma as seen in hypoglycaemia or hyponatraemia. The neurological manifestations may overshadow the other features of these metabolic disturbances.

Other metabolic changes produce more insidious nervous system damage. For example, diabetes mellitus causes peripheral neuropathies, more often if glycaemic control is poor. The gradual accumulation of copper in Wilson's disease produces psychiatric disturbances and a Parkinsonian syndrome.

Toxic

Neurotoxins can affect the central or peripheral nervous system. The most common neurotoxin is alcohol; others include drugs, heavy metals, organic solvents and rarer 'designer' drugs. These substances can produce acute neurological illnesses or subacute or chronic illnesses. Some effects of drugs are common: for example, the extrapyramidal syndromes seen with antipsychotic agents and the cerebellar syndromes seen with phenytoin or carbamazepine toxicity.

Nutritional

Most nutritional deficiencies produce chronic or subacute problems. Vitamin B12 deficiency leads to subacute combined degeneration of the cord and a peripheral neuropathy. Thiamine deficiency leads to Korsakoff's psychosis (marked loss of short-term memory) and Wernicke's encephalopathy (ophthalmoplegia, ataxia and confusion). The metabolic effects of thiamine can be very sudden in their onset.

Immunological

Systemic immunological diseases such as systemic lupus erythematosus or sarcoidosis can affect the nervous system by directly producing destructive inflammatory lesions in the brain, spinal cord or peripheral nerve or by producing vasculitis and vascular lesions.

Endocrinological

Endocrinological diseases particularly affect muscle, for example steroid myopathy.

Vascular

The nervous system can be affected by vascular disease in two ways:

- Haemorrhage – can be within the substance of the brain, in the subarachnoid space, in the subdural compartment or the extradural space.
- Infarction – can be caused by an embolus, thrombosis or arterial disease such as vasculitis.

With the exception of subdural haematoma, these are characterized by a sudden onset.

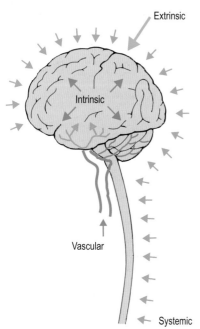

Fig. 1 **Four types of pathological processes.**

Table 1 **Systemic processes**		
Disorder	**Clinical syndrome**	
Metabolic	Hypo- or hyperglycaemia, hyponatraemia, hypoxia, hypercarbia, hyper- or hypocalcaemia } Renal failure	Metabolic encephalopathy
	Liver failure Wilson's disease	Extrapyramidal syndrome
Toxic	Drugs Heavy metals Organic solvents	
Nutritional	Vitamin B12 deficiency	Neuropathy, myelopathy
	Thiamine deficiency	Neuropathy, Wernicke–Korsakoff encephalopathy
Endocrine	Hypothyroidism Hyperthyroidism Addison's disease	Myopathy

Table 2 Extrinsic pathological processes classified according to the level of the nervous system affected

Brain	Trauma
	Hydrocephalus
	Extrinsic tumour (e.g. meningioma)
	Abscess
Spinal cord	Trauma
	Cervical spondylitic compression
	Abscess
	Extrinsic tumour (e.g. meningioma, neuroma)
Nerve root	Lumbar and cervical disc disease
Plexus	Trauma
	Tumour infiltration
	Radiation damage
Peripheral nerves	Compression, e.g. median at wrist, ulnar at elbow

Table 3 Some degenerative diseases of the nervous system

Level of nervous system	Syndrome
Brain	Alzheimer's disease
	Pick's disease
	Huntington's disease
	Parkinson's disease
Brain stem and cerebellum	Progressive bulbar palsy
	Cerebellar degeneration
Spinal cord	Motor neurone disease
	Hereditary spastic paraparesis
Peripheral nerve	Hereditary sensory and motor neuropathies
Muscle	Muscular dystrophies

Extrinsic

In these situations the nervous system itself is normal but is being disrupted by external factors. Management of these conditions depends on correcting the external factor and is therefore usually neurosurgical.

Every level of the nervous system can be affected. Some of the processes are summarized in Table 2.

Intrinsic

These processes can be divided into:

- **m**etabolic
- **i**nfectious
- **n**eoplastic
- **d**egenerative
- **p**aroxysmal
- **i**mmunological
- **g**enetic.

This can be remembered as MIND PIG.

Metabolic

Metabolic diseases that affect the nervous system often have systemic features and so this category overlaps with systemic metabolic problems.

There are a large number of different conditions, usually recessively inherited, that affect the nervous system and usually present in childhood. Commonly there is a combination of developmental delay or regression, intellectual impairment, ataxia and seizures. Specific metabolic disturbances have particular features. All are rare, the most common being phenylketonuria and Hartnup's disease.

Several metabolic conditions can present in adult life; many of these affect muscle, e.g. McArdle's disease (myophosphorylase deficiency). Mitochondrial diseases are being increasingly recognized as the cause of neurological disease in adults; features include seizures, deafness, episodic lactic acidosis and myopathy.

Infectious

The most common infections in the developed world are viral and bacterial meningitis and viral encephalitis. Leprosy, cerebral malaria and tuberculous meningitis are common infections in other parts of the world.

Less-common infections include Lyme disease, human immunodeficiency virus infection and its complications, human T-cell leukaemia virus 1 myelopathy and Creutzfeldt–Jakob disease. These are discussed on pages 98–101.

Neoplastic

Neoplasia can affect the nervous system in three ways:

- primary tumours
- secondary tumours
- paraneoplastic manifestations.

Paraneoplastic syndromes are non-metastatic syndromes related to cancer. These syndromes are thought to be immunologically mediated and include a limbic encephalitis, cerebellar degenerations and a myasthenic syndrome called Lambert–Eaton syndrome.

Degenerative

Degenerative diseases of the nervous system (Table 3) are progressive; some are familial but most are of uncertain aetiology. In some, a genetic cause has been found, for example Huntington's disease. All levels of the nervous system can be affected. These conditions are grouped together for convenience. When the underlying pathophysiology of these conditions is better understood they may be further reclassified as genetic or metabolic diseases.

Paroxysmal

Paroxysmal syndromes include epilepsy and migraine.

Immunological

Immune-mediated disease can be systemic but may be limited to the nervous system, where it can affect every level. Multiple sclerosis can affect any part of the central nervous system; Guillain–Barré syndrome is a generalized inflammatory demyelinating neuropathy; myasthenia gravis results when antibodies block neuromuscular transmission; and inflammation in muscle causes polymyositis.

Genetic

Many neurological conditions are genetically based. In some the underlying metabolic basis is known and other conditions are degenerative, so there is some overlap with other categories.

Pathological processes in neurology

- Pathological processes affecting the nervous system can be classified as systemic, vascular, extrinsic or intrinsic.
- Extrinsic disorders usually require neurosurgical management.
- Intrinsic processes can be divided into infectious, metabolic, immunological, neoplastic, degenerative and paroxysmal.

History taking

Introduction

Taking a patient's history (Fig. 1) is the most important part of the clinical assessment (Box 1). The history is used to find out the nature of the neurological problem, and how it is affecting the patient. It also puts this in the context of previous medical problems, medical problems in the family, occupation and social circumstances, and other aspects of the patient's life. The elements of a neurological history are the same as for any other subject, but because many neurological diagnoses are based solely on the history it carries greater emphasis (Table 1).

The history is usually presented in a conventional way (Table 1) so that doctors being told, or reading, the history know what they are going to be told about next. Doctors often adapt their method depending on the clinical problem with which they are faced. This section is organized in the usual way in which a history is presented, recognizing that sometimes the history can be obtained in a different order.

Basic background information

It is worthwhile establishing initially some basic background information: the age, sex, handedness and occupation, or previous occupation, of the patient.

Handedness is important. The left hemisphere controls language in almost all right-handed individuals, and in 70% of patients who are left-handed or ambidextrous.

Presenting complaint

Give the patient the opportunity to describe the problem in his or her own words. This is best done with an open question such as 'tell me all about it . . .' and then avoiding interrupting. Most patients will describe their problems in less than a minute. It is remarkable how often patients will use the same form of words to describe particular problems. For 'It was like being hit on the head with a bat' read subarachnoid haemorrhage until proved otherwise. 'My hands go dead at night. When I wake it helps if I shake them' suggests carpal tunnel syndrome. 'The pain in my cheek is sudden, like a red hot needle' suggests trigeminal neuralgia.

Frequently patients have trouble describing the feelings or sensations that they have experienced. This will require you to help interpret what they tell you – from everyday language into medical English. Patients find some sensations particularly difficult: for example, dizziness can mean light-headedness, a sensation of rotational vertigo or a feeling of being distant, among others (p. 46); the term numbness can be used by patients to mean weakness, loss of sensation, or stiffness. Your knowledge of the range of symptoms that people feel will help to sort out what the patient means.

After clarifying the nature of the symptoms you need to determine the *time course*. Establish the onset of the symptoms (sudden or gradual), their progression (progressive, stepwise or intermittent) and their duration. If possible some sort of measure should be used: how far could the patient walk at various times, when did the patient start to use a walking stick, and so on. The time course is critical to interpretation of the history. For example, a 50-year-old woman has had an episode of unilateral visual loss:

- If it was of sudden onset ('like a shutter coming down') and resolved over 5 min she has had amaurosis fugax (a retinal transient ischaemic attack).

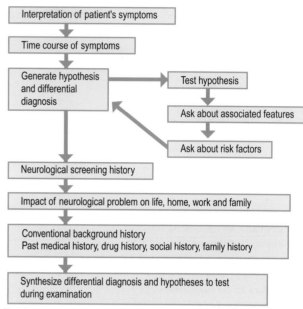

Fig. 1 **How to take a neurological history.**

Interpretation of patient's symptoms → Time course of symptoms → Generate hypothesis and differential diagnosis → Test hypothesis → Ask about associated features → Ask about risk factors → Neurological screening history → Impact of neurological problem on life, home, work and family → Conventional background history: Past medical history, drug history, social history, family history → Synthesize differential diagnosis and hypotheses to test during examination

---

Box 1

Common neurological diagnoses made on the history, with normal examination

Migraine
Tension headache
Epilepsy
Transient ischaemic attack

Table 1 **The neurological history**

Age, sex, handedness, occupation	Drug history
History of present complaint	Family history
Neurological screening questions	Social history
Past medical history	

- If it developed progressively from the centre of the vision over 15 min with bright lights at the edges, resolving after 15 min followed by a headache, it was a migraine aura.
- If there was a gradual loss of vision over 24 h with pain on eye movement and gradual recovery over 6 weeks, it was optic neuritis.

A 60-year-old man has developed a right-sided weakness affecting his face, arm and leg:

- If of sudden onset, he has had a stroke.
- If it developed over 10 days, beginning 10 days after a moderate head injury, it is probably a subdural haematoma.
- If it developed over 4 months it is probably a tumour.

Hypothesis testing

The next stage is to develop hypotheses on the basis of the initial description as to the possible site of the abnormality or type of syndrome. These hypotheses can be tested by:

- Asking about other symptoms that might further help to localize the cause of the symptoms. For example, a 45-year-old man has a slowly progressive weakness and stiffness in both legs and tends to trip on small steps. His symptoms suggest a bilateral upper motor neurone lesion so you should ask about (i) other symptoms of spinal cord lesions – sensory symptoms in the legs and bladder and bowel function; (ii) the upper level of the symptoms – if the arms are affected this suggests cervical cord disease, if there are brain stem symptoms then the lesion must be higher, or there is more than one lesion; (iii) other clues that might suggest the level such as back or neck pain.

- Asking about other recognized symptoms of a particular clinical syndrome. For example, in a patient with suspected Parkinson's disease, asking whether there has been any change in the writing; in suspected multiple sclerosis, asking if symptoms are worse after a bath or in hot weather.
- Asking about risk factors for the condition and associated diseases. For example in a patient in whom you suspect a stroke, asking about vascular risk factors (hypertension, smoking, diabetes) and associated vascular disease (ischaemic heart disease, peripheral vascular disease).

This process may involve testing more than one hypothesis.

Common difficulties in taking a history

- *Too much incidental detail*
  'Do you know Gloucester at all? Well, just behind the bus station there's a chemist . . .'
  Gently redirect the patient to give more relevant history.
- *Lists of medical contacts*
  'So I went to see my doctor, and he said . . . And then the specialist in Oxford thought . . .'
  If you need to know what another doctor did or thought, contact them directly.
- *Forgetting everyday events*
  Most young women taking the oral contraceptive pill do not consider this to be tablets or medicines so you have to ask directly about them.
- *History needed from someone else*
  'The first I knew about it was when I came to in the hospital'
  In patients with blackouts or altered consciousness and impairment of higher function it is important to get

Table 2 **Neurological screening questions**
Do you have, or have you had?
■ headaches
■ memory disturbance
■ dizziness or giddiness
■ blackouts
■ change in taste or smell
■ visual problems
■ double vision
■ difficulty with speech
■ difficulty with swallowing
■ weakness in your arms or legs
■ numbness or tingling

a witnessed account of events from whoever is available – relative, friend or passer-by.
- *History just doesn't seem to make sense*
  This tends to happen in patients with speech problems, memory or concentration difficulties and in patients with non-organic disease. Think of aphasia, depression, dementia and hysteria.

Neurological screening questions

After the investigative phase of history taking, usually one asks further standard screening questions for other aspects of neurological disease (Table 2). If the hypothesis is correct this usually does not throw up any surprises.

Past medical history

This needs to be documented. It is always useful to consider the basis for any diagnosis given by the patient. For example, a patient whose past medical history starts with 'known epilepsy' may not have epilepsy, but once accepted it rarely gets questioned and patients may be inappropriately treated.

Drug history

Current therapy is important. In some conditions, prior exposure to particular drugs can be important: for example, movement disorders can occur following phenothiazine exposure, whether taken for psychiatric indications, sickness or as a vestibular sedative.

Family history

Many of the degenerative diseases of the nervous system are familial. It is important to take a detailed family history when those conditions are being considered. In some circumstances patients can be reluctant to tell you about certain inherited problems, e.g. Huntington's disease. On other occasions other family members can be very mildly affected: for example, in the

hereditary motor and sensory neuropathies some family members will simply be aware that they have high arched feet. This can also be sought in the history.

Social history

The impact of the neurological problem will vary according to the social circumstances of an individual and this will be important in the further management of a patient. For example, the diagnosis of epilepsy will have a dramatic effect on a heavy goods vehicle driver, who will be unable to work because of the driving regulations. The impact of the same diagnosis is less in someone who can take public transport to work.

The home circumstances, housing, family support and finances of a patient with a neurological disability are very important in the management.

How detailed the social history needs to be will vary according to the clinical problem. In a patient with difficulty walking, the home circumstances need to be clearly defined. (Are there stairs? Is there a toilet downstairs? Are there steps between rooms or into the home?) The level of social support available may significantly affect management: a patient with an able-bodied spouse may be able to manage at home with a greater disability than someone living alone. Such details are redundant in a patient who only complains of a headache. Asking about life at home, how things are at work can be helpful in some patients, for example in someone suffering with a tension headache or someone with memory problems, where such questions may provide useful insights into their function as well as risk of job loss.

It is important to try to consider the whole patient and how the neurological problem may affect the patient's life.

> ### History taking
>
> - The history is the most important part of the clinical assessment.
> - The time course of the symptoms give an insight into the pathological process
> - The history should be used to construct and test hypotheses about the diagnosis.
> - The history is used to put the current problems into the context of the patients' previous medical problems, their family history and their social and financial situation.

Examination: introduction

Introduction

In training medical students and doctors how to examine the nervous system there is an entirely appropriate emphasis on technique. It is important to learn how to elicit physical signs correctly. However, this can lead to the students tending to think more about technique and less about what information they are meant to be getting from the examination. Students often dive into the active part of the neurological examination and miss important physical signs that can be seen if looked for, for example the relative facial immobility in Parkinson's disease.

The examination is used, like the history, as a screening test and as an investigative tool (Fig. 1). In patients in whom you anticipate a normal examination (e.g. migraine or epilepsy), a simple screening examination is appropriate (Table 1). The examination is used to investigate the hypotheses generated by the history and to clarify and understand any abnormalities found on the screening examination. For example, sensory examination of the hand will need to be done carefully in a patient with sensory symptoms affecting the hand; this would not be done in the same detail in a patient who presented with blackouts.

When considering the examination as a whole you should try to answer the following questions:

- Are there any abnormalities?
- Can the abnormalities be explained by a single lesion?
- Can the abnormalities be explained by several discrete lesions?
- Do the abnormalities conform to a recognizable syndrome?

These observations then need to be integrated with the history to lead to a diagnosis or differential diagnosis.

The following sections will explore how to examine the nervous system and highlight some of the patterns of abnormality that can be found. These brief descriptions should only be regarded as an outline to be augmented by bedside teaching. Various areas of importance will be further highlighted in a later section, which deals with particular problems.

The type of neurological examination carried out will vary according to the clinical problem. Any description of neurological examination technique will inevitably include brief excursions into blind alleys that are only occasionally

important. In the following sections describing examination, a few conditions will be briefly discussed as they provide specific signs and are not dealt with elsewhere.

General examination

The general examination (Fig. 2) is important for several reasons. It may provide clues to the *cause* of the neurological disorder or uncover risk factors. For example, finding a breast mass in a woman with a progressive hemiparesis suggests there are cerebral metastases; raised blood pressure and hypertensive retinopathy indicate hypertension as a significant risk factor in a patient with a stroke. General examination may reveal *conditions associated* with the neurological problem, for example finding peripheral vascular disease in a patient with transient ischaemic attacks. General examination can also find other *unrelated important diseases* that may affect the management of the neurological condition: for example, a patient with difficulty walking and lumbar canal stenosis who was also found to have significant osteoarthritis of the hip may benefit more from a hip replacement than from lumbar canal decompression.

For most patients with neurological disease the general examination is simply a screening examination. There are exceptions, for example:

- Patients in whom stroke or a transient ischaemic attack is being considered in the differential diagnosis need a careful examination of the cardiovascular system.
- Patients who present with possible metastases need examination to try to identify the likely primary tumour.
- Patients complaining of dizziness need an examination of their ears and hearing.

There are several conditions that come to mind as soon as you see the patient – if they don't come to mind then they can

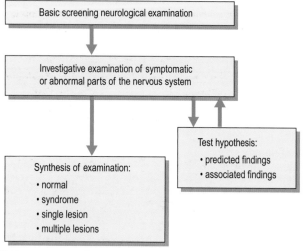

Fig. 1 **Approach to neurological examination.**

Table 1 **Screening neurological examination**
■ Gait
■ Pupils – direct and consensual reactions
■ Test fields to hand movements
■ Fundoscopy
■ Eye movements to pursuit on upgaze and lateral gaze
■ Facial sensation to light touch with finger tip in all three divisions of the trigeminal nerve
■ Facial movement – 'screw up your eyes, show me your teeth'
■ Mouth – 'open your mouth (look at tongue) and say 'arrh' (observe palate). Please put out your tongue'
■ Test neck flexion
■ Arms
– look for wasting
– test tone at wrist and elbow
– observe outstretched arms with eyes closed
– test power (shoulder abduction, elbow flexion and extension, finger extension and abduction and abductor pollicis brevis)
– reflexes (biceps, triceps arid supinator)
■ Legs
– look for wasting
– test tone at hip
– test power (hip flexion and extension, knee flexion and extension, foot dorsiflexion and plantar flexion)
– reflexes (knee and ankle and plantar response)
■ Sensation
– test joint position sense in toes and fingers
– test vibration sense on toes and fingers
– test light touch and pinprick distally in hands and feet
■ Coordination
– test finger–nose and heel–shin

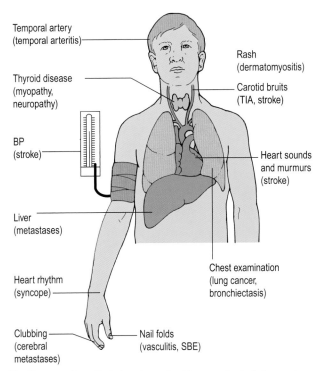

Temporal artery
(temporal arteritis)

Rash
(dermatomyositis)

Thyroid disease
(myopathy,
neuropathy)

Carotid bruits
(TIA, stroke)

BP
(stroke)

Heart sounds
and murmurs
(stroke)

Liver
(metastases)

Chest examination
(lung cancer,
bronchiectasis)

Heart rhythm
(syncope)

Clubbing
(cerebral
metastases)

Nail folds
(vasculitis, SBE)

Fig. 2 **General medical signs important in neurological diagnosis.**

Table 3	**Framework for mental state testing**	
Heading	**Consider**	**Comment**
Appearance and behaviour	Does he or she seem anxious or depressed? Does his or her behaviour seem appropriate? Do moods swing?	Ask relatives and make your own assessment
Mood	Is the patient depressed? Does the patient see any hope in the future?	Ask the patient directly and also form an impression from your own observations
Delusions	Belief, not amenable to argument, not usual in patient's culture	Revealed by the patient in the history Cannot be sought directly
Hallucinations	Classify according to sensory modality affected (visual, auditory, etc.) Elementary or complex?	
Vegetative symptoms	Appetite, weight, constipation, libido	

Table 2	**Presentation of neurological examination findings**
■ General examination	■ Tendon reflexes
■ Mental state	■ Sensory findings
■ Higher function	■ Coordination
■ Cranial nerves in order	■ Gait
■ Limbs (arms then legs), appearance, tone, power	■ Conclusion

be difficult to find. These include hypothyroidism, acromegaly, myotonic dystrophy and Parkinson's disease.

Organization of the examination

Neurological examination findings are presented in a traditional way (Table 2). This has developed because it is easier to make sense of what can be quite a large amount of information if it is provided in a standard way. While most neurologists will examine patients broadly following this conventional order, most have developed their own habits. One I know starts his examination at the feet! You need to develop (and practise) your own order and system of examination.

Mental state examination

The mental state examination is an assessment of the patient's mood and thoughts. This is not undertaken formally on every neurological patient. However, it is important to be aware of the possibility of psychiatric disease while taking the history. Abnormalities of mental state can occur for three reasons:

■ Patients with neurological disease may develop delusions or personality change, for example in dementia or frontal lobe disease.
■ Patients with neurological conditions, particularly chronic and incurable diseases, can develop depression and other psychiatric illness.
■ Patients with psychiatric illness can present with physical symptoms. For example, fatigue, headaches and misery may be the primary presentation of depression.

The mental state examination is conducted along with the history. It is useful to have a mental framework for areas to consider in a patient with an altered mental state (Table 3). In

patients in whom the changes result from neurological disease it is important to obtain independent corroboration of any change in personality, delusions and so on.

The psychiatric diagnoses most commonly seen in neurological practice are neuroses, depression and anxiety. Patients with psychoses, illness characterized by delusions and hallucinations, are usually seen when there is a concern that these reflect an underlying neurological disease, the organic psychoses. Patients with organic psychoses (e.g. dementia, confusional states) have an altered mental state examination. There are associated abnormalities in higher function, which will be considered in the next section.

Personality changes usually result from frontal disease. This can result in two extremes of behaviour, either apathy, loss of interest in appearance and mental slowness or disinhibition, and overfamiliar and at times outrageous behaviour. There is usually little insight into these changes.

Hallucinations can be defined as sensations without a physical basis that are perceived to be real. These need to be distinguished from illusions, where there is a misinterpretation of a physical sensation (the dressing gown on the door in half-light looks like a person). Hallucinations can occur in all sensory modalities. Olfactory, visual and tactile hallucinations are more commonly organically determined. Auditory hallucinations are usually associated with psychiatric disease. A hallucination can be described as being elementary (e.g. a flash of light) or complex (seeing the face of a man). Simple hallucinations are more commonly organic.

Delusions are fixed beliefs not amenable to argument and outside those accepted within the culture of the patient. These usually occur in psychiatric disease, though when they occur in organic disease there are usually other significant higher function deficits.

These more dramatic abnormalities of mental state are rare. In general neurological practice it is important not to miss the opportunity to treat patients who have either a physical presentation of anxiety or depression or have anxiety or depression relating to their neurological problems.

> *Examination: introduction*
>
> ■ General examination can provide information about the aetiology of, or risk factors for, neurological disease.
>
> ■ Some diagnoses are made by looking at the whole patient.
>
> ■ Mental state examination is important in selected patients.

Speech and higher function

Speech and higher function is not formally examined in every neurological patient. This should be undertaken in patients who report difficulties or if an abnormality is suggested by the history. Abnormalities in these areas can explain difficulties in obtaining a clear history. If in doubt, test.

Speech

Speech is required for the patient to give a history and it therefore constitutes the first part of the examination. The processes in language and terms used to describe abnormalities are summarized in Figure 1. Speech processing occurs in the dominant hemisphere. The process of understanding occurs in Wernicke's area in the supramarginal gyrus of the parietal lobe and the upper temporal lobe. This is linked by the arcuate fasciculus to Broca's area in the inferior frontal gyrus where speech output is generated. This then requires motor output involving corticospinal tracts, the basal ganglia and cerebellar inputs. The larynx is innervated by the vagus nerve to produce the voice, and then the tongue and lips, innervated by the hypoglossal and facial nerves, produce articulated speech (Fig. 1).

Aphasia

There are two main types of aphasia, which have been given different names in different classifications.

Fluent aphasia = Wernicke's aphasia = receptive aphasia = sensory aphasia. Patients have impaired understanding and do not answer questions appropriately and do not obey commands. The speech output is fluent but is often meaningless because they cannot edit their own output. This pattern of aphasia results from lesions in Wernicke's area. Patients with a milder fluent aphasia may seem normal superficially, especially on social pleasantries. However, any attempt at more meaningful questioning will highlight the difficulties. This pattern of aphasia is frequently misinterpreted as confusion.

Non-fluent aphasia = Broca's aphasia = expressive aphasia = motor aphasia. Patients have preserved comprehension and will obey commands. Speech is non-fluent with difficulties finding words. In milder deficits this particularly affects less commonly used words. This results from lesions in Broca's area.

These patterns of aphasia can occur in isolation but there is often a mixed picture affecting comprehension and speech production, which, if severe, is referred to as global aphasia. Smaller lesions can produce more subtle speech problems: for example, lesions of the arcuate fasciculus impair repetition; smaller lesions within Broca's area can lead to subtle difficulties in word finding or impaired spontaneous speech; nominal aphasia, difficulty in finding names for objects, occurs in lesions of the angular gyrus.

Assessment

Assessment of aphasias follows the pathway of language processing given above. Establish that patients can hear you. Give instructions of increasing complexity to determine the degree of comprehension. Listen to spontaneous speech (patients may need to be asked to describe something, for example their work) – is it fluent? Are they using the words correctly? Assess word finding ability by asking them to name objects (watch, strap, buckle), to list animals (normally > 18 in 1 min) or words beginning with F or S (normal > 12 in 1 min). Other facets of language can also be tested, e.g. reading and writing. Intriguingly,

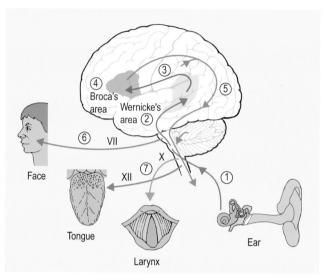

Site	Function	Abnormality
① Ear and auditory nerve	Hearing	Deafness
② Wernicke's area	Understanding	Fluent aphasia
③ Arcuate fasciculus	Repetition	Loss of repetition
④ Broca's area	Language production	Non-fluent aphasia
⑤ Motor output pathways, central: cerebellum Corticospinal tracts	Articulation of speech	Dysarthria
⑥ Motor output pathways, peripheral: facial, hypoglossal, vagus nerves, face and tongue	Articulation of speech	Dysarthria
⑦ Larynx	Voice production	Dysphonia

Fig. 1 **Process of language.**

with dominant occipitoparietal lesions, reading can be lost without losing the ability to write (alexia without agraphia) so patients can write but not read their own writing!

Higher function

Higher function is the term used to include all the processes of thought, memory, interpretation and comprehension of visual, auditory and sensory information. The objectives are:

- to determine if there are abnormalities in higher function
- to determine if these are focal or diffuse
- to assess their severity.

Factors affecting assessment of higher function

1. The testing needs intact speech and attention. If these are affected, testing has to be more limited and interpretation is more difficult. Non-verbal communication can sometimes be used to a limited extent with abnormal speech.
2. The level of premorbid intelligence needs to be considered, and some estimation made of expected level of function.
3. Other neurological deficits such as visual or hearing difficulties affect the results. Formal assessment of higher function needs to be undertaken after conducting a full neurological examination.

4. The mental state of a patient will affect higher function testing. Anxiety or depression can impair performance.

The interpretation of higher-function deficits should incorporate information from the mental state examination. Patients with frontal lesions have marked behaviour changes, with altered personality, apathy or disinhibition and perseveration, but may have relatively modest abnormalities of higher function. Patients with parietal lobe abnormalites have normal mental state examinations but many abnormalities in higher function. Higher function can be divided into the following areas.

Attention and orientation
Attention can be tested using digit span – the number of digits that the patient can repeat both forward and backwards (normal: 7 forward, 5 backwards). Orientation is given in terms of time (time, day, date, month, year), place (ward, hospital, town) and person (what is your name?). Abnormal orientation is non-specific and has no localizing value, it simply indicates an abnormality either of attention or memory.

Memory
Memory is complicated and can be classified in several ways (Fig. 2). The content of the memory can be divided into:

- episodic memory, the recall of particular events
- semantic memory, the knowledge of objects, facts, concepts, words and meanings
- motor or procedural memory, i.e. how to juggle and tie knots.

For bedside testing the following scheme is useful, but is only the beginning of the assessment of memory:

- Immediate memory: tested with digit span or giving the patient a name and address to repeat.
- Short-term memory: ask the patient to repeat the name and address after 5 min.
- Long-term memory: general information is easiest to test and needs to be adjusted according to knowledge that the patient could be reasonably expected to know, e.g. dates of World War II, name of Prime Minister, etc.

Memory is represented bilaterally in the temporal lobes and is usually lost in diffuse rather than focal lesions. Loss of short-term memory occurs in early dementia and rarer amnestic syndromes (e.g. Korsakoff's psychosis). Long-term memory is usually only involved in severe organic brain disease; isolated abnormalities of this are usually functional.

Calculation
This can be tested using serial 7s (taking 7 away from 100 repeatedly), doubling 3s or other simple calculations. This usually reflects a generalized disturbance in higher function but can be involved in isolation in dominant hemisphere abnormalities.

Abstract thought
This is a test of frontal lobe function. Ask the patient to interpret proverbs (e.g. people in glass houses shouldn't throw stones). If the metaphor is not understood this indicates concrete thinking.

See if the patient can give you reasonable estimates of, for example, the weight of an elephant (5 tonnes) or the length of a jumbo jet (70 m). Outlandish estimates and concrete thinking suggest frontal lobe dysfunction.

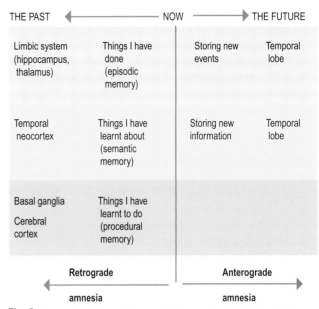

Fig. 2 **Types of memory.** Memory disturbances (pp. 52–55) may be for past events (Retrograde amnesia) or storage of new information (Anterograde amnesia).

Spatial perception
This can be tested by asking the patient to draw a star or clock. Inattention can be revealed when only half the clock is drawn, and inability to draw anything is a constructional apraxia; both indicate a contralateral parietal lobe lesion.

Visual and body perception
Agnosias are abnormalities of perception despite being able to demonstrate that the sensory modality is intact: for example, the inability to recognize faces despite normal vision (prosopagnosia) or an inability to recognize an object put in the hand despite normal sensory testing (astereognosis). These indicate parietal lobe lesions. In some instances the patient fails to recognize half his or her own body (usually the left side) – asomatagnosia. More marked is the phenomenon of neglect when the patient completely ignores one side, again almost always the left side. These too reflect contralateral parietal lobe lesions.

Apraxias
An apraxia is when an action cannot be carried out even though the necessary motor and sensory function is intact. Examples include dressing apraxia (patient cannot organize clothes to allow dressing) or ideomotor apraxia (cannot mime an action, e.g. striking a match). These abnormalites can reflect either frontal premotor or dominant parietal lobe lesions.

> ### Speech and higher function
> - Speech is usually assessed informally while taking the history.
> - Intact speech is needed to test other aspects of higher function.
> - Test speech more formally if there are specific complaints, if there is difficulty getting the history or if there is a suggestion of other higher function deficit.
> - Simple bedside testing can categorize most speech abnormalities.
> - Higher function testing aims to quantify any deficit and distinguish between focal and generalized higher function loss.

The eyes and visual system

An examination of the eyes and the visual system can prove helpful in patients with no visual or ocular symptoms. This section will first describe examination of the eye generally, then examination of the pupils, visual function, acuity, visual fields and fundoscopy. Eye movements are discussed on pages 18–19.

General examination of the eye

Ptosis is common and is often missed (Table 1). Partial ptosis is usually associated with unilateral overactivity of the frontalis. Ptosis is *not* a feature of facial nerve palsy (with a facial palsy the eye does not close).

Exophthalmos is usually a feature of hyperthyroidism but may indicate orbital disease. Enophthalmos is a feature of Horner's syndrome. Lid retraction is seen in hyperthyroidism and in rare upper brain stem lesions.

Remember false eyes can be cosmetically effective – a pitfall in exams.

Examination of the pupils

First look at the pupils. Are they the same size? Examination then aims to assess the afferent (optic nerve) and the efferent (parasympathetic via 3rd nerve constricting and sympathetic dilating) elements of the pupillary reflexes.

Ask the patient to look into the distance and shine a light twice in each eye in turn. First, look at the response in the eye into which you are shining the torch (the direct response), and then at the response in the other eye (the consensual response). Then ask the patient to look at your finger held 15 cm from the patient's face and look at the pupils for brisk constriction – the accommodation response. If no response is obtained from shining a light into the eye, but there is a normal response on accommodation, this is called an afferent pupillary defect and indicates significant optic nerve disease. Other abnormalities are summarized in Table 2.

When a bright light is shone into the eye with an intact optic nerve there is a brisk constriction of both pupils. When an optic nerve is partly damaged the constriction to the same stimulus is less brisk. If the light is moved rapidly from a normal eye to one with an abnormal optic nerve the pupil of the damaged eye continues to dilate. This is because the relatively weaker stimulus to constriction transmitted by the impaired optic nerve does not overcome the relaxation following a powerful stimulation on the other side. This is called a relative afferent pupillary defect.

Horner's syndrome

This is a lesion of the sympathetic innervation of the eye. This can result from central lesions in the brain stem (especially the medulla) and cervical spine, or peripheral lesions in the sympathetic chain, cervical ganglion or carotid. Common causes include brain stem stroke, Pancoast's tumour at the lung apex and carotid dissection. Many are idiopathic.

Holmes–Adie pupil

This idiopathic physical sign is also called the myotonic pupil. It may be associated with areflexia (Holmes–Adie syndrome) and is benign.

Argyll Robertson pupil

This is a classical but very rare sign, which is associated with syphilis but is now more commonly seen in diabetes.

Examination of acuity

This is best done using a Snellen's chart; alternatives include a near-vision chart. Refractive errors are best corrected using the patient's glasses but can be improved using a pin hole. The result of the Snellen's chart is expressed as two numbers: the distance from the chart (usually 6 m or 20 ft) and the distance at which the letter the patient could read should be read at. For example, 6/6 – letter read at the correct distance; 6/60 – the patient could read a letter at 6 m that could normally be read at 60 m. If the patient cannot read any letters, see if he or she can count fingers (abbreviated to CF), see hand movements (HM) or only has perception of light (PL).

Acuity can be affected by lesions anywhere in the visual pathway from ocular causes such as corneal lesions, cataracts and macular degeneration, through optic nerve disease and hemianopias involving the macula, to cortical blindness. Cortical blindness results from bilateral occipital lesions and is associated with normal pupillary responses and a normal eye examination.

Examination of visual fields

The visual fields are described from the patient's point of view. When looking

---

Table 1 Ptosis

Ptosis	Causes	Features
Neurogenic	Homer's syndrome, sympathetic lesion	Partial ptosis, small pupil, enophthalmos, may be altered sweating
	Oculomotor palsy (3rd nerve)	May be complete ptosis, associated reduced adduction and elevation, pupil may be large
Neuromuscular junction	Myasthenia gravis	Variable ptosis that fatigues, may be associated diplopia and facial weakness
Myopathic	Myopathies, especially myotonic dystrophy	Usually symmetrical. Features of associated muscle disease
Mechanical	Aponeurotic dehiscence (common in the elderly)	The tarsal plate is separated from the levator muscle

---

Table 2 Abnormal pupillary responses

Pupillary response	Direct response	Consensual response	Other signs	Conclusion
Large pupil	Normal	Normal	None	Anisocoria
	None	Normal	None	Mydriatic drugs
	None	Normal	Ptosis, eye movements abnormal	Oculomotor palsy
	None	None	Impaired vision, normal accommodation response	Optic nerve lesion
	None	None	Slow reaction to accommodation	Holmes–Adie pupil
Small pupil	Normal	Normal	None	Senile meiosis
	Normal	Normal	Ptosis, enophthalmos	Horner's syndrome
	None	None	Irregular pupils, normal accommodation	Argyll Robertson pupil (rare)

out of the right eye the right half of the vision is the temporal field and the left the nasal field, and vice versa from the left eye.

The visual fields are examined by covering one of the patient's eyes, asking

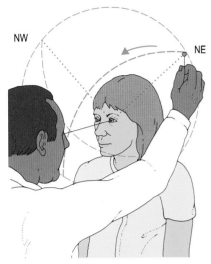

Fig. 1 **Examining visual fields.**

the patient to fixate on your opposite eye and then bringing an object in from the periphery to find the edge of the patient's vision (Fig. 1). This is done slightly differently depending on the type of object at which the patient is asked to look. The visual field for a large moving object is normally much larger than for a small red object. It is easiest to screen the visual fields using a crude stimulus, for example a wiggling finger, and then refine any defect with a smaller object, usually a small red hat-pin head.

Screening examination. While the patient fixates on your eye, bring your finger from outside the expected field towards the point of fixation from the four quadrants – if the vertical plane is north–south, bring the stimulus in from the north-east, south-east, south-west and north-west. Make sure the patient maintains fixation. Determine the edge of the visual fields.

More detailed examination. Keeping the red pin in a plane midway between

yourself and the patient, bring the pin in from the same directions, as described above, starting outside your own field for the red object. Ask the patient to tell you when the object is seen *as red*.

Ask the patient to compare the red colour each side of the point of fixation. Test for the blind spot. This is in the temporal field about 15° from the point of fixation. This should be quite difficult to find and be the same size as your own blind spot. If patients complain of holes in their visual field it is easiest to ask them to find them for you. Holes in the central vision are called scotomas, and are described according to their shape and position.

Examination of the visual field can be recorded using manual or automated perimeters (e.g. Goldman or Humphrey perimeters).

The location of a lesion producing a field defect can be deduced from the anatomy and organization of the visual system (Fig. 2; Table 3) (p. 56).

Any field defect affecting only one eye must be due to a lesion anterior to the optic chiasm. This can result from retinal disease or optic nerve disease.

Field defects affecting both eyes can indicate bilateral ocular or optic nerve disease. They usually occur with lesions at the chiasm, which produce bitemporal hemianopias, or in the optic tract, optic radiation or occipital lobe when they result in homonymous hemianopias or quadrantanopias. A homonymous field defect is one where the loss from both eyes overlaps such that there is a defect in binocular vision. These defects can be identical in both eyes (congruent) or differ (incongruent). The macula can be spared, which is important functionally and needs to be assessed specifically, though this finding is of limited localizing value.

Occipital lobe lesions are associated with highly congruent fields.

Table 3 **Field defects**

	Site of lesion	Possible associations
Unilateral visual field loss	Optic nerve or retina	Loss of pupillary responses, reduced acuity
Bitemporal hemianopia	Optic chiasm	Pituitary abnormalities, hypersecretion with or without hypopituitarism
Superior homonymous quadrantanopia	Temporal lobe	Hemisensory loss, mild hemianopia
Inferior homonymous quadrantanopia	Parietal lobe	Sensory agnosias (p. 13)
Congruent homonymous hemianopia or quadrantanopia	Occipital lobe	Patients often have limited awareness of the defect
Incongruent homonymous hemianopia	Optic tract	

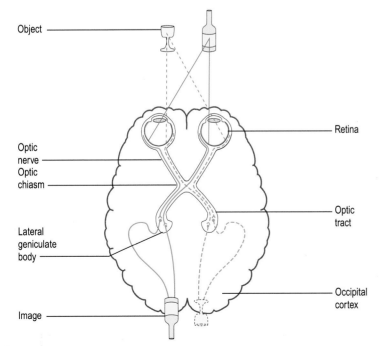

Fig. 2 **Organization of visual tracts.**

> *The eyes and visual system*
>
> - Systematic examination of the visual system and eyes involves general examination of eyes and eyelids, pupils, acuity, visual fields and fundoscopy.
>
> - Ptosis is a commonly missed sign.
>
> - Examination of the visual system and eyes is often informative in patients without visual symptoms.

Fundoscopy

Examining the fundus with an ophthalmoscope is often thought to be particularly difficult. This need not be the case with an understanding of how to use an ophthalmoscope, a clear idea of what is normal and what are normal variants, the appearances of common and important abnormalities and, of course, practice.

Setting up the ophthalmoscope (Fig. 1)

Set focus ring to 0. Remove dust cover. Select beam to plain. Some people remove their own glasses; if so then move the focus ring to correct. Make sure the light works.

Examine the patient's right eye with your right eye, and the left with your left. It takes practice to use your non-dominant eye, but it is important for three reasons:

- you do not rub noses with the patient
- you do not block the vision from the other eye so they lose fixation
- it is often tested in exams.

Useful facts to remember:

- The optic disc is in the same plane as the macula and the point of fixation.
- The optic disc is found 15° medial to the macula.
- Vessels branch as they go *away* from the disc.

Sit the patient comfortably and ask him or her to look at a particular point in the distance. Draw curtains, turn down lights. With your eye in the same plane as the patient's eye and the fixation point, and at 15° from the line between eye and point of fixation (so you are aiming at the centre of the occiput), look at the eye from about 30 cm (Fig. 2). Look at the red reflex. Any lens or vitreous opacity will be seen in silhouette. Gradually move in towards the eye. The disc should come into view. The ophthalmoscope may need focusing. If the disc is not seen, find a vessel and track it from branches to trunk.

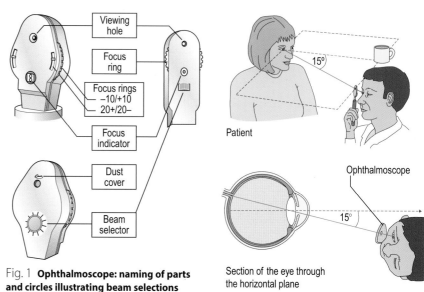

Fig. 1 **Ophthalmoscope: naming of parts and circles illustrating beam selections available.**

Section of the eye through the horizontal plane

Fig. 2 **Approaching the patient.**

Look at the disc (Figs 3 and 4). You may be able to see pulsation in the veins as they turn into the optic disc. This is venous pulsation and is normal and is seen in 70% of normal patients. If present it indicates intracranial pressure is normal. It is lost in raised intracranial pressure, though its absence does not indicate raised intracranial pressure.

Look at the vessels from the disc to the periphery. Look at the background retina (Fig. 3). In patients who have had cataract surgery and not had a lens replacement it is easiest to examine the fundi when their glasses are kept on.

Papilloedema

Papilloedema (Fig. 5) is commonly due to raised intracranial pressure: its absence does not exclude raised pressure. It is also

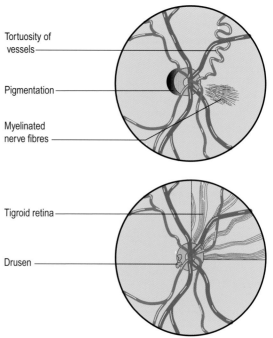

Tortuosity of vessels

Pigmentation

Myelinated nerve fibres

Tigroid retina

Drusen

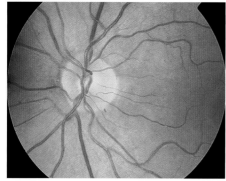

Fig. 3 **Normal fundus.**

Fig. 4 **Normal variants.**

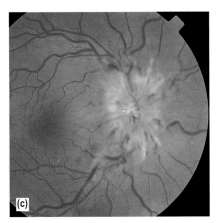

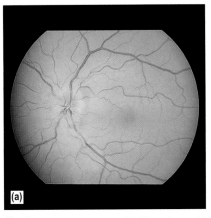
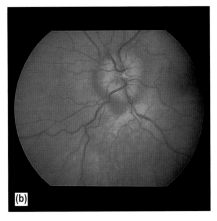

Fig. 5 **Papilloedema. (a)** Mild; **(b)** moderate; **(c)** severe.

Fig. 6 **Optic atrophy.**

Fig. 7 **Glaucoma.**

seen in hypertension and hypercapnoea. Vision is normal in most patients with papilloedema, but long-term chronic papilloedema produces an enlarged blind spot and peripheral field loss. Papillitis has the same ophthalmoscopic appearances but is associated with significant visual loss; this is commonly caused by MS.

Optic atrophy
Optic atrophy (Fig. 6) indicates optic nerve pathology, either prior optic neuritis, optic nerve compression or due to rarer degenerative conditions.

Chronic glaucoma
In chronic glaucoma (Fig. 7) the intraocular pressure is increased, resulting in widening of the optic cup. This produces peripheral field defects.

Hypertensive retinopathy
The appearances are described in Figure 8 and Table 1.

Diabetic retinopathy
In background retinopathy one may find microaneurysms, dot and blot haemorrhages and hard exudates. In proliferative retinopathy one may find cotton wool spots and new vessel formation.

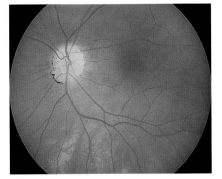
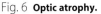

Hypertensive retinopathy

AV nipping

Variable calibre

Mild

More severe

Haemorrhage

Cotton wool spot

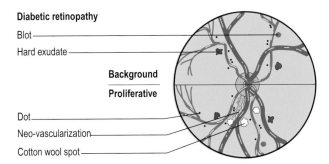

Diabetic retinopathy

Blot

Hard exudate

Background

Proliferative

Dot

Neo-vascularization

Cotton wool spot

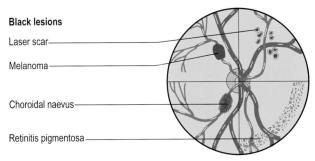

Black lesions

Laser scar

Melanoma

Choroidal naevus

Retinitis pigmentosa

Fig. 8 **Common retinal and vascular abnormalities.**

Table 1 **Fundoscopic appearances of hypertensive retinopathy**

Stage	Appearance
1	Arteriolar narrowing and irregularity
2	Arteriovenous nipping
3	Flame-shaped haemorrhages, hard exudates and cotton wool spots
4	Papilloedema

Fundoscopy

- Fundoscopy allows you to look directly at one part of the nervous system and at blood vessels.
- Competence at fundoscopy can be achieved by following a simple procedure and practice.
- There are a few common normal variants and common or important abnormalities that you need to recognize on fundoscopy.

Cranial nerves 1, 3–6

Traditionally the examination of the cranial nerves is reported according to their numerical order (Table 1). However, during the examination it is easier to group them according to their function – for example, considering the 3rd, 4th and 6th together as eye movements.

Olfactory nerve (1st)

This nerve is usually only tested formally in patients with specific complaints regarding the sense of smell. The examination consists of the presentation of a range of smells such as peppermint, camphor and rosewater to each nostril while closing off the other and asking the patient to identify them. Ammonia is also tested: this is not perceived by the olfactory nerve but is a direct irritant to the nasal mucosa, stimulating the trigeminal nerve. Failure to respond suggests non-organic anosmia.

Olfactory nerve lesions are usually post-traumatic, but can occur rarely in patients with frontal lesions, and subtle abnormalities are found in degenerative conditions such as Parkinson's disease. Anosmia occurs commonly with nasal blockage (e.g. colds).

Eye movements (3rd, 4th, 6th)

Eye movements are controlled in several ways. They can be moved as follows:

- Voluntarily (e.g. look right) – movement is initiated from the frontal eye fields. These are also called saccadic movements.
- On pursuit – following objects (e.g. follow my finger); this is controlled by the occipital lobe.
- Under vestibular control, reflex movements maintain eye posture with head and other movements. This is tested as the vestibulo-ocular reflex, which subserves the doll's head phenomenon.
- Convergence, to look at close objects (rarely of clinical importance).

These movements are integrated in the brain stem with the 3rd and 4th nuclei in the midbrain, and the parapontine reticular formation and 6th nerve nucleus in the pons. These are connected by the median longitudinal fasciculus (MLF).

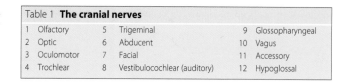

Table 1 **The cranial nerves**					
1	Olfactory	5	Trigeminal	9	Glossopharyngeal
2	Optic	6	Abducent	10	Vagus
3	Oculomotor	7	Facial	11	Accessory
4	Trochlear	8	Vestibulocochlear (auditory)	12	Hypoglossal

Eye movements result from contraction of the extraocular muscles. All but two of the extraocular muscles are supplied by the 3rd nerve, the superior oblique and lateral rectus being supplied by the 4th and 6th nerves, respectively (Fig. 1). Weakness of the extraocular muscles results in double vision in the direction of movement of that muscle. The image that is further out arises from the affected eye. Get the patient to look in the direction where diplopia is maximal and then cover each eye in turn to find which eye sees the outer image. The relative position of the two images is helpful: if the images are horizontally displaced but parallel this indicates a weakness in the lateral, or occasionally the medial, rectus. If the images are at an angle then other muscles are affected.

In simple terms, examination of eye movements involves answering the following questions:

- What is the position of the eyes at rest looking straight ahead (in primary gaze)?
- Does each eye move to all positions of gaze (Fig. 1)?
- Is there double vision in any direction of gaze?
- Do the eyes appear to move together in each direction of gaze?
- Can the eyes converge when looking at a close object?

Infranuclear lesions

Double vision usually results from a 3rd, 4th or 6th nerve palsy and these are illustrated in Figure 2.

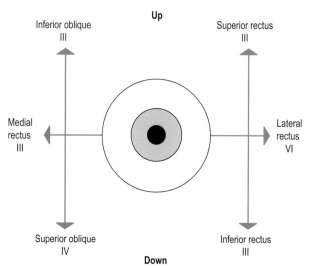

Fig. 1 **Muscles involved in eye movement.**

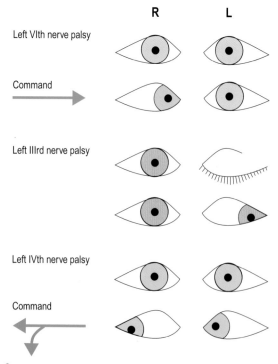

Fig. 2 **Single nerve palsies.**

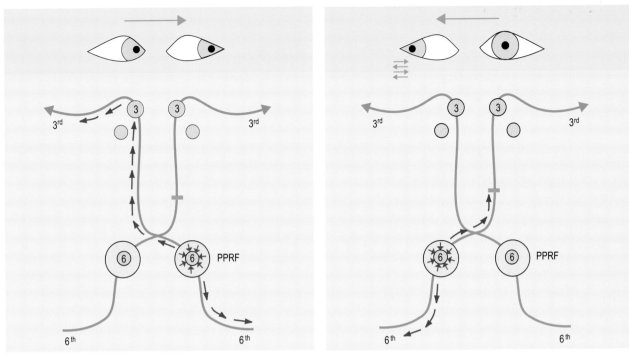

Fig. 3 **Internuclear connections. (a)** Normal; **(b)** internuclear ophthalmoplegia (INO). PPRF = Parapontine reticular formation.

If double vision does not conform to a single cranial nerve then consider neuromuscular junction failure, as in myasthenia gravis, or muscle disturbance, such as ocular myopathies, or mechanical distortion as in thyroid eye disease. Associated ptosis is seen in myasthenia and ocular myopathies.

Internuclear and nuclear lesions
- Lesions of the MLF (Fig. 3) usually do not produce double vision.
- Lesions of the nucleus for lateral gaze lead to lateral gaze palsies; this is where neither eye can look in one direction.
- Inability to look up (upgaze paresis) or look down (downgaze paresis) results from upper and lower brain stem lesions, respectively.
- Lesions to the MLF lead to an internuclear ophthalmoplegia (INO) (Fig. 3). The lateral gaze nucleus in the pons stimulates the ipsilateral 6th nerve nucleus, causing the ipsilateral eye to abduct; however, the message fails to reach the opposite 3rd nerve nucleus and the contralateral eye does not adduct. This is associated with nystagmus in the abducting eye, so called ataxic nystagmus.

Supranuclear abnormalities of eye movements arise when there is an abnormality of voluntary or pursuit movements yet the eye movement can be produced using the doll's head manoeuvre. These are rare.

Nystagmus
Nystagmus is rhythmic to-and-fro movements of the eyes. This should be watched for during testing of eye movements, paying attention to the direction of gaze in which the nystagmus occurred and the direction of the fast phase. Be careful not to consider the normal nystagmoid jerks found on extreme lateral gaze as nystagmus. Nystagmus is normal in certain situations, such as looking out of the window in a moving train.

The following patterns can be seen:

- *Pendular nystagmus.* This is symmetrical nystagmus in primary gaze, and indicates impaired fixation. It occurs in albinism and, classically but now rarely, coal miners.
- *Unidirectional jerk nystagmus.* This can be classified as first degree if it occurs only on looking in the direction of the fast phase, second degree if occurring on primary gaze, and third degree if looking away from the direction of the fast phase. This can occur in central or peripheral vestibular syndromes. Peripheral lesions are associated with vertigo while central ones may not be.
- *Multidirectional jerk nystagmus.* This indicates a central vestibular syndrome, for example phenytoin toxicity.
- *Vertical nystagmus.* Up or downbeat nystagmus indicates central brain stem lesion but has poor localizing value.
- *Ataxic nystagmus.* This occurs with internuclear ophthalmoplegia – see above.

Vestibular syndromes are discussed further on pages 46–47. Other abnormal eye movements are rare and include opsoclonus or dancing eyes and chaotic movements of the eyes.

> ### Cranial nerves 1, 3–6
> - Anosmia is usually due to blocked nostrils.
> - Neurogenic anosmia is usually due to prior head trauma.
> - Diplopia is most commonly due to lesions of the oculomotor (3rd), abducens (6th) and rarely trochlear nerves (4th).
> - Myasthenia gravis is a cause of complicated and variable eye movement abnormalities with ptosis, fatiguability and normal pupils.
> - Nuclear and supranuclear lesions produce abnormalities that can be recognized on clinical examination.

Other cranial nerves

Face, motor and sensory

Trigeminal nerve (5th)

Facial sensation is supplied by the trigeminal nerve (Fig. 1), which has three branches:

- the ophthalmic, supplying forehead to vertex and tip of the nose, and including the cornea
- the maxillary, supplying the cheek to the angle of the jaw and the inner aspect of the mouth and upper palate
- the mandibular, supplying the lower jaw but not the angle of the jaw.

The sensation to pinprick, light touch and temperature can be tested in each division. The afferent component of the corneal reflex is the ophthalmic branch of the trigeminal nerve.

Trigeminal motor function is rarely abnormal. This can be tested by getting the patient to clench the teeth and feeling the masseter and temporalis.

Facial nerve (7th)

Look at the patient's face for asymmetries. Compare the blink rate.

To test facial nerve function, ask the patient to look up at the ceiling (look at the frontalis), screw up the eyes (look at the orbicularis oculi), to whistle and show the teeth. Three patterns of abnormality are seen (Fig. 2):

- Lower motor neurone (LMN) 7th: all facial muscles are affected; if severe, the patient is unable to close the eye and the eye is seen to roll up on attempted closure (Bell's phenomenon) (common cause is Bell's palsy, see Box 1). Reduced blink rate.
- Upper motor neurone 7th: relative sparing of the frontalis.
- Extrapyramidal weakness: limited spontaneous movement, full voluntary movement.

Bilateral facial weakness is difficult to spot. The facial nerve also supplies (1) the stapedius, so LMN 7th can lead to hyperacusis (noises sound particularly loud); (2) taste to the anterior two-thirds of the tongue, so LMN 7th can lead to altered taste; and (c) the lacrimal and parotid glands, so aberrant recovery can lead to crocodile tears (crying when hungry).

The corneal reflex is carried out by touching the cornea (not the conjunctiva) with cotton wool; the normal response is a brisk contraction of both orbicularis oculi. A lesion to the afferent (ophthalmic branch of the 5th) produces loss of the reflex. Lesions to the efferent (7th) can impair the reflex on that side but not on the other side.

Hearing and vestibular function (8th)

Hearing can be tested at the bedside in several ways. The volume of a sound can be compared between ears, for example using a whisper, a tuning fork or a ticking watch. If the hearing is impaired unilaterally the Weber and Rinne tests will determine whether this is conductive or sensineural (Box 2).

Vestibular function is assessed by looking at eye movements, gait and coordination.

Box 1

Bell's palsy

This is a common condition (25 per 100 000 per year) of unknown aetiology. The patient develops a unilateral facial weakness, often with pain behind the ear, altered taste on one side of the tongue and hyperacusis. It usually improves spontaneously, but patients may be left with some facial weakness or aberrant renervation. Treatment with oral steroids may hasten recovery. The most important task is to protect the cornea from trauma and abrasions (artificial tears, patching eye closed).

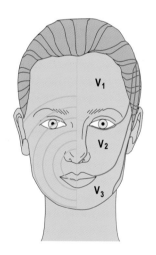

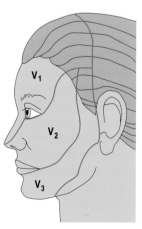

Fig. 1 **Facial sensation is supplied by the trigeminal (V) nerve.**

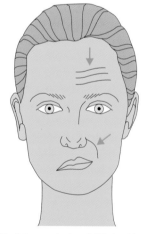

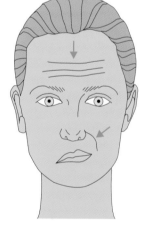

(a)   (b)

Fig. 2 **Facial nerve lesion. (a)** Right-sided lower motor neurone weakness; note droopy mouth, loss of nasolabial fold and eyebrow lines; **(b)** right-sided upper motor neurone lesion; note weakness in lower face with sparing of forehead muscles – especially when asked to look up.

Box 2

Weber and Rinne tests

Rinne test. Hold a tuning fork (512 Hz) in front of the patient's ear, then transfer it to the mastoid process behind the ear. Ask which is louder. Conduction in air should be louder than that in bone.

Weber test. Place the tuning fork on the vertex. Ask where the sound is heard. Normally it is heard in the centre of the head.

Patterns of abnormality
- Bone conduction is better than air conduction
  - Weber test lateralizes to the affected ear = conductive hearing loss
  - Weber test lateralizes to the other ear = a complete sensineural deaf ear, with bone conduction appreciated from the good ear.
- Hearing diminished but air conduction better than bone conduction
  - Weber test lateralizes to the other ear = sensineural hearing loss.

Mouth, tongue and palate (9th, 10th, 12th)

The glossopharyngeal nerve (9th) supplies sensation to the posterior pharynx. This is tested as part of the gag reflex. Touching this area is normally appreciated and provokes pharyngeal movement (vagus nerve, 10th). This is rarely affected in isolation. There is no clinically relevant motor output.

The vagus nerve has many functions: the parasympathetic supply to the stomach, upper gastrointestinal tract and heart, the supply to the larynx, muscles of deglutition and the palate. Palatal movement can be assessed by asking the patient to say 'Ahh'. The uvula normally lifts centrally; unilateral weakness causes the uvula to be pulled to the good side, and bilateral lesions mean the uvula does not lift (Fig. 3).

Laryngeal function can be tested by asking the patient to speak and to cough. In dysphonia speech is a whisper, and the cough is weak. This is usually due to laryngeal disease. Neurological causes include recurrent laryngeal or vagal nerve lesions and myasthenia gravis. Neurological dysphonia is usually associated with a bovine cough as a result of failure of laryngeal closure. Dysphonia may be non-organic and then the cough is usually normal.

The tongue is supplied by the hypoglossal nerve (12th). Look at the tongue for wasting; ask the patient to put out the tongue and move it quickly from side to side watching the speed of tongue movement. Lower motor neurone lesions lead to wasting and weakness of the tongue; upper motor neurone weakness tends to make the tongue slow moving. If the tongue is bilaterally wasted with fasciculations this is usually a sign of progressive bulbar palsy, a form of motor neurone disease.

Fasciculation of the tongue is an important sign. The tongue should only be assessed when relaxed in the mouth; there is often the appearance of fasciculation when a normal patient puts out the tongue. It is important to be absolutely sure before saying there is tongue fasciculation.

Dysarthria

Dysarthria is a distortion of the articulation of speech. Listen to speech for a variation in tone, melody and rhythm. Phrases such as 'yellow lorry' test the lingual sounds, while 'baby hippopotamus' tests the labial sounds. The abnormalities are classified in Table 1.

Accessory nerve (11th)

This nerve supplies the sternocleidomastoid (SCM) and trapezius muscles, which can be tested as follows. SCM: (1) ask the patient to flex the neck and resist the movement with a hand against the forehead; (2) place a hand on the patient's right temple and ask the patient to turn the head to the right – watch the left SCM. Trapezius: ask the patient to shrug the shoulders.

'Ahh'

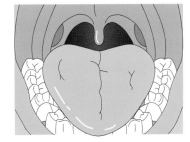

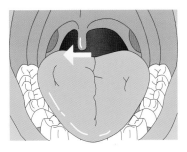

Weak left side

Fig. 3 **Palatal weakness.** The palate is pulled to the normal side.

Table 1	**Type of dysarthria**
	Clinical features
Spastic	Laboured speech, with slow tongue and lip movements
Cerebellar	Slurred as if drunk; staccato with loss of normal variation of emphasis, as if scanning a poem
Extrapyramidal	Quiet and monotonous, running out of steam before the end of the sentence
Lower motor neurone, neuromuscular junction and muscle	Normal rhythm, difficulty with sounds depends on affected muscle groups: tongue – sound t; face – sound b (think ventriloquist); palate – sound c or k (as if patient has a bad cold)

Other cranial nerves

- Trigeminal nerve abnormalities are usually sensory and rarely motor.
- Bell's palsy is the commonest, but not the only, cause of lower motor neurone facial weakness.
- Hearing loss can be classified as conductive or sensineural on bedside clinical testing.
- Dysarthria can be clinically categorized into spastic, cerebellar, extrapyramidal or lower motor neurone in type.

Limbs: motor

Examination of motor function is divided into:

- position and posture
- muscle inspection
- tone
- power testing
- tendon reflexes and plantar response.

As with all parts of the examination, attention needs to be paid to the hypotheses thrown up by the history.

Position and posture

Patients with different types of motor disease assume typical positions. It is worth looking at the position of the patient before examining the limbs at closer quarters. For example, a patient whose arm is held with a flexed elbow, wrist and fingers and whose leg is extended at the knee and ankle has a contralateral hemisphere lesion, typically a stroke. The myasthenic patient has an extended neck to overcome the ptosis, and a droopy jaw. The patient with Parkinson's disease is stooped with flexed elbows.

Muscle inspection

Look at the bulk of the muscles. Is the bulk normal, decreased (atrophied) or increased (hypertrophied)?

Muscle atrophy is most commonly seen distally in the small muscles of the hands and in the feet and tibialis anterior. Muscle atrophy can be confined to one muscle group or be more generalized. Atrophy usually reflects lower motor neurone abnormalities, though muscles do atrophy from disuse, for example in a longstanding upper motor neurone lesion, or with severe muscle disease.

Muscle hypertrophy is much rarer than atrophy. The calves are most commonly affected. This is seen in the Duchenne and Becker muscular dystrophies.

Fasciculations are small movements within the muscle and reflect contraction of a motor unit. These usually indicate a lower motor neurone abnormality. They are widespread in anterior horn cell diseases, typically motor neurone disease. They can occur in the absence of neurological disease, and are quite commonly observed in the calves of people without neurological disease.

Tone

This is usually assessed at the wrist, elbow, hip and knee (Fig. 1). The joint is moved through its range, initially slowly and then at increasing speeds.

There are four patterns of abnormality (Table 1). Rigidity is usually easiest to find at the wrist and elbow. Spasticity is best found at the extension of the elbow or pronation and supination of the forearm and is more marked as the joint is moved more rapidly.

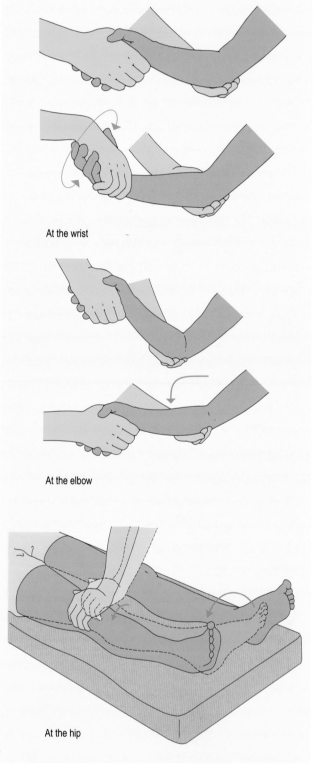

At the wrist

At the elbow

At the hip

Fig. 1 **Testing tone.**

Table 1	**Abnormalities of tone**			
	Reduced tone	**Rigid tone**	**Spastic tone**	**Gegenhalten tone**
Features	Floppy	Increased through whole range: with breaks – cogwheel, smooth – lead-pipe	Increased in tone with sudden increase or 'spastic catch'	Patient seems to push voluntarily against examiner
Causes	Lower motor neurone disease Muscle disease, Cerebellar disease	Extrapyramidal disease, e.g. Parkinsonism	Upper motor neurone disease	Diffuse frontal disease

Power testing

Although traditionally called power testing, what is actually being measured, using your arms and hands as strain gauges, is force. It is important to develop a systematic approach to testing the different muscles and movements described here. As you test, try to think of the nerve root and peripheral nerve innnervation of each muscle. The muscles routinely tested are shown in Figures 2–8 and 10–14 (pp. 24–25) and the less commonly tested muscles in Figure 9 (p. 24).

It is important to isolate the muscle or muscles that you want to test to avoid trick movements. Usually the joint across which the muscle acts needs to be held.

The amended Medical Research Council scale is used to record power and indicates the maximal power achieved, no matter how briefly (Table 2).

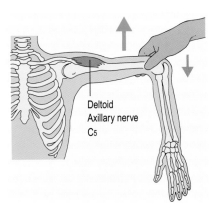

Fig. 2 **Testing shoulder abduction.**

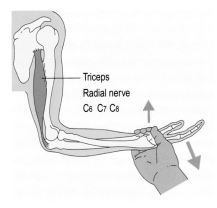

Fig. 3 **Testing elbow extension.**

Table 2 **Medical Research Council grades for muscle power**	
5	Full power
4+	Submaximal movement against resistance
4	Modest reduction of movement against resistance
4–	Some movement against resistance
3	Moves against gravity but not resistance
2	Moves with gravity eliminated
1	Flicker of movement
0	No movement

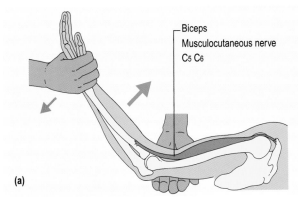

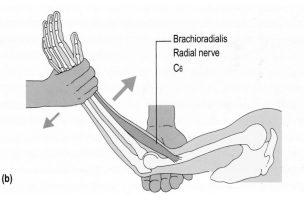

Fig. 4 **Testing elbow flexion. (a)** Biceps; **(b)** brachioradialis.

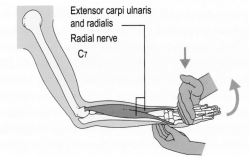

Fig. 5 **Testing wrist extension.**

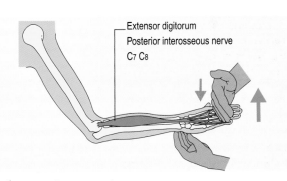

Fig. 6 **Testing finger extension.**

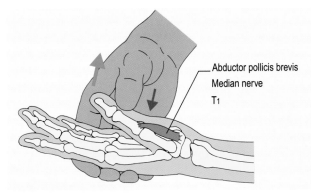

Fig. 7 **Testing thumb abduction.**

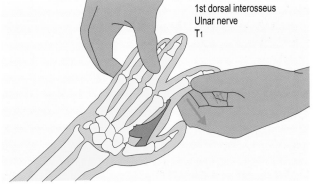

Fig. 8 **Testing finger abduction.**

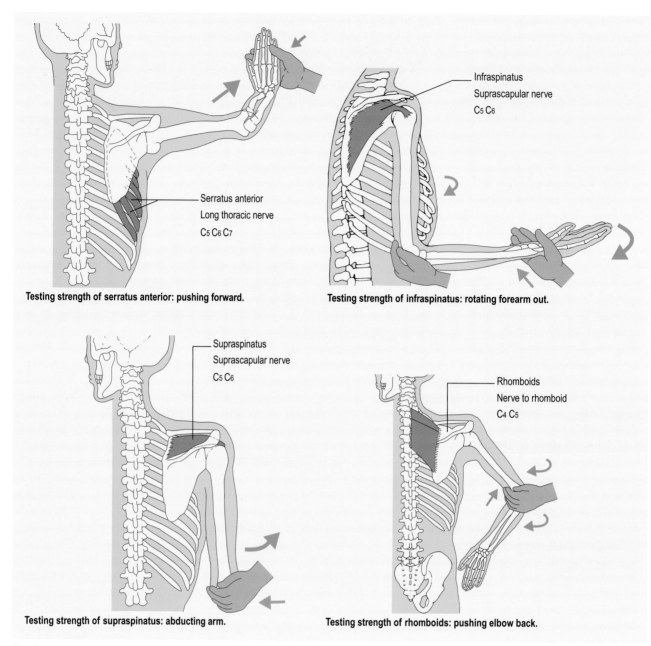

Serratus anterior
Long thoracic nerve
C5 C6 C7

Testing strength of serratus anterior: pushing forward.

Infraspinatus
Suprascapular nerve
C5 C6

Testing strength of infraspinatus: rotating forearm out.

Supraspinatus
Suprascapular nerve
C5 C6

Testing strength of supraspinatus: abducting arm.

Rhomboids
Nerve to rhomboid
C4 C5

Testing strength of rhomboids: pushing elbow back.

Fig. 9 **Less commonly tested muscles in the shoulder.**

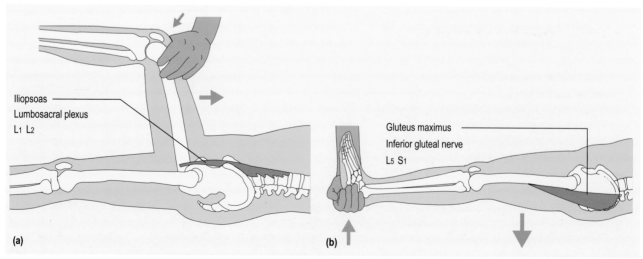

Iliopsoas
Lumbosacral plexus
L1 L2

Gluteus maximus
Inferior gluteal nerve
L5 S1

(a)

(b)

Fig. 10 **Testing hip flexion (a) and extension (b).**

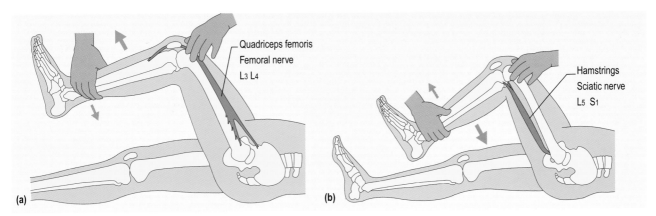

Quadriceps femoris
Femoral nerve
L3 L4

Hamstrings
Sciatic nerve
L5 S1

(a) (b)

Fig. 11 **Testing knee extension (a) and flexion (b).**

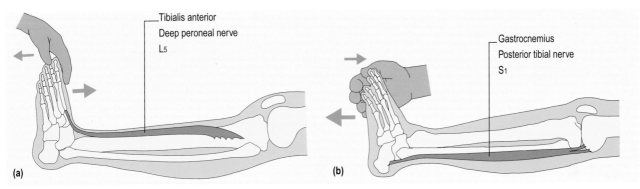

Tibialis anterior
Deep peroneal nerve
L5

Gastrocnemius
Posterior tibial nerve
S1

(a) (b)

Fig. 12 **Testing dorsiflexion (a) and plantarflexion (b) of the foot.**

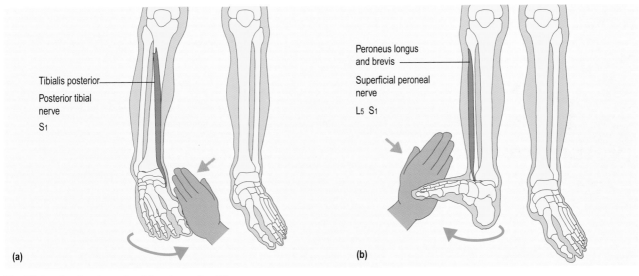

Tibialis posterior
Posterior tibial nerve
S1

Peroneus longus
and brevis

Superficial peroneal nerve
L5 S1

(a) (b)

Fig. 13 **Testing foot inversion (a) and eversion (b).**

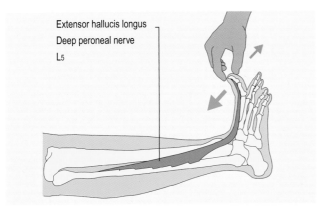

Extensor hallucis longus
Deep peroneal nerve
L5

Fig. 14 **Testing toe extension.**

Limbs: motor

■ Examination of tone provides useful information about the cause of a motor abnormality.

■ It is important to develop a systematic and reliable approach to motor examination.

Limbs: reflexes and sensation

Examining reflexes

Tendon reflexes are single synapse reflexes. A rapid stretch of the muscle stimulates the muscle spindles and this message is conveyed via the sensory root to the spinal cord at the segmental level of the muscle stimulated. This synapses with the motor neurone that supplies the muscle and leads to contraction of the muscle.

If this is interrupted, by either peripheral sensory or lower motor neurone lesions, the reflex is reduced or lost. Reflexes are reduced in muscle disease. If there is an upper motor neurone lesion, the reflex is increased because inhibitory factors have been removed.

Tendon reflexes are important because they provide an objective sign indicating abnormality and some indication as to the level of the abnormality.

Reflexes can be graded as absent, obtainable with reinforcement (see below), reduced, normal, increased and increased with clonus.

How to elicit tendon reflexes

The patient needs to be relaxed, with the muscle to be tested in the middle of its range of movement (Figs 1–3). The tendon hammer is swung to hit the

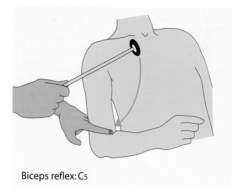

Biceps reflex: C5

Fig. 1 **Testing reflexes in the arm.**

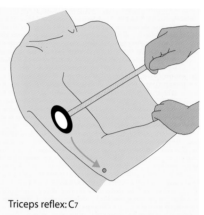

Triceps reflex: C7

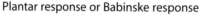

Supinator reflex: C6

tendon or, for the biceps and supinator reflexes, a finger on the tendon. The muscle is watched for movement in response to this. If the reflex is not obtainable then the patient is asked either to clench the teeth or make a fist – reinforcement – which may allow the reflex to be found. When testing the reflexes it is useful to remind yourself of the segmental level being tested.

Clonus is the rhythmic contraction of a muscle when it is stretched. This is most commonly found at the ankle (up to three beats is normal) and is occasionally found at the knee. Clonus indicates an upper motor neurone lesion.

Plantar response or Babinske response

This neurological sign has attained almost mythical status. An extensor plantar response is when the hallux extends and the other toes spread out in response to a stimulus. This stimulus is usually stroking the lateral part of the sole, though there are numerous alternatives, with different eponyms. This extensor response indicates an upper motor neurone lesion. Difficulties arise from false-positive results, especially when the patient withdraws or when there is a 'dystonic toe' in extrapyramidal disease, and too great an emphasis being put on the sign. False-negative responses

arise when there is sensory loss on the sole or profound weakness of toe extension. An extensor plantar response needs to be interpreted within the context of the rest of the motor examination.

Abdominal reflexes

These reflexes are not stretch reflexes. The muscles of the abdominal wall contract in response to a scratch of the skin of the same segmental innervation. The abdomen is usually considered in four quadrants. A response is normal. In upper motor neurone lesions, after multiple abdominal operations or multiple pregnancies, the response is lost. It is invisible in obesity.

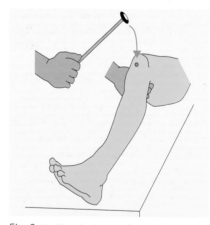

Fig. 2 **Testing the knee reflex: $L_{3/4}$.**

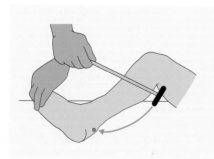
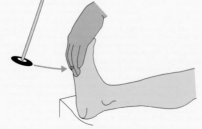
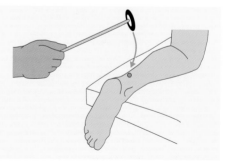

Fig. 3 **Testing the ankle reflex: S_1.**

Sensory examination

This section will describe some background and the techniques of sensory testing. The findings and their interpretation are discussed on pages 60–61.

There are five commonly tested modalities of sensation. These are subserved by particular-sized axons and run in particular tracts.

Joint position sense (proprioception) and vibration sense are carried in large myelinated fibres and then run in the posterior columns of the spinal cord. These remain on the same side until the medulla, where they cross over.

Pain, which is tested by using pinprick, and temperature are conveyed in small fibres, including unmyelinated fibres and they run in the spinothalamic tracts. These cross over and synapse within one or two levels of entry into the spinal cord.

Light touch is conveyed to a degree in both systems. Loss of joint position sense and vibration sense is frequently dissociated from loss of pain and temperature; light touch is not usually helpful in this situation.

How to examine sensation

Sensory examination requires the patient's cooperation, understanding and often patience. The degree of detail depends on whether there are sensory symptoms or other signs that make sensory examination important. It is easiest to start with the modalities that are easiest to test.

Remember that you need to *teach* the patient about the test, then undertake the *test* and have a system to *check* the validity if you are in doubt.

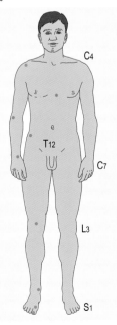

Fig. 4 **Sites for testing vibration sense (*) and key dermatomes to remember.**

Vibration sense

Use a 128 Hz tuning fork.

- *Teach:* Set off the tuning fork and apply this to the sternum to allow the patient to experience the feeling of vibration.
- *Test:* Ask the patient whether the vibration is felt when it is applied to the bony prominences (Fig. 4). If this is perceived distally there is no need to proceed proximally.
- *Check:* Apply the tuning fork, having stopped it vibrating, and ask the patient if vibration is still felt.

Joint position sense

When testing joint position sense, hold the joint so that your grip is perpendicular to the direction of joint movement (Fig. 5). Normally, small movements are perceived. Testing patients without neurological problems allows you to establish a 'normal range'.

- *Teach:* Move the joint with the patient's eyes open, indicating which way is up and down.
- *Test:* With the patient's eyes closed, move the joint up and down, asking the patient to tell you the direction of movement. Start with large movements and gradually reduce them until the patient makes errors.
- *Check:* Repeat the test for the lowest amplitude movements perceived. (See also Romberg test, p. 28.)

Pinprick

Use a slightly blunted pin, preferably a pin developed for this purpose. Do *not* use hypodermic syringe needles, which puncture the skin and leave a dotted line of marks.

- *Teach:* Touch an area of clinically unaffected skin with a pin and inform the patient that 'this is a pin'.
- *Test:* Start distally or in a clinically affected area. Work proximally. Ask the patient to close the eyes and tell you when the pin feels sharp; if abnormal, map out the affected area.
- *Check:* Occasionally use a blunt stimulus, such as the opposite end of the designed testing pins, which the patient should recognize as blunt.

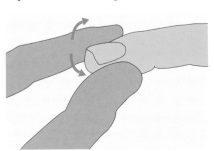

Fig. 5 **Testing joint position sense.**

Temperature

This can be tested at the bedside using a tuning fork, which feels cold. More formal testing requires matched dry test tubes filled with warm and cool fluids.

- *Teach:* Touch the patient on an unaffected area with the side of the tuning fork so that the patient knows how cold the fork is.
- *Test:* Touch the affected area and map out any area of altered sensation.
- *Check:* This can only be done using hot and cold test tubes by varying the order of application of the tubes.

Light touch

This can be tested using cotton wool or a fingertip.

- *Teach:* Show the patient what the stimulus feels like on an unaffected area.
- *Test:* Start distally or in a symptomatically affected area. Ask the patient to tell you when the sensation is felt and whether the sensation feels normal.
- *Check:* Vary the frequency of testing.

Special situations

Inattention, agraphaesthesiae or astereoagnosia are all signs of contralateral parietal lesions. Before testing, check that there is normal superficial and posterior column sensation.

Inattention. Ask the patient to close the eyes and tell you which side you are touching: touch one side, then the other and then both. Patients with inattention will correctly recognize the side on single stimulation, but only one side on bilateral stimulation.

Agraphaesthesiae. Write a letter or number with your finger on the palm of the patient's hand. Normally this is readily recognized. If not there is agraphaesthesiae.

Astereoagnosia. Ask the patient to identify an object, such as a coin or key, put in the hand.

> ### Limbs: reflexes and sensation
>
> - Tendon reflex changes are 'hard' neurological signs.
> - The plantar response is very helpful but needs to be treated with caution when the result is 'surprising'.
> - Sensory examination needs concentration and patience from both patient and examiner. This may need repeating.

Gait, coordination and abnormal movements

When examining gait and coordination, the results must be interpreted in the light of any motor or sensory findings in the rest of the examination. Patients with significant weakness or posterior column sensory loss will have some loss of coordination. There may be additional incoordination, and assessment of this is difficult and is based on a judgement as to whether the incoordination is disproportionate to the weakness or sensory loss.

Gait

Ask the patient to walk and observe whether the gait is broadly symmetrical. If it is symmetrical, look at the posture – stooped or erect; the step size – normal or shortened; the distance between the feet – normal, wide-based or scissoring; how high the knees are lifted – normal or high-stepping gait; the arm swing – normal or reduced; and if there are any abnormal movements. If the gait is asymmetrical, look at whether this is due to pain (antalgic gait), an orthopaedic problem such as a shortened limb, or weakness (a hemiplegic gait or unilateral foot drop).

Heel–toe walking

Ask the patient to walk placing their heel directly in front of their toe. This is normally done relatively easily. This is a sensitive test for ataxia.

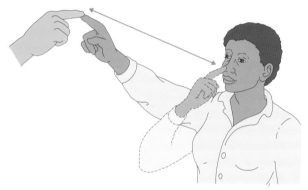

Fig. 1 **The finger–nose test.**

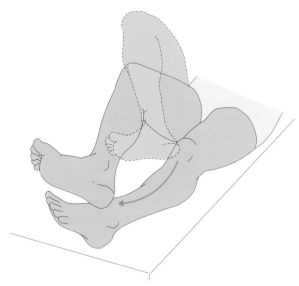

Fig. 2 **The heel–shin test.**

Romberg test

This is a test primarily of posterior column sensation. Ask the patient to stand with the feet close together. Once balanced, tell the patient to close the eyes. If the patient is steady with eyes open but falls with eyes closed, the Romberg test is positive. If the patient is unable to stay still with the eyes open then the test cannot be completed.

Coordination

In testing coordination, look for smoothness and accuracy of movement. The standard manoeuvres used for bedside testing are finger–nose coordination (Fig. 1), fast repeated movements and heel–shin testing (Fig. 2). Other parts of the examination afford an opportunity to observe coordination, e.g. the way the patient gets dressed and undressed and does up buttons.

Finger–nose coordination (Fig. 1)

Hold out your finger about 50 cm in front of the patient's face. Ask the patient to touch your finger with his or her finger and then touch the nose. Ask the patient to repeat this.

Repeated movements

Ask the patient to tap one hand on the back of the other. Then ask the patient to tap the same spot first with the palm of the hand and then quickly turning the hand over to touch with the dorsum of the hand. When this is done slowly and clumsily it is referred to as dysdiadokokinesia. Listen out for the 'slappy' sound it produces.

Heel–shin testing (Fig. 2)

Ask the patient to lift the heel up and put it on the opposite knee and then run it accurately down the front of the shin.

Other repeated movements

There are several other movements used, though not primarily as a test of coordination. Fast movements, particularly relatively simple ones, may be slowed in extrapyramidal and upper motor neurone lesions. Movements that are often tested are: rapidly bringing the index finger and thumb together; pronation and supination of the wrist; tapping a finger on a table; foot tapping, as if listening to fast music. In upper motor neurone lesions these movements are slow and deliberate, and in extrapyramidal disease the movements start slowly, becoming slower and smaller in amplitude.

Abnormal movements and posture

The diagnosis of patients with movement disorders is primarily syndromic and depends on the clinical classification of their movement disorder. There is considerable overlap between the movements and classification of some movements can be difficult, and in some patients this is a subject of dispute between experts (Fig. 3). However, the most common types of abnormal posture and movement are relatively easily identified.

Abnormal posture

The patient can have an abnormal posture as part of a generalized movement disorder, e.g. the stooped posture of a patient with Parkinson's disease, with arms flexed and an

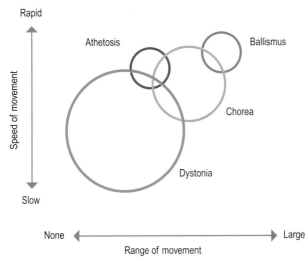

Fig. 3 **Types of abnormal movement.**

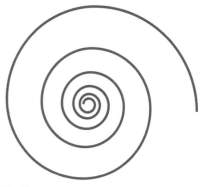

Fig. 5 **Archimedes spiral.**

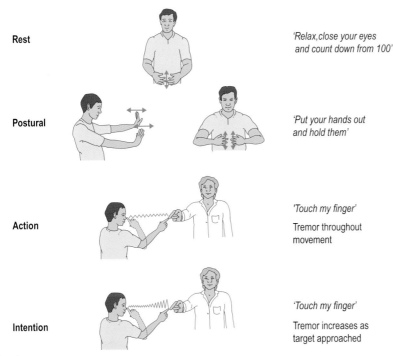

Fig. 4 **Classification of tremor.**

'Relax, close your eyes and count down from 100'

'Put your hands out and hold them'

'Touch my finger'
Tremor throughout movement

'Touch my finger'
Tremor increases as target approached

immobile face. The abnormal posture may be the only abnormality, such as in focal dystonia where agonist and antagonist muscles co-contract and maintain an abnormal position. The most common focal dystonia is torticollis or cervical dystonia (p. 92).

Abnormal movements

Tremor

Tremor is a rhythmical movement that can be described in terms of:

- amplitude – fine, moderate and coarse
- frequency – measured in Hertz
- the situations in which it occurs – rest, position, action or on intention.

Some tremors have a particular character, such as the 'pill-rolling' tremor

of Parkinson's disease. Examination of tremor aims to distinguish these features. Observe patients at rest; they may need to be distracted to bring out the rest tremor – ask them to say the months of the year backwards or count down from 100. Ask the patient to hold the hands out in the positions (Fig. 4). Observe to see if the tremor develops (postural tremor). Test finger–nose coordination – the tremor can appear as the finger moves (action tremor) or increase as it gets closer to the target (intention tremor). Asking the patient to draw an Archimedes spiral (Fig. 5) is a useful way to document a tremor.

Rest tremor is commonly seen in extrapyramidal disease, and intention tremor as part of cerebellar syndromes (p. 63).

Dystonia, chorea, athetosis and ballismus

These abnormal movements have considerable overlap and can be usefully thought of as a spectrum rather than distinct entities (Fig. 3).

Dystonia, described above, is associated with abnormal posture but may also be associated with slow movement or may occur during a particular movement. It is described by its distribution (focal or generalized) and whether it is related to one action (e.g. writing, as in writer's cramp) when it is a task-specific dystonia.

Chorea is a fidgety, semi-purposeful movement that can vary in amplitude of movement and frequency of occurrence. Patients are often adept at hiding it by converting some of the abnormal movements into apparently intentional movements. Its causes are discussed on page 93. Athetosis refers to a more distal writhing movement. It is almost always seen in association with chorea, which is used instead so the term has gone out of fashion.

Ballismus is a much more dramatic movement (it means throwing) where the limbs are thrown about violently. They are usually unilateral – hemiballismus.

Tics

These are relatively stereotyped movements, often affecting the face (blink or grimace) or hands.

> ### Gait, coordination and abnormal movements
>
> - Abnormalities in coordination need to be interpreted in the light of any motor or sensory deficits.
> - Classification of abnormal movements depends on description using specialized terms. Even experts disagree . . .

Neuroradiology

The central nervous system is encased in bone, the skull and the spinal canal. Until the 1970s it could be visualized only indirectly by means of changes in bony structures visible on X-ray or by means of contrast media introduced to the cerebrospinal fluid (ventriculography or myelography) or into the circulation (angiography). The advent of X-ray computerized tomography (CT) has revolutionized neuroradiology, with soft tissue visible directly. The development of magnetic resonance imaging (MRI) has added a new dimension to the sensitivity and anatomical resolution. MRI is the best technique for imaging most CNS pathology of both the brain and spinal cord.

Contrast media may be used to enhance diagnosis of CT and MRI scans, particularly highlighting defects in the blood–brain barrier (BBB). While different agents are used in each (iodine-based preparation for CT, gadolinium for MRI), the principle is the same. They are injected into a vein, usually in the arm, and become concentrated in vascular structures or where the blood–brain barrier is disrupted, making these areas appear brighter. For example, a tumour is vascular with an impaired BBB and will therefore enhance, while the centre of the tumour is necrotic with no circulation and will not enhance, giving a characteristic pattern of 'ring-enhancement' with contrast on the scan (Fig. 1).

Computerized axial tomography

CT scan is the most commonly available form of neuroimaging in the UK (Fig. 2a). The patient lies with the head in a ring which contains both X-ray emission and detection apparatus. Images are formed one slice at a time, as the head is moved through the ring. The dose of X-rays is relatively large and CT is contraindicated in pregnancy except in emergencies. CT scan remains the method of choice, however, for the demonstration of acute intracranial haemorrhage and intracranial calcification. CT is relatively insensitive at detecting pathology of the spinal cord but can detect most herniated lumbar intervertebral discs and is useful in delineating bony abnormalities.

Magnetic resonance imaging

X-rays are intuitively easy to understand because the denser the tissue, the less penetration by X-ray. MRI is a more complicated imaging technique and the following is a simple (perhaps simplistic) account of some features. The MRI scanner uses the interaction of a strong magnetic field and a pulsed electric field to alter the energy state of protons in the patient's tissues. This energy is released again after each pulse and is used to form the image. The rate of energy release depends on how tightly the protons are bound, hence on the chemical composition of the tissue. Since by far the greatest number of protons is in water, this forms the major contrast of the image. The scans can be reconstructed in axial, sagittal or coronal planes.

There are two commonly performed types of scan.

- T1 – water is dark and anatomical resolution is optimized (Fig. 2b).
- T2 – water is bright and pathological tissue is often highlighted, but with some loss of anatomical resolution (Fig. 2c).

CSF is chemically close to water so to tell whether an image is T1 or T2, see if the ventricles are bright or dark.

MRI parameters may be set to detect blood flow and MRI may thus be used as a non-invasive form of angiography (MRA) (Fig. 3), of both arterial and venous circulations. MRI can be tailored so that tissues alter appearance according

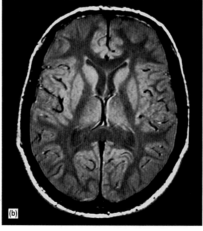
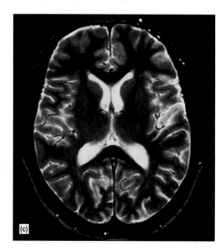

Fig. 1 **CT scans before (a) and after contrast (b) showing a ring-enhancing lesion.**

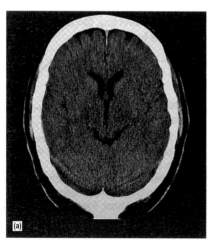
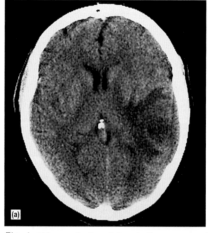
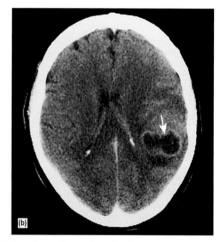

Fig. 2 **Normal axial images of the brain. (a)** CT scan; **(b)** MRI, T1 axial; **(c)** MRI, T2 axial.

to scan parameters (e.g. suppressing signal from fat), and it is the combination of appearances on different types of scans that leads to the diagnosis.

MRI may also be used to detect atoms and molecular species other than hydrogen, if in high enough concentrations. Magnetic resonance spectroscopy is the term given to this technique that may give some information of regional brain chemistry in vivo. It is still largely a research tool.

MRI does not involve high doses of ionizing radiation. However, despite this, MRI is relatively contraindicated in the first trimester of pregnancy because of uncertainty about toxicity. Patients may find the procedure claustrophobic and noisy. **MRI is contraindicated in patients with pacemakers, metallic foreign bodies in their eyes or intracranial implants of certain metals, because of the effect of the magnetic field.**

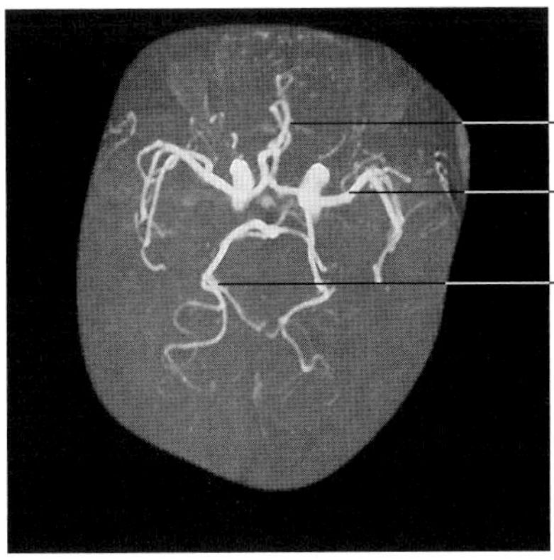

Anterior cerebral artery

Middle cerebral artery

Posterior cerebral artery

Fig. 3 **Magnetic resonance angiogram showing the vessels viewed from above.**

Myelography

Myelography is still used for imaging the spinal cord and roots in centres where MRI is not available or contraindicated. A lumbar puncture is performed and water-soluble contrast medium is introduced into the CSF. This is run up and down the spinal column by tipping the patient. Compression is detected by indentation of the column of fluid or by blockage of flow. The contrast medium also outlines the nerve roots, and compression here (e.g. by a disc) can be seen as failure of the nerve root sheaths to fill with contrast medium.

Myelography may cause severe headache. Rare complications include introduction of infection (meningitis) and subdural haematoma. Older contrast agents that were never completely cleared from the subarachnoid space were associated with a chronic, progressive inflammation of the meninges, 'chemical arachnoiditis'.

Angiography

This is still the 'gold standard' test for imaging blood vessels intracranially and in the neck (Fig. 4). Advances in MRA may replace this technique for diagnostic purposes in the future. A

cannula is inserted into the femoral artery under local anaesthetic, manoeuvred into the aortic arch and into the carotid or vertebral arteries. Contrast is injected and X-rays are taken. Delayed X-rays allow visualization of the venous system. The examination is relatively safe, major complications such as stroke occurring in 0.5%. Transient neurological deficits due to vasospasm are seen occasionally. Bruising may occur at the site of arterial puncture and bleeding is occasionally severe. Most units monitor pulse and blood pressure very closely for several hours after angiography.

Recently, interventional angiographic treatment techniques have been developed, for example insertion of glue or coils into aneurysms and other vascular malformations, and balloon dilatation of carotid and vertebral artery stenosis. These developments can be used in conjunction with or as an alternative to surgery. They are the subject of ongoing trials.

Functional neuroimaging

A variety of techniques are becoming available to explore regional cerebral function. These are generally research

techniques. The most widely available is single photon emission computed tomography (SPECT) (Fig. 5). This utilizes radioactive isotopes whose distribution mirrors cerebral perfusion. Regional uptake of these isotopes is determined by CT detection of radioactive decay emissions. This has very limited temporal and spatial resolution.

Positron emission tomography (PET) uses rapidly decaying substances that are attached to metabolic molecules (such as glucose) to detect metabolically active regions, or attached to water which maps blood flow. These substances emit positrons which are detected by CT using a specialized detector. The substances decay so rapidly that their activity disappears within minutes and they have to be produced by an on-site linear accelerator, restricting the technique's use. It is more sensitive than SPECT and can be used to detect neurotransmitter activity, with appropriate isotopes, as well as local metabolism.

Echo-planar MRI is a variation of MRI technique and can be used to detect variations in oxyhaemoglobin and deoxyhaemoglobin, which relate to tissue oxygen uptake and, therefore, to metabolic rate.

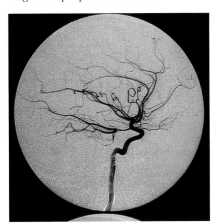

Fig. 4 **Normal digital subtraction carotid angiogram.**

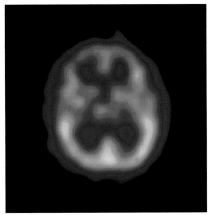

Fig. 5 **Normal SPECT scan.**

Neuroradiology

- Plain radiography gives little useful information regarding the CNS and should be restricted to assessing bony structures.

- The investigation of choice for acute intracranial haemorrhage, e.g. trauma, is CT.

- The investigation of choice for most other brain and spinal imaging is MRI.

- MRI can be tailored to different purposes.

- Myelography has an occasional role.

- Angiography remains the best way to visualize the intracranial circulation.

Neurophysiological investigations

The electroencephalogram

The electroencephalogram (EEG) records the electrical activity of the brain. Its major use is in the diagnosis and characterization of epilepsy. An EEG is usually recorded between seizures (interictal) but sometimes during seizures (ictal). The diagnosis of epilepsy is clinical and a normal interictal EEG does not exclude a diagnosis of epilepsy. The EEG is also useful in the diagnosis of encephalitis, coma and dementia, especially if rapidly progressive. It is complementary to imaging techniques such as CT and MRI and should not be used to look for structural pathology.

Method

The patient rests back and 20 electrodes are attached over the scalp with glue (Fig. 1). These are connected to a multichannel recorder, which generates a paper tracing or a computer record. This is often synchronized with a video recording of the patient. A skilled technician monitors the recording throughout, to detect and eliminate artefacts. The EEG is recorded with the patient's eyes open and closed and several methods may be used to enhance sensitivity of the technique, routinely including forced hyperventilation for 3 min and stroboscopic photic stimulation at 1–50 Hz. Another technique to increase sensitivity is to deprive the patient of sleep before the EEG, then allow the patient to fall asleep during the recording.

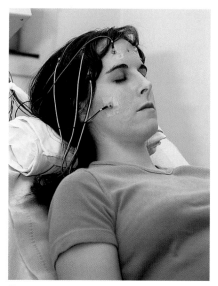

Fig. 1 **EEG leads on a patient.**

EEG interpretation

There are two features in the interpretation of the interictal EEG: background rhythm and paroxysmal EEG changes. Normal background rhythm in waking adults is 8–13 Hz 'alpha' activity, best seen over the occipital cortex when the individual's eyes are shut. It varies with the age of the patient, changing especially in children as the brain matures. In sleep the EEG is slower and varies according to the stage of sleep.

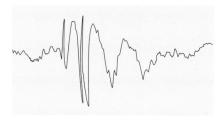

Fig. 2 **Spike and wave.**

Abnormalities of background rhythm

Focal slow waves may represent focal structural lesions (tumour, infarct, etc.) and a brain scan is usually indicated. Widespread slow waves are seen as part of diffuse encephalopathic processes, often due to metabolic disturbance such as renal or hepatic failure, drug intoxication, encephalitis, advanced degenerative processes, or sometimes thalamic or brain stem lesions that affect arousal. Faster background rhythms are usually due to drugs, especially benzodiazepines or barbiturates.

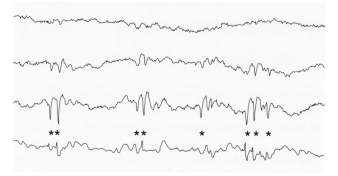

Fig. 3 **Focal EEG disturbances.**

Paroxysmal interictal EEG changes

During the EEG, much briefer discharges may be seen. Spikes (< 70 ms) and sharp waves (70–200 ms) are brief, near-simultaneous discharges of large numbers of neurones.

Spikes and sharp waves may be focal (affecting only part of the brain) or generalized (simultaneously affecting all parts of the brain) (Figs 2 and 3). Focal spikes suggest epilepsy due to a focal disturbance and imply a focal structural cause; neuroimaging should be considered. Generalized spikes are seen as part of the generalized epilepsies, which usually start in childhood or adolescence (pp. 74–75). The EEG shows normal background rhythms with frequent paroxysmal spike discharges. Photic stimulation triggers the discharges in about 5% of patients with primary generalized epilepsy (PGE) but rarely in other forms of epilepsy. Other generalized patterns may be seen in children with an abnormal background EEG who have a poorer prognosis and are associated with mental retardation or structural pathology such as tuberose sclerosis.

Sensitivity and specificity of paroxysmal interictal EEG discharges

The EEG has a relatively low sensitivity and a higher specificity for the diagnosis of epilepsy. The results depend heavily on the population being tested. The false-positive rate of epileptiform interictal EEG abnormalities (epileptiform EEG changes in individuals who definitely do not have epilepsy) is 0.5–2% of randomly selected individuals and 5–10% of first-degree relatives of patients with epilepsy. The first EEG may show epileptiform changes in 50% of patients with definite epilepsy. A sleep-deprived EEG increases the diagnostic yield to 75% and repeating the EEG up to 80%. As many as 15% of patients with epilepsy consistently have a normal interictal EEG.

Table 1 **EEG abnormalities**	
Herpes simplex encephalitis	Very regular sharp wave (e.g. 1 Hz) activity over one or both temporal regions with underlying slow activity called periodic lateralized epileptiform discharges (PLEDs)
Metabolic encephalopathy	Generalized slow activity. Triphasic waves typically seen in hepatic encephalopathy
Creutzfeldt–Jakob disease (CJD)	Widespread rhythmic triphasic waves at 0.5–2 Hz, often associated with near-simultaneous myoclonic jerks (may be absent in new variant CJD)

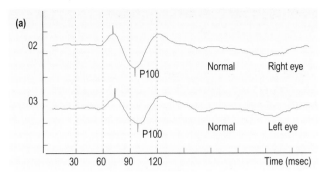

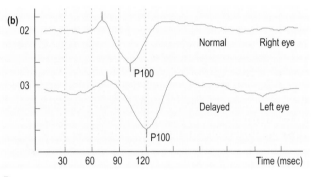

Fig. 4 **Visual evoked potential. (a)** Normal; **(b)** delay in the left eye indicating optic nerve demyelination.

Ictal EEG

None of the interictal EEG changes in themselves makes the diagnosis of epilepsy, but diagnostic changes can be seen if the patient has a seizure during the recording. This can usually be achieved in absence epilepsy, where the typical 3 Hz spike and wave discharges can almost invariably be triggered in untreated patients by vigorous hyperventilation. Other seizures are seen more rarely.

The electrographic appearance of a focal seizure is characterized by an evolving seizure discharge. Normal rhythms are replaced by rhythmic activity which may be spikey, slow or fast but increases in prominence during the ictus and then subsides, to be replaced by slow activity, for minutes to hours until the EEG returns to its usual interictal appearance. Nearly all seizures can be detected on ictal scalp EEG.

With the increase in surgical treatment for epilepsy, it has become more important to define the region of seizure generation with EEG. Prolonged EEG monitoring using portable EEG equipment with video monitoring of the patient is commonly used to detect seizure discharges in presurgical evaluation.

Important non-epileptic EEG patterns

Some non-epileptic EEG patterns are listed in Table 1.

Evoked potential studies

Evoked potential studies are a method of testing the integrity of sensory pathways from end-organ to cerebral cortex. They are useful in identifying subclinical sites of nervous system involvement, providing evidence of multiple lesions in CNS demyelination. The optic nerve is a particularly common site of subclinical involvement in multiple sclerosis (MS) and the visual evoked potential (VEP) is generally the most useful test (Fig. 4). VEPs give a relatively poor indication of the site of disease along the sensory pathway and they have become less important in the diagnosis of MS since the advent of MRI scanning. Indications for evoked potentials are summarized in Table 2.

Method

Recordings are made from the scalp with EEG electrodes. A stimulus is delivered repeatedly and the EEG is averaged over many trials to eliminate random background activity, leaving just the electrographic effects of the stimulus. The stimuli used are clicks to the ears for auditory evoked potentials, a patterned chequerboard to assess VEP and electrical stimuli to the lower limbs for somatosensory evoked potentials. The output is the latency of different waveforms.

An evoked potential may be delayed (slowed conduction, implying demyelination) or reduced in amplitude (implying loss of axons). These need to be interpreted in conjunction with the clinical picture and other investigations, including imaging studies.

Central motor conduction time

The motor cortex can be stimulated by an external magnetic coil. The delay to motor nerve action potentials in the nerve roots and to the muscle action potential can be measured, reflecting central and peripheral conduction times. This is largely a research tool.

Table 2 **Indications for evoked potentials**	
Investigation	**Possible indications**
Visual evoked potentials	Monocular visual loss, optic nerve disease, multiple sclerosis
Auditory evoked potentials	Unilateral hearing loss, multiple sclerosis
Somatosensory evoked potentials	Spinal cord lesions, radiculopathy, multiple sclerosis

Neurophysiological investigations

- EEG is an aid to diagnosis of epilepsy but a normal EEG does not exclude the diagnosis.
- The EEG may help to define the patient's epilepsy syndrome: partial or generalized.
- The EEG may help in the diagnosis of encephalitis, coma and dementia.
- Evoked potential studies are of value in the diagnosis of sensory pathway disturbances, especially in the confirmation of the diagnosis of multiple sclerosis.

Nerve conduction studies and electromyography

Nerve conduction studies

Nerve conduction studies (NCS) can be used to study the motor and sensory function of the large myelinated fibres of selected accessible nerves. The main measurements are of conduction velocity and amplitude.

Sensory studies

Sensory nerves are studied by stimulating the nerve at one point along it, for example the index finger, and recording at a distant site along the nerve, for example the median aspect of the wrist (Fig. 1a). By recording the time difference for the action potential to appear at two sites along the nerve and measuring the distance between them, the mean conduction velocity can be calculated across the segment of nerve between the two recording points. The amplitude of the action potential can be recorded from the oscilloscope screen. Sensory nerves can be studied orthodromically (distal to proximal) or antidromically (proximal to distal).

Motor studies

Motor studies involve stimulating the motor nerve at distal and proximal sites and recording the muscle action potentials (Fig. 1b). The amplitude of the muscle response (compound muscle action potential, CMAP) to supramaximal nerve stimulation can be measured. The time from the distal site of stimulation to the onset of the CMAP is the terminal or distal motor latency. This measure includes components of nerve conduction, neuromuscular transmission and muscle activation times. The difference in time to CMAP between the two sites of stimulation and the distance between is used to measure conduction velocity.

Interpretation of nerve conduction studies

There are two types of abnormality detected by nerve conduction studies:

- slowing due to demyelination
- reduction in amplitude of response due to loss of axons.

A survey of appropriate nerves can establish the pattern of peripheral nerve involvement. This can be:

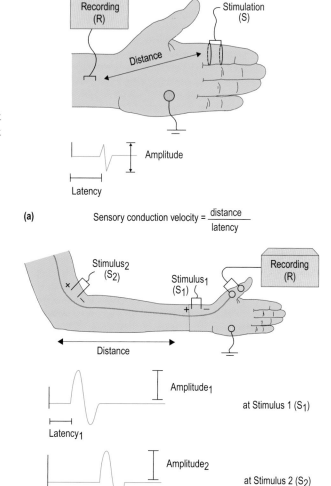

(a) $$\text{Sensory conduction velocity} = \frac{\text{distance}}{\text{latency}}$$

(b) $$\text{Motor conduction velocity} = \frac{\text{distance}}{(\text{Latency}_2 - \text{Latency}_1)}$$

Fig. 1 **Method of nerve conduction studies. (a)** Sensory; **(b)** motor.

Table 1 **Typical patterns of neurophysiological abnormality**				
Condition	**Sensory conduction**	**Motor conduction**	**EMG**	**Comments**
Demyelinating neuropathy	Slow, normal amplitude	Slow, normal amplitude or dispersed	Reduced recruitment, normal MUP	Widespread changes with no denervation of muscle. Prolonged F-waves, with proximal denervation and conduction block
Axonal neuropathy	Normal velocity, reduced amplitude	Normal velocity, reduced amplitude	Reduced recruitment, giant MUP	Widespread changes with muscle denervation
Local nerve entrapment	Delayed or reduced in severe cases	Delayed or reduced in severe cases	Normal or denervation changes in severe cases	Abnormality restricted to muscles innervated by that nerve conduction may show focal reduction at site of pressure
Motor neurone disease	Normal	Normal velocity, amplitude reduced	Fasciculations, fibrillations and giant MUP	Denervation with normal nerve conduction studies and with bulbar and upper motor neurone signs
Radiculopathy	Normal	Normal	Myotomal pattern of denervation changes	May have denervation of proximal muscles (paraspinal) and abnormal dermatomal evoked potentials
Myopathy	Normal	Normal	Reduced interference pattern and small motor units	May have some spontaneous fibrillations, especially in inflammatory myositis
Myasthenia gravis	Normal	Normal	Electrodecrement on repetitive stimulation	Increased jitter on single-fibre EMG
MUP, motor unit potential				

Table 2 Special techniques in peripheral neurophysiology

Technique	Method	Significance
F-wave	Supramaximal nerve stimulation causes antidromic anterior horn cell stimulation and a rebound wave down the motor neurone	Measures delay in proximal conduction, affected in demyelinating neuropathies and radiculopathies
H-wave	Electrophysiological equivalent of the tendon reflex; stimulation of motor neurone via sensory input	May be affected by proximal sensory disturbance or motor neurone dysfunction
Single-fibre electromyography	A measure of the time difference of activation of two muscle fibres, innervated by branches of the same nerve, by using two very fine concentric electrodes	Great variability in the time difference ('increased jitter') is seen in disorders of neuromuscular transmission, e.g. myasthenia gravis
Thermal threshold	Measure patient's ability to detect small temperature changes, produced by heating a small patch of skin, measured by a thermistor	Measure of small unmyelinated fibre function
Sympathetic skin response	Laser Doppler measurement of nailbed blood flow response to temperature change	Measures small unmyelinated sympathetic fibres

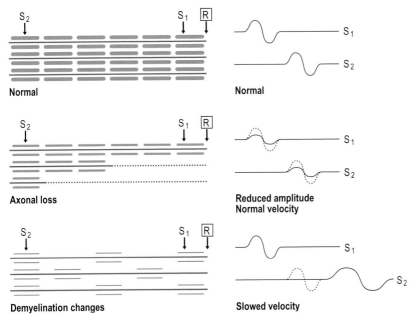

Fig. 2 **Waveforms of normal, demyelinating and axonal neuropathy.**

- *Focal:* where a single nerve is affected, e.g. the median nerve at the wrist in carpal tunnel syndrome.
- *Multifocal:* where there are multiple focal areas of abnormality. If this affects named nerves, it is mononeuritis multiplex; if not, it is a multifocal neuropathy.
- *Generalized neuropathy.* This can be further characterized as axonal, if responses are small with normal velocity, or demyelinating, if there is prominent slowing of motor conduction (Fig. 2). The two changes can coexist. Typical patterns of abnormality are given in Table 1.

Some peripheral nerve diseases are not detectable on routine nerve conduction studies; these include:

- nerve root disease (any disease proximal to the dorsal root ganglion cell)
- unmyelinated fibres, 'small fibre' neuropathies and autonomic neuropathies, for which other tests may be valuable (p. 115)
- inaccessible nerves.

Some more specialist techniques are given in Table 2.

Electromyography

Inserting a fine concentric needle into the muscle allows the study of muscle function. It can be used to determine the type of abnormality affecting a muscle and the distribution of muscles affected. The electrical activity is displayed on an oscilloscope screen and transduced to an auditory signal via a loudspeaker.

There are three parts to the electromyographic examination of a muscle.

Spontaneous activity

The normal muscle at rest is electrically silent. The electromyogram may record abnormal spontaneous activity:

- fasciculations: spontaneous discharges of motor units, usually indicative of denervation
- fibrillations: spontaneous muscle fibre discharges, indicative of denervation or inflammatory muscle disease
- more complex discharges, for example, myotonic discharges are heard as a 'dive-bomber' sound on the loudspeaker.

Motor unit analysis

The structure of the motor unit can be examined during gentle muscle contraction. Motor units are smaller and amplitude is of shorter duration in muscle disease. In lower motor neurone lesions the amplitude is larger and discharges are more prolonged.

Recruitment of motor units and interference pattern

These are examined as the muscle is contracted with increasing force. A full interference pattern with limited force suggests a myopathy, as pathologically some fibres in each motor unit are affected, so motor units are small. A few motor units firing at high rates suggests a lower motor neurone lesion, because in denervation there is axonal sprouting of remaining axons to take over denervated muscle fibres, so the remaining motor units are fewer but larger.

Other situations

Neuromuscular junction disorder resulting from myasthenia gravis causes a failure of neuromuscular transmission with increasing use (p. 110). The electrophysiological equivalent of fatiguability is the decline in amplitude of the compound motor action potential on repetitive stimulation of the motor nerve. Single-fibre electromyography may also help in diagnosis (Table 2).

Nerve conduction studies and electromyography

- Nerve conduction studies can define the pattern and nature of peripheral nerve abnormalities.
- Electromyography can detect denervation, the distribution of denervation and abnormalities in muscle disease.
- Some patterns of peripheral nerve disease can only be detected indirectly using neurophysiology.

Neurogenetics

Introduction

Individual genetic disorders are rare but there are many of them so that together their cumulative morbidity is significant. Some are particularly important as they are treatable. In recent years, new insights have been made into these diseases and this field is changing rapidly. This section will describe some aspects of clinical neurogenetics, and discuss the principal patterns of inheritance and some of the clinical problems posed by the more common neurological conditions.

Molecular genetic techniques have enabled identification of genes for inherited conditions, which allows:

■ Identification of gene products, enhancing understanding of pathophysiology and potentially allowing the development of treatments.
■ Increased understanding of the relationships between phenotype and genotype.
■ Improved diagnosis for the affected patient and for patients at risk. This has improved both preconceptual and antenatal advice.

In this section we will explore the clinical approach to patients with genetic or suspected genetic disease and consider the ways in which the newer genetic tests are used.

Clues to diagnosis

Family history of neurological disease. The pedigree helps to define the pattern of inheritance. However, in some situations a positive family history may be lacking (e.g. autosomal recessive and X-linked recessive illnesses, and dominant illnesses with partial penetrance).

Parental consanguinity (marriage between relatives). This makes autosomal recessive disorders more likely. Certain small racial groups have particularly high rates of autosomal recessive disease, e.g. Tay–Sachs disease in Askenazi Jews.

Mildly affected relatives. Dominant illnesses may have variable penetrance (variable disease expression) such that some affected members never come to medical attention, e.g. tuberous sclerosis. They may have to be seen to establish whether they are affected.

Evidence of longstanding disease. Inherited neurological illnesses usually cause a slowly progressive neurological deficit, with a variable age of onset. There may be a history of delayed developmental milestones, even if the patient only comes to medical attention in adult life.

Multiple system involvement. Dominantly inherited conditions especially tend to affect several systems, e.g. myotonic dystrophy or tuberous sclerosis.

Patient with unusual appearance. Unusual facial appearance is a common indicator of genetic abnormality, e.g. Down's syndrome. An excessively large or small head points to abnormal CNS development and other skeletal abnormalities may suggest failure of neural guidance of development, e.g. small stature or pes cavus. These could also represent congenital disease or sometimes an insult in early postnatal life. Retinitis pigmentosa is virtually always due to inherited disease and some conditions are associated with typical skin lesions such as tuberous sclerosis and neurofibromatosis.

Disease definition and genetic testing

The clinical definition of inherited diseases is crucial in the identification of their underlying defects. However, as genes underlying diseases are being identified, it is becoming apparent that the link between phenotype and genotype is less clearcut than had been anticipated. The phenotype of the same gene defect may be very different in different individuals, presumably because of other constitutional and environmental factors. This means that although a diagnosis

Table 1 **Some important autosomal dominant conditions**		
Condition	**Clinical features**	**Genetic defect**
Huntington's disease	Progressive dementia with chorea	Huntington, chromosome 4
Myotonic dystrophy	Progressive myotonia and weakness, with multisystem disease (p. 112)	Myotonin protein kinase, chromosome 19
Hyperekplexia (startle disease)	Falls with injury on being startled. Responds to clonazepam	Glycine receptor
Torsion dystonia (some families)	Generalized dystonia (p. 92)	Chromosome 9
Dopa responsive dystonia	Generalized dystonia, very responsive to levodopa	Defects of tyrosine hydroxylase and coenzymes
Hereditary motor and sensory neuropathy I	Progressive demyelinating neuropathy with pes cavus and champagne bottle legs	A: PMP 22 gene B: PO protein C: 20% unknown

Table 2 **Some rare but important treatable autosomal recessive disorders**		
Condition	**Clinical features**	**Genetic defect**
Wilson's disease	Movement disorders and psychiatric illness. Liver disease in children (p. 92)	Copper-binding ATPase
Phenylketonuria	Developmental delay, retardation, hypopigmentation, emotional disturbance. Treated by diet. Routine screening at birth	Phenylalanine hydroxylase
Galactosaemia	Failure to thrive, retardation, liver and renal disease, hypoglycaemia. Treatment is avoidance of all milk products	Galactose-1-phosphate uridyl transferase
Vitamin E deficiency	Progressive ataxia, with myelopathy, ophthalmoplegia and neuropathy. Treatment is with vitamin E supplements	Abetalipoproteinaemia

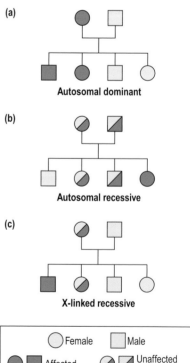

(a) Autosomal dominant

(b) Autosomal recessive

(c) X-linked recessive

○ Female   □ Male

● ■ Affected   ◑ ◪ Unaffected carrier

Fig. 1 **Common types of genetic inheritance.**

Table 3 **Risk associated with common inherited disorders**		
Condition	**Risk in general population**	**Risk in first-degree relatives**
Multiple sclerosis	0.2%	5–15%
Epilepsy	0.5%	5% (some types much higher)
Alzheimer's disease	< 1% at age 60 years (p. 54)	Three times age-matched controls
Parkinson's disease	0.5% over age 70 years	1.5% (higher if younger onset)

can be made, it is sometimes difficult to give a prognosis, making it difficult to give clear advice. Equally the same clinical syndrome may be due to several gene defects, some unidentified, and a genetic diagnosis can only be made in a proportion of similarly affected individuals. For example, in hereditary sensory and motor neuropathy type I, only 80% of patients have identified mutations. Thus a normal genetic test does not exclude the diagnosis. In any one family, however, the genetic defect should be in the same locus in all affected individuals.

Selected inherited diseases

Chromosomal abnormalities

Chromosomal abnormalities may cause disease if there is too much or too little genetic material: duplications or deletions. These large defects are often associated with severe mental retardation and epilepsy. Down's syndrome (trisomy 21) is the most common and is due to replication of chromosome 21, resulting in three copies of the chromosome.

Single gene abnormalities

Autosomal dominant disorders. Males or females are equally affected, transmission is from mother or father and 50% of offspring are affected (Table 1; Fig. 1a).

Trinucleotide repeat expansions. In several neurological diseases the underlying mutation has been identified as consisting of repeat sequences of redundant trinucleotides. Normal individuals may have some repeats, and disease sufferers usually have increasing numbers. In general, the more repeats, the earlier the onset and the more severe the disease. Successive generations tend to have larger numbers of trinucleotide repeats and are affected earlier and more severely: the phenomenon of 'anticipation'. Huntington's disease and myotonic dystrophy are two common examples (dominant), other examples are fragile X syndrome, bulbospinal neuronopathy (Kennedy's syndrome) (X-linked), Friedreich's ataxia (recessive) and other spinocerebellar degenerations.

Autosomal recessive disorders. Males and females are equally affected, often

without a family history, as parents are asymptomatic carriers; 25% of offspring are affected (Fig. 1b). Autosomal recessive disorders are often due to single enzyme defects, raising the possibility of therapeutic metabolic manipulation (Table 2).

X-linked recessive disorders. These diseases almost exclusively affect males; females are carriers (Fig. 1c). The disease may appear to skip generations. Each son of a carrier is at 50% risk and each daughter is at 50% risk of being a carrier. Daughters of affected males may be carriers, but sons can never be affected. In the female, every cell contains only one active X-chromosome: which one is inactivated varies between cells. If the abnormal chromosome is active in some cells important in the disease process (e.g. muscle cells in Duchenne muscular dystrophy), the female may suffer some disease symptoms. Duchenne (DMD) and Becker (BMD) muscular dystrophies are both due to abnormalities of the same gene, encoding the protein 'dystrophin' (p. 112). In DMD the protein may be absent, whereas in BMD it is deficient. Clinical features of muscular dystrophy are summarized on page 112. Fragile X syndrome (30% of female carriers affected) is a common cause of mental retardation.

Mitochondrial diseases

Many mitochondrial proteins are encoded in the nuclear DNA and their disorders are transmitted as autosomal traits. Some mitochondrial respiratory proteins are encoded in DNA within the mitochondrion itself. This DNA is passed from mother to child via mitochondria in the ovum; the sperm does not contribute any mitochondria. Consequently, defective DNA can only be passed from mother to child, although either sex may be affected: 'maternal inheritance'. There are many mitochondria in the ovum, some of which may be normal.

The clinical pattern and the severity of the disease are very variable because they depend on the number of abnormal mitochondria, the nature of the chemical defect and where the abnormal mitochondria end up in the

offspring. Several typical syndromes are recognized, e.g. Kearn–Sayres syndrome (progressive external ophthalmoplegia), Leber's optic atrophy, mitochondrial encephalomyopathy and stroke-like episodes (MELAS), and myoclonic epilepsy and ragged red fibres (MERFF).

Polygenic inheritance (Table 3)

In some common conditions, relatives of sufferers are more frequently affected than the general population. The increased risk is small and cannot be attributed to a simple gene defect. This may be because a combination of several genes and environmental factors are required for the disease and having some of the abnormal genes puts the individual at increased risk. This needs to be differentiated from disease in which the majority of cases are sporadic, e.g. motor neurone disease (MND), but with a clear minority of familial cases (familial MND).

Ethical issues of the new genetics

Being able to establish that an individual carries a gene defect raises ethical problems. These are highlighted by Huntington's disease (autosomal dominant), which causes late-onset chorea with dementia (p. 93) with complete penetrance. Finding the gene in clinically normal people means that they will develop the disease and that their children are at 50% risk. This knowledge places a considerable burden, especially for those who have seen the decline of relatives affected with this devastating illness. Adults may not want to know their genetic status, but if their teenage child wishes to be tested and find they carry the gene, they know that their parent must also develop the disease. It is, therefore, important that patients understand fully the implications of any test they undergo, both for themselves and their families. Counselling should be undertaken by specialized clinical geneticists, and ideally should involve the whole family.

Neurogenetics

- Accurate clinical diagnosis is needed for antenatal advice as well as treatment.

- The family history points to the pattern of inheritance, but in some disorders, especially recessive disorders, there may be no affected relatives.

- Clinical clues point to a longstanding illness in many cases.

- Patients should be counselled by a clinical geneticist before genetic testing.

Cerebrospinal fluid and lumbar puncture

Anatomy and physiology

The brain and spinal cord are surrounded by three layers of meninges: thick dura mater, trabeculated arachnoid mater and thin pia mater. The trabeculae of the arachnoid traverse the subarachnoid space, which contains cerebrospinal fluid (CSF). The CSF is essentially an ultrafiltrate of plasma with some differences: for example, 80% of proteins are transudated and 20% are synthesized locally. In order to reach CNS tissue, substances must cross one of two relative barriers: blood–brain barrier (BBB) and blood–CSF barrier (BCB).

The CSF is clear in colour and its total volume is 140 ml. The rate of CSF production is 500 ml per day: 70% from the choroid plexuses within the lateral, third and fourth ventricles and 30% from the capillaries and metabolic water. CSF circulates from the lateral ventricles to the third ventricle, through the aqueduct of Sylvius to the fourth ventricle. From here it enters the subarachnoid cistern around the medulla. It is then reabsorbed in the arachnoid villi because of the pressure difference between CSF and venous blood in the superior sagittal sinus and venous circulation. CSF is freely interchangeable with CNS extracellular fluid and is under a pressure of 100–200 mmH$_2$O in the supine individual. The normal CSF contains no red cells and very few leucocytes. Plasma proteins are present in inverse proportion to their molecular size, consistent with an ultrafiltration process. Ions are present in very similar concentrations to plasma and the glucose concentration is about 60% of that in plasma. The problems related to intracranial pressure are discussed on pages 48–49.

Abnormalities of CSF constituents

Routine tests

Microscopy. Microscopy is performed on a fresh, spun CSF specimen. Excess leucocytes may be present in infection, malignancy and inflammatory conditions, e.g. sarcoidosis. A high neutrophil count (often > 800/ml) is usually due to acute bacterial meningitis. Excess mononuclear cells are seen in chronic meningitis (e.g. tuberculous or fungal), viral meningoencephalitis, partially treated bacterial meningitis, chronic inflammation and malignant meningeal infiltration. Special stains may be used to identify microorganisms: Gram stain, Ziehl–Neelsen for acid-fast bacilli and fungal stains. Abnormal cells may be seen in malignant meningeal infiltration, but the sensitivity of cytology in proven malignant meningitis is only about 50% and repeated lumbar puncture may be required. Red cells are seen in subarachnoid haemorrhage but may represent a traumatic CSF tap. Xanthochromia confirms subarachnoid haemorrhage.

Glucose. Glucose levels in the CSF are compared with those in blood measured at the same time. CSF glucose is normally 60% of blood glucose levels. It is profoundly reduced (often < 1 mmol/l) in acute bacterial meningitis and tuberculous meningitis. Milder reductions are seen in viral infections, malignant meningitis and inflammatory conditions.

Total protein. Total protein is elevated in many situations, including most causing CSF cellularity. A rise without an increased cell count is seen in inflammatory neuropathies, especially Guillain–Barré syndrome ('albuminocytologic dissociation') and in blockage to CSF flow of any cause. Elevated protein is a non-specific manifestation of diabetes mellitus.

Specialized tests

Oligoclonal bands. Oligoclonal bands are visible as an increased concentration of restricted bands of IgG after isoelectric focusing and immunofixation of IgG. A serum sample is taken at the time of the lumbar puncture as oligoclonal bands may be present in CSF alone or CSF and blood. If present in both, they may represent systemic infection, autoimmune disease, sarcoidosis or neoplasia. Local CNS synthesis implies local CNS disease, especially multiple sclerosis but sometimes other CNS inflammation, infection or neoplasia. The sensitivity in clinically definite multiple sclerosis is above 95%.

Polymerase chain reaction (PCR). DNA amplification is available for increasing numbers of infections, including Herpes simplex encephalitis and *Mycobacterium tuberculosis* meningitis. The sensitivity and specificity of PCR is improving and it may become the diagnostic test of choice for these otherwise difficult to diagnose infections.

Immunodetection of antigen. This may be helpful in diagnosing infections, for example partially treated bacterial meningitis, where few organisms are present and do not multiply in culture.

Spectrophotometry. Measurement of blood breakdown products can be used to confirm subarachnoid haemorrhage.

Table 1 **The contraindications of lumbar puncture**

- Focal symptoms or signs attributable to intracranial disease*
- Symptoms of raised intracranial pressure, including confusion*
- Papilloedema (may be absent in raised intracranial pressure)*
- Neuroimaging evidence of obstruction to CSF flow
- Bleeding diathesis
- Local sepsis, e.g. sacral sores

* In some situations, LP may be deemed safe after neuroimaging has excluded obstruction to CSF flow

---

Table 2 **Examples of abnormal cerebrospinal fluid (CSF) results**

Indication	CSF picture	Significance
Acute headache	Increased red cells, xanthochromia and raised protein	Recent subarachnoid haemorrhage Spectrophotometry for xanthochromia
Acute meningitis	Neutrophil leucocytosis elevated protein, very low CSF glucose	Acute bacterial infection, early tuberculous meningitis
Chronic meningitis	Mononuclear leucocytosis elevated protein, low sugar	Tuberculosis, fungal or neoplastic; meningitis
Acute or chronic meningoencephalitis	Mononuclear leucocytosis, elevated protein, normal sugar	Viral meningitis or meningoencephalitis, neoplastic meningitis, inflammatory conditions, e.g. sarcoidosis
Demyelinating neuropathy: acute or chronic	Elevated protein, normal cell count	Supports inflammatory cause, e.g. Guillain–Barré syndrome
Inflammatory CNS disease	Isolated oligoclonal bands in CSF not blood	Localized CNS inflammatory response; supports multiple sclerosis, sometimes tumours or infection
Inflammatory CNS and systemic disease	Oligoclonal bands in blood and CSF	CNS inflammation as part of systemic disease, e.g. viral infection or sarcoidosis

How to do a lumbar puncture

The potential indications for and contraindications of lumbar puncture (LP) are summarized in Tables 1 and 2. Following appropriate guidelines, LP under these circumstances is a safe and invaluable procedure. If an LP is performed when contraindicated, in the presence of obstructive hydrocephalus, permanent disability or death may result from herniation of the intracranial contents.

Technique (Fig. 1)

1. Position the patient carefully in the left lateral position (for a right-handed operator) on a firm couch. The patient's back is initially right at the edge of the couch, next to the operator, then the patient curls up as much as possible. Ensure that the right shoulder remains exactly above the left shoulder and place a single pillow under the head. The patient's legs are curled up with the knees separated by another pillow.
2. *Choose the site of the LP.* Find the anterior superior iliac spine; vertically beneath this is the L3–L4 interspace.
3. Sterilize the skin (iodine).
4. Inject lidocaine (2%) subcutaneously and anaesthetize deeper tissues.
5. Insert needle pointing towards the umbilicus.
6. The supraspinous ligament provides the first dense resistance, within 1 cm in a thin person. The interspinous ligament provides the next slight resistance. About 3–5 cm deep, there is a further resistance, which is the dura.
7. Once through it, there should be a backflow of CSF when the stylet is removed.
8. Remove the stylet from the cannula and replace with a three-way tap, connected to a manometer. Measure the CSF pressure. When the flow of CSF ceases to rise up the manometer, the height of the CSF column in the manometer is equal to the CSF pressure in millimetres of water.
9. The sample in the manometer can be used for analysis and at least two further 5 ml samples should also be taken. Take a sample into a fluoride bottle for glucose estimation.
10. Take a simultaneous blood glucose sample and serum sample for oligoclonal bands, if indicated.
11. Reinsert the stylet into the cannula and remove the cannula. A plaster can be applied; no superficial dressing will make any difference to the hole in the meninges. After the LP, the patient should rest until recovered from the procedure, but prolonged bedrest is not required.

Problems with lumbar puncture

Failed tap

Failure to obtain CSF is usually due to technical difficulties. This is more common with degenerative spine disease (narrow disc spaces), obesity (difficulty in identifying landmarks), kyphoscoliosis, ankylosing spondylitis (bamboo spine calcified throughout) and rarely infiltrative intraspinal lesion causing a 'dry tap'.

Bloody tap

The differential diagnosis lies between a subarachnoid haemorrhage and a traumatic tap. After subarachnoid haemorrhage, the CSF is uniformly blood-stained in all bottles and haemoglobin breakdown products (xanthochromia) appear 12 h after onset. Spectroscopy may help define xanthochromia.

With a traumatic tap, a cannulation of venous plexus, the cell count falls in successive bottles as the proportion of CSF increases and there is no xanthochromia.

Complications

The most common complication of LP is headache. This is due to continued leakage of CSF after the procedure causing a decrease in CSF pressure. When present it is made worse by standing or sitting, which reduce intracranial pressure. Remaining supine after the procedure does not prevent headache. The headache usually resolves spontaneously. In refractory cases, 10 ml of the patient's own venous blood can be introduced into the lumbar epidural space to seal the hole: 'autologous blood patch'. The risk of headache is reduced by using smaller needles (22G rather than 18 or 20G) and by using a bullet- or pencil-pointed needle rather than a traditional bevelled needle. Thirty per cent of patients develop a headache if a bevelled 20G needle is used, compared with 7% when a 22G bullet or pencil point is used. Serious complications are very rare. Persistent dural leak is treated as above, but very rarely may result in intracranial subdural haematoma. Introduction of infection, causing meningitis, can occur.

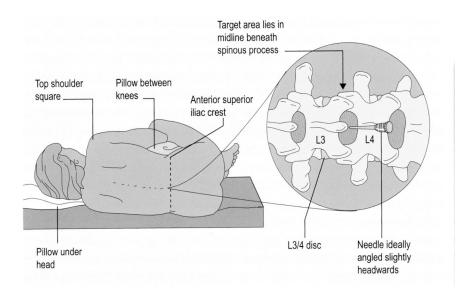

Target area lies in midline beneath spinous process

Top shoulder square

Pillow between knees

Anterior superior iliac crest

L3 L4

Pillow under head

L3/4 disc

Needle ideally angled slightly headwards

Fig. 1 **Posture of patient undergoing lumbar puncture.**

> ## Cerebrospinal fluid and lumbar puncture
>
> - Cerebrospinal fluid is a modified ultrafiltrate of plasma.
> - Raised intracranial pressure may be due to masses, brain swelling or altered CSF reabsorption.
> - The CSF contents help in the diagnosis of infection, neoplasia and inflammation, especially multiple sclerosis.
> - Any evidence of focal intracranial disease or raised intracranial pressure is a contraindication to LP until neuroimaging has been performed.
> - Positioning of the patient is crucial in performing LP.
> - The risk of post-LP headache depends mainly on the type of needle used.

Headache

Headache is common. Almost everyone has a headache at some time in life. Headache accounts for 2% of general practice visits and 20% of neurological outpatients. Headaches are only very rarely sinister. However, it is important to recognize certain *dangerous* headaches, and the major types of *safe but unpleasant* headaches (Table 1).

Table 1 **Types of headaches and estimate of incidence**			
Dangerous headaches	**Per 100 000/year**	**Safe but unpleasant**	**Per 100 000/year**
Subarachnoid haemorrhage	15	Tension-type headache*	250
Temporal arteritis	5	Migraine	250
Meningitis	10	Trigeminal neuralgia	5
Encephalitis	2		
Raised intracranial pressure	~10		
* Severe enough to seek help			

History

The history is the most important diagnostic tool in patients with a headache; in most patients the physical examination is normal. The key points in the history are:

- Length of history.
- Pattern – when and how often do they occur?
- Duration – how long does each headache last or is it there all the time?
- Progression – is it getting worse?
- Site – whereabouts in the head does it occur?
- Quality of the pain – what does it feel like?
- Associated symptoms – does anything else occur with the headache, e.g. flashing lights, numbness, sickness or a runny nose? Are there any other neurological symptoms suggesting focal neurological disease?
- Triggers – does anything seem to bring the headache on, particularly bending, coughing or straining?

The different features of the common but unpleasant and the rare but dangerous headaches are summarized in Figures 1 and 2.

Examination

General and neurological examination is normal in most patients with headache. Hypertension is usually an incidental finding; occasionally, headache can be attributed to severe hypertension. Points of particular significance in this clinical setting are fever, rash and neck stiffness in patients with recent-onset headaches, scalp tenderness in older patients and fundoscopy in all patients. It is especially useful to see retinal venous pulsation on fundoscopy as this indicates that the intracranial pressure is normal.

Dangerous headaches

These headaches are *single* episodes of headache that develop in seconds to weeks. All are uncommon.

Subarachnoid haemorrhage (Fig. 1a)

These patients classically present with a sudden severe headache: 'like being hit by a baseball bat'. There may be associated loss of consciousness and focal neurological signs. The subarachnoid blood provokes neck stiffness. Currently up to 50% of patients who present with subarachnoid haemorrhage are misdiagnosed by the first doctor who sees them. A high threshold of suspicion is needed (p. 72).

Meningitis (Fig. 1b)

Meningitis is characterized by progressive headache developing over hours or days. There is an associated fever and neck stiffness, and there may be a rash and impaired consciousness. As early treatment favours a good prognosis a high threshold of suspicion is needed (p. 98).

Temporal arteritis (or giant cell arteritis) (Fig. 1c)

This is a vasculitis that affects middle-sized arteries. It is dangerous because the arteritis can affect retinal vessels and cause blindness. It occurs in patients aged over 50 years and the incidence increases with age (1 in 100 000 aged over 50 years and 800 in 100 000 over 80 years). Women are affected twice as commonly as men.

The headache is insidious in onset and may be unilateral or more generalized, though it usually produces bitemporal pain. The scalp is often tender. A specific symptom is 'jaw claudication', the development of pain in the muscles of mastication on chewing. Twenty-five per cent of patients also have generalized joint and muscle aching typical of polymyalgia rheumatica.

The erythrocyte sedimentation rate (ESR) is elevated, usually strikingly (60–100), as are other serological inflammatory markers such as plasma viscosity and C-reactive protein. The diagnosis is confirmed by a biopsy of a temporal artery; however, this may be negative as the arteritic lesions are patchy. If the diagnosis is suspected, treatment is with steroids, to which there is usually a brisk response. The treatment is monitored using the ESR. Treatment can usually be stopped within 2 years.

Raised intracranial pressure (ICP) (Fig. 1d)

The headaches of raised intracranial pressure (ICP) (p. 48) are generalized and made worse or brought on by manoeuvres that increase ICP such as coughing, bending or lying down; for this reason they are worse on waking in the morning and tend to clear within a short time of getting up. They may be associated with vomiting. There may be false localizing signs such as 6th or 3rd nerve palsies and signs of raised ICP such as papilloedema. There may be associated focal signs and altered consciousness depending on the cause of the raised ICP. In only 20% of patients with intracranial tumours is headache the presenting feature.

The time course of the headache will depend on the cause. Acute hydrocephalus following obstruction of CSF flow can develop rapidly over hours or days. A slow-growing meningioma can produce a headache increasing over weeks or months. The headache is progressive.

Idiopathic intracranial hypertension

Idiopathic intracranial hypertension (IIH) is also called benign intracranial hypertension and pseudotumour cerebri. It presents with the syndrome of raised intracranial hypertension, often with an associated machinery noise in the ears. It almost exclusively affects young obese women. The aetiology is uncertain and there are probably several causes, including

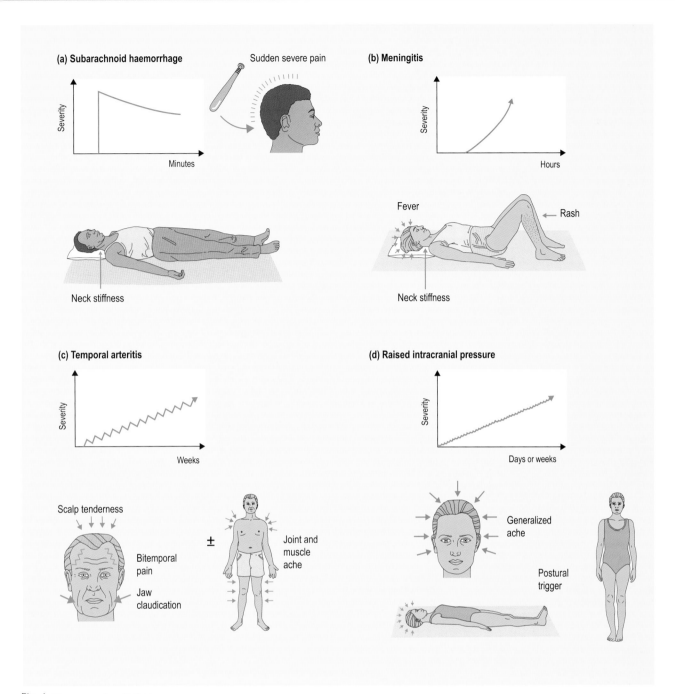

Fig. 1 **Dangerous headaches.**

tetracycline. Venous sinus thrombosis produces a similar clinical picture and is associated with the oral contraceptive pill and ear infections. It is diagnosed by magnetic resonance venography.

Diagnosis depends on demonstrating no structural cause for the raised ICP and measuring the increased ICP on lumbar puncture, usually over 30 cm CSF, with normal CSF constituents. The importance of the diagnosis is that, untreated, the raised ICP puts the optic nerve at risk and can result in significant visual field defects. Treatment is by lumbar puncture, acetazolamide (decreases CSF pressure) and weight loss. Visual field measurement documents progress. Occasionally, surgical drainage is required, using lumboperitoneal shunting.

Sinusitis
Tender painful sinuses, especially the frontal and maxillary sinuses, associated with fever and nasal discharge can usually be readily diagnosed. More insidious infections may present with diagnostic difficulties, which may require imaging of the sinuses and ENT intervention. Most patients who say they get sinus headaches have migraine.

Arterial dissection
Carotid or vertebral dissection can present as sudden-onset neck or head pain. Carotid dissections may be associated with ipsilateral Horner's syndrome. There may be associated stroke or transient ischaemic attacks (pp. 64–71).

Safe but unpleasant headaches (Fig. 2, p. 42)
These headaches are common and produce significant pain and distress to individual patients and are of considerable economic importance, interrupting work in 6% of the workforce.

The aetiology of these headaches is uncertain, with the exception of trigeminal neuralgia.

Migraine and migraine with aura (Fig. 2a)

Migraine is an episodic headache, associated with nausea and a dislike of light (photophobia) and sound (phonophobia). This may be preceded by focal neurological symptoms (aura). The headaches are the same regardless of the presence of the aura.

About a third of patients have premonitory symptoms for a day or so before the attack. These consist of mood swings, hunger and drowsiness.

An aura occurs in about a third of migraine patients. The aura is most commonly visual with either flashes of light or more complicated zigzag fortification spectra which shimmer and enlarge over 5–30 min. About 5% have sensory symptoms, usually paraesthesiae; others have aphasia and rare, more complicated auras, including body distortion. Auras tend to last 10–30 min.

The headache is usually unilateral, but is bilateral in a third of cases. The pain is mainly over the temples but can affect the occipital regions. The headache is usually throbbing; it typically lasts hours, but may last days. It is usually made worse by activity and helped by sleep. The nausea associated with this can be debilitating. Surprisingly patients often report their headaches improve if they vomit. The frequency of the attacks varies widely, though medical help is usually only sought with particularly frequent or severe attacks.

The attack may be triggered by dietary factors such as cheese, chocolate, coffee or red wine. There is a significant trigger in about 20% of cases. Sleep, particularly lying in at the weekend, can also trigger attacks. Relaxation and relief of stress can be a trigger, further increasing the attacks at weekends. In women, hormonal factors seem to be important.

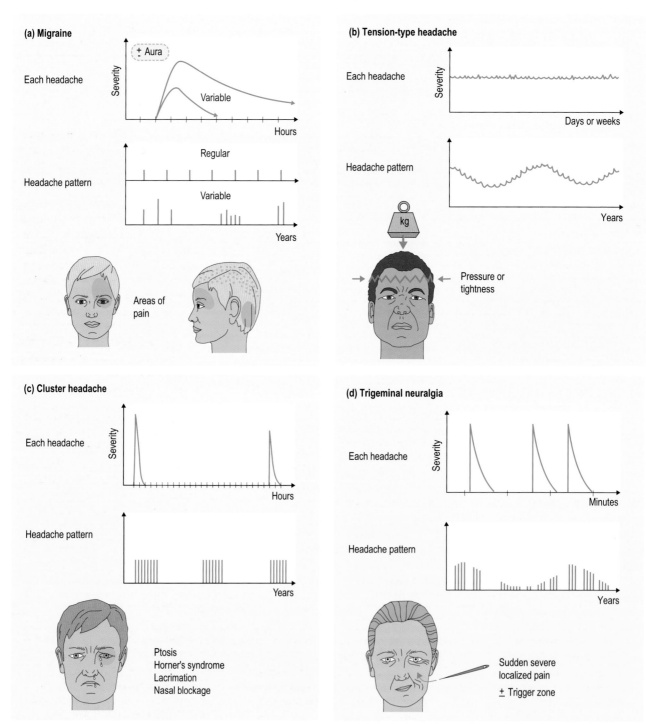

(a) Migraine

(b) Tension-type headache

(c) Cluster headache

Ptosis
Horner's syndrome
Lacrimation
Nasal blockage

(d) Trigeminal neuralgia

Sudden severe localized pain
± Trigger zone

Fig. 2 **'Safe' but unpleasant headaches.**

The oral contraceptive can trigger attacks; attacks are more common with menstruation and migraine often changes at the time of the menopause.

There is usually a family history. In some rare types, such as hemiplegic migraine (where hemiplegia can follow migraine), there is a strong genetic element.

Occasionally patients may develop the migraine aura without the migraine, so-called migraine equivalents. This can cause diagnostic difficulties.

Treatment of migraine is at three levels:

- Identification and removal of triggers. This can include dietary manipulation, avoidance of late nights or lying in and change of contraceptive method.
- Treatment of acute attacks. Most patients respond to simple analgesics such as paracetamol or aspirin or to over-the-counter proprietary combination drugs. In some patients antiemetic treatment is more important than analgesia; metoclopramide or prochlorperazine are commonly used drugs. More specific drugs include serotonin agonists (e.g. sumatriptan), which can be given orally, intranasally or subcutaneously, and ergotamine preparations which can be given orally, rectally or sublingually. The daily and weekly ergotamine dose is limited.
- Prophylaxis. For patients with frequent attacks, prophylaxis can be helpful. Commonly used agents include beta-blockers (propranolol and atenolol), pizotifen, amitriptyline and sodium valproate. Recently topiramate has been demonstrated to be helpful.

Tension-type headache (Fig. 2b)

Tension-type headache is the most common form of headache. The headache can be continuous or episodic and is described as pressure or a tight band around the head. The pain usually responds relatively poorly to analgesics but the patient continues to take them. The pain may be related to stress or fatigue, though can lack any clear trigger.

The pathophysiology of these headaches is not known. In spite of the frequency, the available treatments are rather disappointing. Amitriptyline is helpful, as are relaxation exercises. Helping the patient with any other associated problems may be helpful.

Many patients have a mixture of headaches with features of both migraine and tension-type headaches. These patients can be treated both on the basis of migraine or tension-type headache.

Medication overuse headache

Patients with chronic headache often consume large amounts of analgesics. If they are taking codeine-based analgesia or ergotamine-based drugs regularly they may be experiencing headaches from the withdrawal of the drug, which they then treat by further dosage, as well as their original headache type. In some patients the original headache has resolved. Treatment is to switch to non-codeine-based analgesics and try to stop analgesia altogether by using prophylactic treatment.

Cluster headache (Fig. 2c)

This is a very characteristic uncommon syndrome that has had many names: migrainous neuralgia, Horton's neuralgia, ciliary neuralgia. It affects men six times more commonly than women. The bouts of severe orbital pain last from 15 min to 3 h and are associated with conjunctival injection, lacrimation and blockage of the nostril. Occasionally a ptosis and Horner's syndrome develops. They occur frequently, once or more per day, for several weeks before subsiding to recur later, again in clusters. Occasionally the headaches occur almost exactly every 24 h. During the headache the patient is restless and walks about, quite unlike a patient with migraine who will lie still. Alcohol may trigger an attack.

The acute attack can be treated with oxygen, sumatriptan by injection or ergot. Treatment to abort the cluster is preferable and steroids and verapamil are usually effective.

Trigeminal neuralgia (Fig. 2d)

Trigeminal neuralgia is a sudden severe pain (like a red hot needle) and lasts seconds to minutes, and may be followed by a dull aching pain. It occurs in bouts, often many times each day. It can be triggered by touch, movement or cold, sometimes preventing the patient eating or drinking even to the point of dehydration. Trigeminal neuralgia is usually caused by compression of the trigeminal nerve by an ectatic blood vessel. It can also occur in multiple sclerosis.

Treatment with carbamazepine is usually effective. Phenytoin or sodium valproate can also be used. If these agents are not effective, glycerol injection or electrical lesion of the trigeminal ganglion can be effective, though may lead to trigeminal sensory loss. Definitive treatment is by surgical decompression of the trigeminal nerve from the compressing vessel.

Atypical facial pain

This occurs in women. It is a unilateral, chronic, unpleasant, aching facial pain. Usually the pain is thought to come from the teeth and often patients have had unsuccessful dental procedures (including extractions). Analgesics are usually ineffective. Amitriptyline and some other tricyclics may be helpful.

Other head pains

There are a large number of other headache syndromes: the international headache society classification runs to a short book. Here are a few of the more common or characteristic ones:

- Ice pick headache – brief sudden severe pain occurring at various sites around the head. A migraine variant, responding to migraine prophylaxis.
- Benign coital or exertional cephalalgia – recurrent sudden severe headache arising at the point of orgasm (coital) or on severe exertion (exertional). Main differential diagnosis is subarachnoid haemorrhage; once this is excluded the condition responds to migraine prophylaxis.
- Low-pressure headache (pp. 39 and 49).
- Thunderclap headache (p. 72).
- Temporomandibular pain – pain from the temporomandibular joint can manifest as headache spreading from the joint up the side of the head. It is triggered by jaw movements, especially grinding of the teeth at night (bruxism). This usually responds to interventions from the oral surgeon.

Headache

- Headache is a very common symptom; most are benign but unpleasant, few are dangerous.
- A clinical diagnosis of headache can be made in most patients.
- Dangerous headaches are rare and are usually single rather than recurrent.

Blackouts and 'funny do's'

Blackouts are one of the most common presentations in neurology, accounting for 18% of new neurological outpatients. The most common causes are seizures or syncope. While a list of possible causes is long, the clinical history, particularly with an account from a witness, will usually define the nature of the attack and direct investigations.

History

'Blackout' is a term that is usually used to mean episodes of loss of consciousness but some patients use it to mean episodes of altered consciousness. Other patients can mean a range of other things including dizzy feelings, memory loss or occasionally even episodes of weakness without impaired consciousness. It is important to find out what they mean. To help you do this, the range of feelings most often included within the term are discussed below. Other key aspects of the history include a detailed description of the blackout – what the patient was doing, any precipitating factors and the time course of the blackout, including any prodromal symptoms, aura immediately before the blackout, features of the blackout (ictus) itself and any post-ictal effects – are all important in making the diagnosis. A *witnessed account* of what happened is *essential*.

Examination

The examination is usually normal in patients with blackouts of all causes. Examinations of the cardiovascular system and the nervous system are particularly important – look for pulse irregularity, evidence of cardiac failure, murmurs, extracranial bruits, erect and supine blood pressures and any focal neurological signs.

Types of blackouts and 'funny do's'

Episodes with collapse

Generalized seizure (Fig. 1). These may occur at any time and in any position. The patient may have a warning (aura), such as a smell or taste or simply a strange feeling (see below). The aura is usually brief (a few seconds). There may be no warning. The patient may be observed to go blank or be lip smacking before losing consciousness. The patient then goes stiff and lets out a grunt. The arms and legs go stiff for a period and the jaw is clenched tight. This may be followed by a jerking of the limbs. This usually goes on for 2–3 min. The patient usually goes into a deep sleep. On coming round, the patient is muddled. Patients frequently bite their tongue and pass urine.

Syncope (Fig. 1). Syncope results from a fall in blood pressure leading to cerebral hypoperfusion. Syncope is usually preceded by a feeling of lightheadedness, dimming of vision, a sweaty feeling and a feeling of becoming distant. This may be brief but usually lasts minutes. Some patients get no warning. The patient is then observed to go pale and to slump to the ground occasionally falling more stiffly. They then lie still, or there are often a few small twitching movements. The period of unconsciousness is usually brief, less than 30 s, and is followed by a rapid recovery. Incontinence of urine does occur. Tongue biting is very rare. Syncope in older patients or those with known ischaemic heart disease, or occurring on exertion, suggests a significant cardiac cause.

NB. A patient who has a syncopal event but is kept upright or who has a prolonged cerebral hypotensive episode for

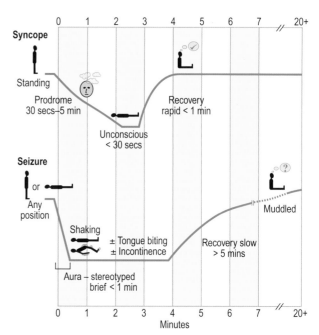

Fig. 1 **Time course of syncope and generalized seizure.**

some other reason may go on to have a generalized seizure (see above). This is a provoked seizure.

There may be factors in the situation of the blackout that suggest syncopal episodes:

- If it occurred after prolonged standing, in a hot place or after some distress such as the sight of blood. All these suggest a vasovagal syncope.
- If it is preceded by a palpitation – suggesting arrhythmia.
- If it occurred on standing – suggesting postural hypotension.
- If it occurred in particular situations, e.g. micturition (micturition syncope) or cough (cough syncope).
- Syncope can be physiologically induced, for example by hyperventilation or Valsalva manoeuvre. Patients may be unaware that they are hyperventilating. In these patients there may be a sensation of breathlessness and tingling in the arms and legs.
- Syncope can occur recurrently, which may reflect carotid hypersensitivity or malignant vasovagal syndrome.

Rarer causes of collapse

Subarachnoid haemorrhage. This may present with sudden severe headache followed by loss of consciousness.

Intermittent hydrocephalus. This may present with sudden loss of consciousness often without warning. This is a 'classical' (meaning very rare but everyone remembers it) presentation of the rare colloid cyst of the third ventricle.

Drop attack. In this condition the patient suddenly drops to the ground. Often it is not clear whether the patient has lost consciousness. This may be a form of seizure, cardiac arrhythmia or may reflect structural brain disease. Most commonly it is seen in older women and no cause is found.

Sleep. Narcolepsy is a disease of unknown aetiology associated with HLA DR2/DQW1 histocompatibility antigen. There are two features that enter the differential diagnosis of blackouts: a tendency to fall asleep suddenly and unexpectedly; and episodes of loss of muscle tone at times of high emotion, such as laughter or tears: cataplexy. Treatment is with dexamphetamine or modafinil.

Hypoglycaemia. Hypoglycaemia presents with lightheadedness, sweating and often a feeling of fear. The patient becomes dizzy. This usually presents no diagnostic problems in diabetics. However, if there is a coexistent autonomic neuropathy, then prodromal symptoms are lost. Hypoglycaemia is also common in alcoholics (poor dietary intake and reduced hepatic glycogen stores combined with the hypoglycaemic effect of alcohol). Insulinomas are very rare causes.

Non-epileptic attacks, pseudo-seizures and psychogenic seizures. These present a difficult diagnostic problem. The attacks are usually different from epileptic seizures: they are variable, longer lasting and fluctuate during the attack. Movements often seem more purposeful or semi-purposeful and they more often resist those attending them: 'It took five people to hold me down'. There is no associated cyanosis or respiratory changes. The differential diagnosis is with frontal seizures and rare intermittent movement disorders.

Episodes without collapse

Absences. Absences typically occur in children as a manifestation of primary generalized epilepsy. The child is still and stares. The eyelids may flutter and there may be some mouth movement. They are usually very brief but may last minutes. They occur frequently. An EEG shows 3 Hz spike and wave discharges.

Partial seizures and complex partial seizures. These are focal onset seizures either with (complex partial seizures) or without (partial seizures) loss of consciousness. The prodromal sensations that occur are the same in either situation whether or not consciousness is lost. The manifestations depend on the site of onset of the seizure. Either type of seizure may go on to a secondary generalized seizure so these may constitute the aura of a generalized seizure.

Common patterns include:

- all are brief (usually seconds or very occasionally minutes)
- a smell or taste often associated with an unpleasant feeling in the stomach (temporal lobe onset)
- a feeling of déjà vu (temporal lobe onset)
- a sensation of numbness or tingling (parietal lobe onset)
- jerking of one limb or head turning, or occasionally more stereotyped movements, e.g cycling (frontal onset)
- a flash of light (occipital lobe onset).

A witness will describe patients with complex partial seizures as going glassy-eyed. They may describe colour change or lip smacking or semi-purposeful movement. The patient is often confused afterwards.

Transient ischaemic attacks. The sudden onset of loss of any function of the nervous system can arise from vascular causes. Only rarely is consciousness lost (p. 70).

Transient global amnesia. This is a moderately common condition in adults aged over 40 years. For a period of 2–6 h, there is almost total failure to acquire new information and patients appear confused. They characteristically ask the same question again and again, ignoring any answers. Otherwise they can do quite complicated things such as driving. The recurrence rate is about 10%. The condition is associated with migraine, but not epilepsy or cerebrovascular disease.

Migraine. Migraine may cause focal neurological symptoms of gradual onset over about 15–30 min. Typically these are visual symptoms, though numbness, tingling or speech disturbance can occur. The typical headache usually follows (p. 42), but may not, which may lead to consideration of other differential diagnoses (Table 1).

Investigation

This is directed by the history. No investigation may be needed (e.g. vasovagal attacks or micturition syncope). If the patient is thought to have had a syncopal attack, the following investigations may be considered: fasting glucose, electrocardiogram, 24 h tape, echocardiogram or tilt table test. If the patient is thought to have had a seizure, the following investigations could be considered (see p. 74 for discussion): MRI or CT brain scan, EEG, 24 h EEG or calcium. If the diagnosis is uncertain, investigation should be directed towards both syncope and seizure, concentrating particularly on treatable options.

Management

Management will depend on the cause. Patients who have had a blackout need to be advised about the regulations relating to driving (Box 1) and commonsense advice about lifestyle; to avoid any situation that could put them or anyone else at risk, for example swimming; showering instead of taking a bath.

Table 1 **Pattern of sensory and other symptoms in different types of attack**

Diagnosis	Typical duration	Symptoms
Partial seizure	Seconds to 3 minutes	Positive
Migraine	10–30 minutes	Positive and negative
Transient ischaemic attack	Minutes to hours	Negative

Box 1

Regulations in relation to driving

This is a summary of some of the driving regulations in the UK in relation to ordinary driving licences. It is the doctor's responsibility to make the patient aware of the regulations and to contact the Driving and Vehicle Licensing Authority (DVLA). Special licences, such as those required to drive heavy goods vehicles, have more stringent regulations.

Situation	Rule
Single seizure or blackout with seizure markers	Licence revoked for 1 year
Single provoked seizure	Dealt with by DVLA on an individual basis. Must inform DVLA
Recurrent seizures	Licence revoked until seizure-free for 1 year
Seizures in sleep only	May drive despite continuing seizures, providing all seizures have been in sleep for at least 3 years
Transient ischaemic attacks	Usually can drive 1 month after a single episode
Transient global amnesia	No effect on driving
Simple faint	No effect on driving

Blackouts and 'funny do's'

- The diagnosis of blackouts depends almost entirely on the history.
- The history from a witness is essential.
- The cause of single unwitnessed blackouts is often uncertain.
- The relevant driving regulations must be explained to the patient after they have had a blackout.

Giddiness

Giddiness or *dizziness* are terms used by patients to describe a wide variety of sensations. It is crucial to obtain a precise understanding of the patient's presenting complaint in order for clinical evaluation to proceed along appropriate lines. Table 1 summarizes the symptoms commonly described as 'giddiness'.

Vertigo

Vertigo is an incorrect perception of relative motion between the individual and the environment. The sensation may be of rotation (semicircular canal dysfunction) or an undulation like being on the deck of a ship (otolith dysfunction) and it may be in any direction. The patient may feel that they or their surroundings are moving. This usually causes postural instability and the patient has to sit or lie down. It is the sensation we normally feel on getting off a playground roundabout. Vertigo causes nausea and sometimes vomiting and there may be associated fear, sweating and pallor. Vertigo is due to a mismatch between sensory inputs involved in maintaining posture. These are the visual, proprioceptive and vestibular systems. In practice, vertigo is usually due to dysfunction of the peripheral vestibular apparatus or its central pathways.

Causes

Seventy per cent of vertigo is caused by four syndromes: benign paroxysmal positioning vertigo (BPPV), vestibular neuritis, Ménière's disease and phobic vertigo. These can be diagnosed clinically, with minimal investigation. If not falling into one of these categories, then the key anatomical differentiation is between peripheral vestibular dysfunction arising from the vestibular structures in the ear and lesions affecting central vestibular connections within the brain stem.

Clinical assessment

Key features in the clinical assessment are:

- *Timing:* is the vertigo intermittent or sustained and what is the duration of intermittent epsiodes?
- *Head movement:* is vertigo triggered by certain head positions? This usually signifies a peripheral lesion, most commonly BPPV.

Table 1 Symptoms commonly described as giddiness

Symptom	Clinical interpretation	Comment
Feeling of relative movement (usually spinning) of self and environment	Vertigo	Peripheral or central vestibular disturbance
Feeling of lightheadedness and impending faintness	Presyncope	See page 44
Feeling of altered awareness and impaired consciousness	Altered consciousness	Consider complex partial seizures, absence attacks
Unsteadiness with a clear head	Ataxia	Cerebellar or proprioceptive

- *Auditory dysfunction:* is there deafness or tinnitus? This points to a disturbance of the labyrinth or vestibulocochlear nerve. Once in the brain stem, auditory and vestibular function are separate.
- *Medication:* anticonvulsant toxicity causes vertigo and aminoglycosides cause irreversible vestibular damage.
- *Eye movements:* nystagmus without vertigo generally points to a CNS cause.
- Signs of CNS involvement (ataxia, dysarthria, sensory and motor signs in the limbs) point to an intracranial cause.

Types

Intermittent vertigo

Positional. BPPV is much the most common cause and is easily recognized. It may follow viral infection or head trauma. There is often a period of a few days when patients are bed-bound, because rising triggers disabling attacks of vertigo and vomiting. They then suffer brief attacks of vertigo, for up to 60 s, each time they put their head into a particular position, usually on lying down. This settles over a period of weeks but may recur. Hallpike's test shows characteristic responses (see below). Other causes of positioning vertigo include alcohol and anticonvulsant intoxication, perilymph fistula (often post-traumatic and usually with a hearing deficit) and, rarely, central oculomotor disorders with failure of vestibulo-ocular reflexes (see below and p. 18).

Non-positional. Ménière's disease is the most common cause of peripheral, non-positional vertigo but is overdiagnosed. Middle-aged patients typically suffer episodes lasting hours with associated tinnitus and a hearing deficit. During the episode there is spontaneous nystagmus and between episodes there is a decline in hearing. Other peripheral causes include

otosclerosis, hyperviscosity syndromes, syphilitic labyrinthitis and Cogan's syndrome (autoimmune).

CNS causes are often associated with symptoms of brain stem dysfunction; diplopia, ataxia, cranial nerve or limb deficits. Vertebrobasilar migraine (VBM) occurs mainly in children, with episodes lasting minutes to hours with headache and often a visual aura. In young adults, multiple sclerosis causes episodes lasting hours to weeks, and vertebrobasilar ischaemia (VBI) is an occasional and overdiagnosed cause of brief attacks in older adults. The idea that neck movement interferes with vertebral artery flow to cause dizziness has been proven false.

Loss of consciousness does not usually occur with vertigo, although patients with VBM or VBI may blackout with their attacks. Very rarely, episodic vertigo may be due to vestibular epilepsy of the temporal lobes, in which there may be other epileptic features such as oroalimentary automatisms or convulsions.

Sustained vertigo. Peripheral disease is usually idiopathic vestibular neuritis, which is believed to be due to infection. There is an acute onset of vertigo, which persists for several weeks and gradually subsides. There is gaze-evoked nystagmus, with a rotatory component. There is canal paresis on caloric testing (see below). Many other acute vestibular lesions also produce this picture, including trauma, infarction (hyperviscosity syndromes), tumours (especially acoustic nerve tumours and Schwannomas) (p. 96) and infections. Important identifiable infections causing this syndrome include syphilis, tuberculosis and Lyme disease. Herpes zoster virus causes acute vertigo, unilateral hearing loss, ipsilateral facial paresis, severe pain, malaise and characteristic herpetic vesicles around the external auditory meatus: 'Ramsay Hunt syndrome'. It responds to aciclovir.

Brain stem lesions may cause sustained vertigo, especially multiple sclerosis, infarction and tumours. The clue is other associated brain stem deficits.

Phobic vertigo. Phobic vertigo is usually characterized by a more vague sensation of unsteadiness that often fluctuates rather than being continuous or coming in discrete attacks. There may be associated symptoms of hyperventilation; difficulty catching breath and paraesthesiae and symptoms may be reproduced by hyperventilation. It is sometimes due to failure of compensation following previous vestibular disturbance or may be a primary psychogenic disturbance.

Specialized clinical tests
Hallpike's manoeuvre may elicit the typical abnormality of BPPV. The patient is lowered down rapidly into the position which elicits vertigo (Fig. 1). There is:

- a delay of several seconds before the onset of the nystagmus
- a rotatory component towards the lowermost ear
- mild nystagmus and severe vertigo, both passing off rapidly
- successively milder responses on repeat testing.

Other causes of positional vertigo may produce severe nystagmus of immediate onset and mild vertigo, neither of which habituates.

Vestibulo-ocular response (VOR) tests 'doll's eye movements' pathways between the vestibular system and the nuclei controlling eye movements. The patient sits in a rotating chair and fixes their eyes on a distant object. The chair is rotated at approximately 30° per second and the patient's eyes rotate at an equal and opposite rate to maintain fixation. Any nystagmus or failure to maintain fixation, which may occur in only one direction, implies a lesion of the VOR.

If there is central otolith malfunction, the patient's perception of the direction of gravity may be abnormally tilted. This is seen especially in lateral medullary lesions, such as infarction of the posterior inferior cerebellar artery. Patients compensate by holding the head tilted. With the head held in the horizontal position, one eye may appear to be above the other: 'skew deviation'.

Investigations
- *Caloric tests.* Water is introduced into one external auditory canal at 32°C and 41°C. This normally causes nystagmus with specific latency and duration that can be measured. **C**old causes the fast phase of the nystagmus to the **O**pposite side and **W**arm to the **S**ame side (COWS).
- *Auditory evoked potentials* measure delay in central auditory pathways, especially in multiple sclerosis (p. 33).
- *Audiometry.* Tests of hearing threshold provide evidence of function of the auditory component of the 8th cranial nerve.
- *MRI scan* is the investigation of choice in central vestibular disturbance. A CT brain scan may miss posterior fossa lesions, especially small acoustic Schwannomas, and will miss demyelination.

Treatment
Treatment can be symptomatic or specific, and is directed at the underlying cause.

Symptomatic
In the acute phase of vertigo associated with nausea and vomiting, vestibular sedatives are indicated:

- Antihistamines, e.g. betahistine and cinnarizine. These are sedative, and patients should not operate machinery or drink alcohol.

- Dopaminergic antagonists, e.g. prochlorperazine and metaclopramide. These are mildly sedative but extrapyramidal side-effects occasionally occur acutely and are common in long-term use (> 6 months).
- Anticholinergics, e.g. hyoscine. These cause dry mouth, constipation and sometimes urinary retention or confusion.

After the acute phase, it is important to encourage compensatory mechanisms to allow recovery of central vestibular function. Vestibular sedatives may delay this process and should be stopped. Patients are taught graded exercises to move their head into all positions, including the one they find uncomfortable, to facilitate retraining of central mechanisms.

Specific
Benign positional vertigo. Positioning manoeuvres have been demonstrated to be effective. This syndrome is caused by debris within the semicircular canals. Positioning so as to remove this is curative, and can be done using several different manoeuvres, such as the Epley manoeuvre, or using Brandt–Daroff exercises.

Vestibular neuronitis. Treatment is symptomatic as this resolves spontaneously.

Ménière's disease. This is an episodic illness so acute treatment is symptomatic only. Acetazolamide can be used as a prophylactic agent. ENT surgeons usually manage these patients. Surgical procedures to decompress the endolymph have been used.

Phobic postural vertigo. This has been demonstrated to improve after a detailed explanation of the presumed basis for the syndrome, a misinterpretation of mismatched vestibular syndromes. This may be a form of cognitive therapy resulting from a reattribution of the causation of the dizziness.

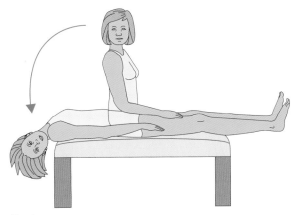

Fig. 1 **Hallpike's manoeuvre.**

> ### *Giddiness*
> - What patients mean by giddiness varies and needs to be clarified.
> - Most cases of vertigo are due to peripheral labyrinthine disease and can be diagnosed with minimal investigation.
> - Key clinical features include the timing of vertigo (continuous or episodic) and associated symptoms and signs.
> - MRI should be performed if there is unilateral hearing loss or there are neurological signs.
> - Vestibular sedatives should only be used in incapacitating vertigo or to control nausea.

Intracranial pressure

Before considering coma and unconsciousness it is useful to understand intracranial pressure and brain herniation. The intracranial compartment is a fixed box containing brain, blood and CSF. The dynamics of CSF flow are illustrated in Figure 1. Pressure may be increased by:

- intracranial masses, either intrinsic (e.g. glioma) or extrinsic (e.g. extradural haematoma)
- diffuse brain swelling following severe hypoxia, liver failure or hypertensive encephalopathy
- impaired circulation or absorption of CSF.

Hydrocephalus and ventricular dilatation occur if CSF is under increased pressure relative to the surrounding brain. This may be due to blocked flow (obstructive) or failure of reabsorption (communicating). Excess CSF production due to a tumour of the CSF-producing choroid plexus is a rare cause of communicating hydrocephalus.

There are two semi-rigid sheets, the falx cerebri and the tentorium cerebelli, which almost divide the brain into separate compartments with relatively small apertures between them (Fig. 2). When the pressure rises in one compartment, the brain may herniate through the apertures into adjacent compartments. The cerebellar tonsils and fourth ventricle may also be forced down through the foramen magnum. These are life-threatening complications that further block CSF flow, causing a vicious circle of rising intracranial pressure, resulting in coma (see below).

Failure of CSF reabsorption may occur because of thrombosis in the sagittal sinus, increased venous pressure reducing the pressure gradient across the arachnoid villi, or because the function of the arachnoid villi is damaged by the contents of the CSF: excessive cellularity (chronic meningitis), subarachnoid haemorrhage or very high protein content (some tumours and inflammatory conditions).

In some circumstances, such as benign intracranial hypertension (BIH), no cause may be found (p. 40).

Raised intracranial pressure

Raised intracranial pressure is a medical emergency. It causes headache, ataxia, confusion, drowsiness and coma. Papilloedema is usually present if the raised pressure has been longstanding, but because it takes time to develop, may be absent. Sixth nerve palsy is a common, false localizing sign due to compression of the 6th nerve as it passes over the petrous ridge. Other signs include 3rd nerve palsy in temporal lobe herniation, failure of upgaze, due to midbrain compression, a rise in systolic blood pressure and a fall in pulse due to medullary involvement.

Intermittent obstruction of CSF flow can cause sudden headache with loss of consciousness. For example intraventricular tumours may block CSF flow on sudden manoeuvres such as coughing or straining.

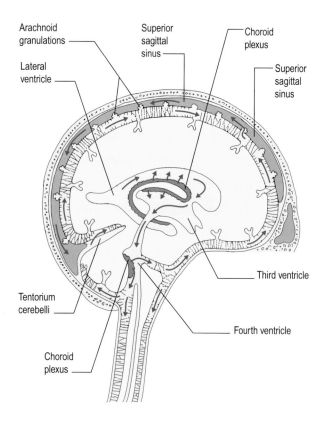

Fig. 1 **CSF production and flow.**

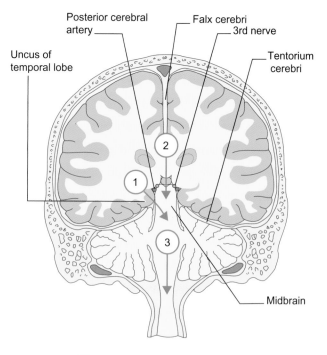

① Asymmetrical tentorial herniation

② Symmetrical tentorial herniation

③ Foramen magnum herniation

Fig. 2 **Tentorial herniation.**

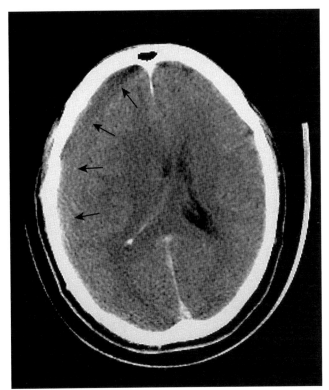

Fig. 3 **An isodense right-sided subdural (arrows) haematoma which presented with symptoms and signs of raised intracranial pressure.**

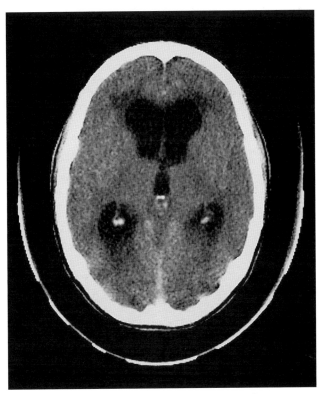

Fig. 4 **Acute hydrocephalus with enlarged lateral and 3rd ventricles.**

In children who develop raised intracranial pressure, usually a result of hydrocephalus, before closure of the skull sutures, presentation may be with a rapidly enlarging head size and minimal neurological compromise.

Low intracranial pressure
Reduced CSF pressure is usually due to CSF leakage through torn meninges. The most common causes are trauma, iatrogenic (neurosurgery, lumbar puncture and inadvertent puncture of the subarachnoid during epidural anaesthesia) and tumours. Spontaneous leaks are rare. It may present with headache on standing or with CSF rhinorrhoea. Leakage from the nose is especially associated with recurrent meningitis.

Herniation
There are two major sites of cerebral herniation.

The tentorium (Fig. 2)
Here the brain herniates through the space between the cerebrum and the cerebellum surrounded by the tentorium cerebri. This can be symmetrical or asymmetrical. Asymmetrical is more common. The uncus of the temporal lobe is squeezed through this space. This compresses:

- the 3rd nerve, leading to unilateral 3rd nerve palsy involving the pupils
- the midbrain, leading to coma and pupillary changes bilaterally with a tetraparesis
- the posterior cerebral artery, leading to occipital infarction, increasing supratentorial pressure and increasing the herniation.

Symmetrical herniation produces compression of the whole of the midbrain as it is forced through the tentorium cerebra, producing bilaterally dilated pupils, coma and tetraparesis.

Foramen magnum herniation
This is rarer and the syndrome results from compression of the reticular formation, respiratory centres and motor tracts. This leads to severe neck pain, erratic breathing, progressing tetraparesis and coma.

Both of these processes progress to death if uninterrupted.

Treatment
Treatment will depend on the cause. There may be readily treatable surgical causes, such as subdural (Fig. 3) or extradural haematoma, or hydrocephalus (Fig. 4). These would be treated with drainage or shunting.

In patients with brain swelling, mannitol, the osmotic diuretic, will briefly reduce the intracranial pressure. However, this is only short lived and is thus of limited use. Steroids will reduce cerebral oedema, though usually not cytotoxic oedema (brain swelling resulting from swelling of dying cells). Hyperventilation of ventilated patients will reduce ICP. In some clinical circumstances surgical decompression can be used.

Intracranial pressure

- Increased intracranial pressure occurs with space-occupying lesions, diffuse brain swelling or abnormal CSF circulation or reabsorption.

- Raised intracranial pressure is a medical emergency, presenting with progressive headache, ataxia and drowsiness.

- Herniation of the brain through the tentorium cerebelli or the foramen magnum leads to brain stem and cranial nerve compression that is fatal if untreated.

Coma and alteration of consciousness

Coma is a common and important medical emergency, accounting for 3% of acute hospital admissions. This section discusses the terminology used in this field, which is often confusing, then considers the aetiology and pathogenesis of coma, then outlines a pragmatic approach to these patients.

Terminology

There are many different terms used to describe different types of altered consciousness, e.g. coma, stupor, confusion or obtundation. Unfortunately these mean different things to different people and so are of limited use. This in part reflects the complicated nature of consciousness, making it unsurprising that this cannot be summed up in a single word. It therefore is more useful to try and quantify consciousness individually using specific descriptions or scales (see below). Altered consciousness and coma are a spectrum. The differential diagnosis and management varies according to the level of consciousness. Within that spectrum, however, coma can be recognized as being very much at one end. Coma can be practically defined as unrousable unconsciousness and is discussed in this section.

Aetiology and pathogenesis

Consciousness depends on the intact functioning of the reticular activating system in the brain stem and the cerebral cortex. Coma and altered consciousness arise from disturbance of these elements (Table 2). This can arise from:

■ infratentorial lesions that disrupt the reticular activating system directly
■ supratentorial lesions – large enough to cause herniation (p. 48) or large enough to disrupt the cortex
■ diffuse cerebral insult that affects the function of the cortex and reticular activation system.

Coma

The clinical assessment of coma is outlined in Box 1. Coma is usually readily recognizable. Potential differential diagnoses include:

■ **'Locked in syndrome'.** This results from a high midbrain lesion or a severe generalized neuropathy, which prevent the patient from all movement despite having a normal consciousness.
■ **Catatonia.** This is a psychiatric state of unresponsiveness.
■ **Vegetative state.** In patients with diffuse bihemispheric disease but normal brain stem function, this may lead to a vegetative state. This is not usually relevant to the acute diagnosis of coma.

The next issue is to determine the cause so as to direct future management of the coma (Box 1). This can be broadly divided into the following categories:

Box 1

Assessment of patients with coma

1. **History.** It is important that this be obtained from anyone that may help – ambulance personnel, passers-by. Silent witnesses, such as a wallet or bracelet, are often very informative.
2. **Examination.**
   ■ General – vital signs – pulse, blood pressure, temperature, respiration and blood glucose
   ■ External signs of trauma, including Battle's signs (as on p. 79), evidence of injections, bitten tongue or neck stiffness
   ■ Neurological examination
     – Glasgow Coma Scale (p. 122)
     – pupillary examination (Table 1)
     – doll's head eye movements
     – fundoscopy
     – signs of any other neurological abnormality
     – look for facial asymmetry and asymmetry of limbs
     – tone, posture or response to pain
     – asymmetry of reflexes or plantar responses may be useful.

Table 1 Pupillary responses in coma

Pupils equal	Pinpoint		Opiate overdose, pontine lesion
	Small	Reactive	Metabolic encephalopathy
	Mid-sized	Unreactive	Midbrain lesion
		Reactive	Metabolic encephalopathy
	Large		Drugs: cocaine, ecstasy, antidepressants, cholinesterase inhibitors
Pupils unequal	Large	Unreactive	3rd nerve palsy (ptosis and deviated pupil)
	Small	Reactive	Horner's syndrome with partial ptosis

Table 2 Some causes of coma

Site of disease	Causes
Infratentorial	Infarct
	Haemorrhage
	Tumour
	Inflammatory lesion
Supratentorial	Subarachnoid haemorrhage
	Extradural or subdural haematoma
	Intracranial haemorrhage
	Tumour
	Infarct
Diffuse	Metabolic
	Hypoglycaemia, hyperglycaemia, hyponatraemia, hypernatraemia, hypoxia, acidosis, hypothyroidism, hepatic failure
	Toxic
	Drugs
	Alcohol
	Epilepsy
	Multiple sedative drugs, in particular benzodiazepines and other sedative drugs
	Hypothermia
	Infections
	Meningitis, encephalitis

■ Coma with neck stiffness. This can arise from meningitis, subarachnoid haemorrhage and, rarely, as a result of foramen magnum herniation.
■ Coma with focal signs. It is especially important to detect signs of herniation. Other causes include supratentorial and infratentorial lesions.

- Coma without focal signs, relating to diffuse cerebral lesions.

Management of coma
Coma is a medical emergency requiring resuscitation. There are two main strands of treatment: (1) supportive treatment applicable to all patients with coma, and (2) specific treatment of the underlying cause.

Supportive
Supportive treatment is aimed at avoiding the complications of unconsciousness. Key elements include:

- protecting airways
- maintaining blood pressure – intravenous fluids or inotropes as needed
- emptying the stomach contents using a nasogastric tube
- avoidance of deep venous thrombosis using TED stockings
- maintaining homeostasis, particularly the blood gases and electrolytes
- urinary catheterization
- nursing with regular turning or use of an air mattress to avoid pressure sores.

Identification and treatment of specific underlying causes
This is in large part going to be dictated by the clinical situation.

Coma with neck stiffness
With fever. Give broad spectrum antibiotics to cover likely meningitic organisms. Undertake a brain scan followed by lumbar puncture, if there is no contraindication on scanning. Further treatment would depend on CSF findings (p. 38).

Without fever. Arrange a CT brain scan. If diagnostic of subarachnoid haemorrhage, management is as described on page 72. If no blood is seen or the scan is not diagnostic, proceed to lumbar puncture.

Coma with focal signs
This requires cerebral imaging to determine the underlying cause. Frequently this can be anticipated on the basis of the history. These patients may require manoeuvres to reduce their intracranial pressure, which include:

- mannitol infusion
- dexamethasone
- intubation and hyperventilation to reduce intracranial pressure.

Further management would depend on the underlying diagnosis.

Coma without signs or neck stiffness
The history is likely to be the most useful aspect in establishing the underlying cause. This may be sufficiently clear cut, e.g. overdose, alcohol excess or post-ictal state. However, there are situations where other investigations are essential.

Investigations include: glucose, urea and electrolytes. Blood gases and a toxicology screen may be important. In some circumstances liver function tests, ammonia, group and even red cell transketolase screening (for low vitamin B1) can be useful. If these do not yield useful information, cerebral imaging needs to be undertaken. Lumbar puncture should be considered as encephalitis can often be difficult to diagnose. An EEG can be helpful in this and in the diagnosis of epilepsy and encephalitis.

Treatment will depend on the underlying cause. For example, a metabolic disturbance should be corrected. NB: A low sodium should be corrected slowly to avoid complications such as central pontine myelinolysis. Antiviral agents can be used in encephalitis.

Specific treatments
These include:

- hypoglycaemia – glucose
- opiate overdose – naloxone
- benzodiazepine overdose – flumazenil
- Wernicke's encephalopathy – thiamine (rare)
- Addisonian crisis – steroids (rare).

Prognosis in coma
This depends on the underlying cause. The outcome from traumatic coma is considered on page 79. Prognosis depends on the cause and duration of coma. Patients with focal signs, especially pupillary signs, do particularly badly.

Criteria for brain stem death are used to determine when ventilatory and other support can be discontinued (Box 2).

Coma due to drug overdosage usually has a good outcome. A hypoglycaemic coma, if short-lived, usually leaves no sequelae.

Other causes of medical coma have a worse prognosis, with an overall recovery rate of only 15%.

Box 2

Diagnosis of brain stem death in the UK
The diagnosis of brain death relies on three elements:

1. The cause of failure of brain function is known to be irreversible.
2. The absence of cerebral function and the patient is unresponsive and unreceptive.
3. There is an absence of brain stem function.

Before testing, metabolic abnormalities should be corrected and time allowed for sedative medications to clear.

Brain stem tests
Tests for brain stem function are undertaken by two senior physicians on two occasions. No response must be found to any of the following:

- pupillary responses
- doll's head eye movements
- eye movements on caloric testing
- corneal responses
- gag responses
- response to painful stimuli
- respiratory response to hypercapnoea after preoxygenation giving a high oxygen flow, and then turning the ventilator off to allow the pCO_2 to rise to 8 kPa.

An EEG is not required to make the diagnosis.

Coma and alteration of consciousness

- Coma is a medical emergency.
- Coma arises from lesions directly affecting the reticular activation system in the brain stem or a generalized process affecting the whole cortex.
- The commonest causes of coma are drug overdose and head trauma.
- Hypoglycaemia needs to be considered early and treated quickly.
- Management involves a systematic assessment and investigation running in parallel with resuscitation.

Confusion and delirium

Introduction

This is an area of difficult terminology because most of the medical terms used are in everyday usage. In this chapter the term delirium will be used to avoid confusion (see what we mean). Some synonyms and alternative titles include:

- acute organic brain syndrome
- acute confusional state
- organic psychosis
- toxic/metabolic encephalopathy.

Delirium is common, occurring in up to 20% of medical ward patients with estimates of up to 50% of elderly hospital patients over the age of 65 years.

The principal abnormality in these patients is an alteration in arousal. Arousal is a prerequisite to normal consciousness. Normal consciousness is manifest by a clear awareness of the environment.

The manifestation of any confusional state or delirium depends on the premorbid state of the patient. A patient with a pre-existing higher function deficit will be more prone to florid delirium than someone with normal higher function.

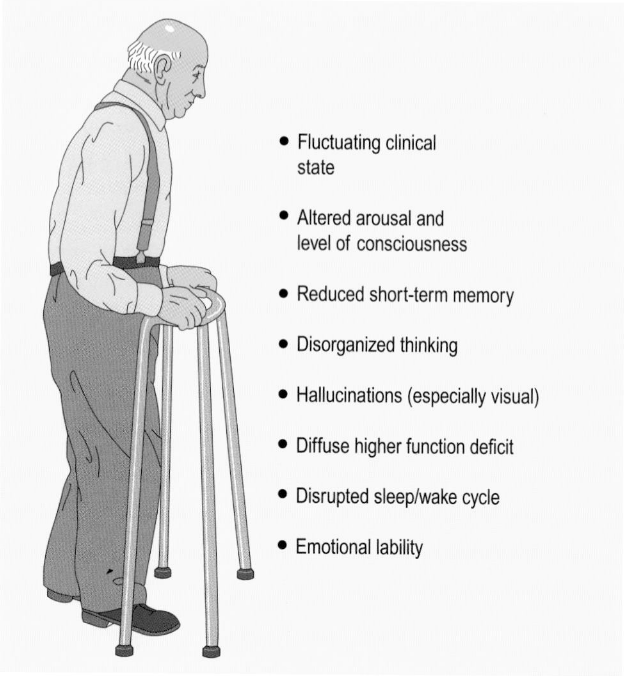

- Fluctuating clinical state
- Altered arousal and level of consciousness
- Reduced short-term memory
- Disorganized thinking
- Hallucinations (especially visual)
- Diffuse higher function deficit
- Disrupted sleep/wake cycle
- Emotional lability

Fig. 1 **Clinical features of delirium.**

Clinical features (Fig. 1)

Delirium comes on within hours to a few weeks. There is a prominent fluctuation in symptomatology. Patients are distractible and disorganized in thinking. They are slow to respond and may find it difficult to answer questions without going off at a tangent. Their speech may be slurred. They may report hallucinations which are often visual, florid and menacing. Their sleep pattern becomes disrupted with sleeping in the day and waking at night. Most patients become physically slowed. They usually have a prominent loss of short-term memory, reflecting their poor attention. Patients become emotionally labile, being tearful or frightened, or become angry and agitated relatively easily. Some patients can become hyperactive and very agitated.

Differential diagnosis

When you see a patient in this state ask yourself:

It it delirium? The differential diagnosis of delirium includes the following.

Dementia

Demented patients usually have normal arousal, although arousal can become altered in dementia. The major difference however, is the onset, which is years for dementia and days to weeks for delirium. A corroborated history is essential.

NB. Delirium is much more prominent in patients with a pre-existing dementing illness.

Aphasia

Patients with aphasia can be thought to be confused, particularly with fluent aphasia. Careful testing of speech usually clarifies the diagnosis.

Schizophrenia

Attention is usually normal in schizophrenia, though testing may be difficult. Hallucinations are usually auditory and delusions tend to be systematic rather than chaotic.

Causes of delirium

In many patients, particularly elderly patients, there may be more than one cause for the delirium (Table 1).

Assessment

Assessment is made difficult by the limited history that is obtainable directly from the patient. It is important to obtain a history to establish:

- Timing of the onset of the confusion.
- Prior level of mental function and pattern of behaviour. Were there any clues to suggest an impaired premorbid intellect?

Table 1	**Causes of delirium**	
Systemic	Metabolic	
		Hyper- or hyponatraemia
		Hypercalcaemia
		Hypoglycaemia
		Hepatic failure
		Hypothyroidism
	Toxic	
		Drugs, especially antiparkinsonian medications and illicit drugs
		Toxins – alcohol or alcohol withdrawal
	Infections	
		Septicaemia, urinary tract infections, pneumonia
Intrinsic	Infectious	
		Meningitis, encephalitis, malaria
	Paroxysmal	
		Epilepsy, ictal or post-ictal
	Immunological	
		Lupus
Vascular	Post-stroke	
	Subarachnoid haemorrhage	
Extrinsic	Subdural haematoma	
	Post-traumatic	
	Hydrocephalus	

- Any coexistent medical problems, particularly diabetes, epilepsy, Parkinson's disease, cardiac or respiratory problems.
- Drug usage, including over-the-counter remedies and illegal drugs. Any recent change in medication.
- Alcohol intake and diet.

- Any history of trauma, particularly head injury, in recent weeks.
- Any history of recent collapse or prior history of seizures.
- History of foreign travel – this broadens the differential diagnosis of infectious causes.

This will often be available from the spouse, another relative or carer. If there is no-one with the patient who can give the essential background information then it needs to be sought from neighbours, the local doctor or anyone else who might be able to provide it, or from any previous medical records. Figure 2 illustrates an important investigative tool used in this process.

General examination may provide clear indications as to the likely diagnosis: for example, signs of infection, liver failure, cardiac or respiratory failure, diabetes, drug usage. Meningitis can present with confusion so be alert for the meningococcal rash and for neck stiffness, especially in younger patients. Stiff neck can also be due to subarachnoid haemorrhage, another potential cause of confusion. The finding of a bitten tongue is useful as this is an indicator of recent seizure. In elderly patients with pre-existing higher function deficits, minor infection, particularly of the urinary tract, can lead to prominent confusion so general

examination must include testing the urine.

Neurological examination usually reveals no focal signs. The Glasgow Coma Scale is a standard way of recording level of consciousness (p. 129). Focal signs, especially in the elderly, raise the possibility of a chronic subdural haematoma. There may be signs in keeping with pre-existing neurological disease such as Parkinson's disease. Fidgeting and picking at objects that are not there is common in delirium, especially relating to alcohol withdrawal. Very occasionally a confused patient will have stereotyped movements of limb or face, which are a manifestation of recurrent complex partial seizures or non-convulsive status epilepticus (continuous absence or complex partial seizures).

Bedside higher function testing (pp. 12–13) documents the pattern of disturbance. Disorientation is particularly prominent with marked abnormal measures of attention, for example digit span. Usually the most useful documentation is specific observation regarding behaviour. Simple scales such as the Mini-Mental State score can be useful if somewhat crude.

Investigations

Further investigations will be led by the clinical assessment of the history and examination, and may include:

- metabolic screen – glucose, sodium, urea, calcium, liver function tests, gamma GT, drug screen, blood gases, red cell transketolase
- infection screen – full blood count and viscosity, blood cultures, urine microscopy and culture, chest X-ray
- neurological investigations – brain scan, CT or MRI, lumbar puncture if

CT is normal and no other cause found or features suggest meningitis or encephalitis, EEG (the diagnostic test for non-convulsive status and useful in encephalitis).

Management

General measures
This involves supporting the patient both physically and psychologically. The patient should have adequate nutrition and fluid intake. Steps should be taken to monitor and maintain physiological measures such as hydration, electrolytes, glucose and oxygenation.

Keeping patients in a standardized environment, with people known to them looking after them as much as possible, will tend to calm their agitation. They are usually best nursed in a well lit area. They should be allowed to move around in a safe environment. Distractions should be limited. Providing cues to help orientation is useful; for example, information about where they are and day and date.

Drugs should be avoided as patients are often particularly sensitive and can occasionally provoke surprising reactions. Sedatives such as haloperidol and chlorpromazine can be useful, especially in severely disturbed or aggressive patients. Benzodiazepines, such as chlordiazepoxide or lorazepam, can help in patients with alcohol withdrawal.

Specific treatment
Specific treatment will depend on the cause. This can involve correction of the underlying metabolic defect, treating the infection or associated medical conditions or controlling pain.

Old notes

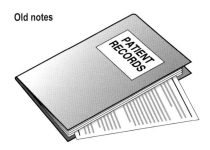

Phone

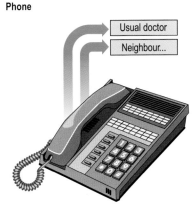

Fig. 2 **Important instruments in the investigation of a confused patient.**

Confusion and delirium

- Delirium is common.
- Delirium needs to be distinguished from dementia, aphasia and schizophrenia.
- A history from spouse, carer or other observer is important in the assessment of delirium.
- It is important to establish the cause of delirium to allow specific treatment.

Dementia

Introduction

Dementia can be defined in several ways but all include the following elements:

- an acquired loss in multiple domains of higher mental function
- a progressive decline
- occurring in clear consciousness.

The incidence is 50 per 100 000 population but is strongly age-related, being rare under the age of 60 years. The most common causes are neurodegenerative conditions, especially Alzheimer's disease (AD), Lewy body disease (LBD) and diffuse cerebrovascular disease. An unusual cause should be suspected in patients under 55, where progression is rapid or if other features are present (Table 1). Most neurodegenerative conditions can only be diagnosed with certainty by neuropathological examination. Most of these conditions progress slowly over many years so the prevalence and social burden of the condition are very high.

The role of the clinician is to identify less common treatable conditions, to advise regarding prognosis and to identify the rare familial diseases for which counselling may be important. The clinician forms part of a multidisciplinary team that coordinates care. Medical treatment may be helpful in the management of some associated problems, such as Parkinsonism, seen in some conditions, and complications such as behavioural abnormalities.

The approach to a patient with suspected dementia

Dementia may be considered immediately if the patient or family members complain of altered higher function. It is more difficult when the patient is alone and has different concerns. Dementia should be considered particularly when there are inconsistencies in the history.

The history, examination and investigation are all aimed at the following questions:

- Is there a deficit of higher function?
- Is it focal or diffuse?
- Is it progressive?
- Are there any other associated features?

History

A history from the patient can often be relatively uninformative. Patients may be unaware of their difficulties. A history from a family member or longstanding contact, a workmate or a neighbour, for example, is essential. The aim is to establish which areas of higher function are causing problems with memory, concentration, reading, daily activities, getting lost and so on. In addition, the history seeks evidence of the progressive nature of the problems.

Examination

Bedside neurological testing of higher function (pp. 12–13) seeking to measure the deficits is combined with a detailed neurological examination. The latter usually only finds non-specific features, such as frontal release signs (snout, grasp reflexes), but may find evidence of associations such as Parkinsonism or focal signs that may point to alternative disease (frontal lesions) (Table 1). Awareness of the mental state is important because depression is one of the most treatable differential diagnoses.

Investigations

These include formal psychometry for the documentation of deficits and as a baseline in patients with subtle defects to allow repetition to demonstrate progression. Other causes can be sought with brain imaging (CT or MRI) and a blood screen, including vitamin B12, thyroid function and syphilis serology (Table 2).

The aim of these assessments is to identify treatable causes and to attempt to characterize the pattern of dementia in neurodegenerative dementias. The latter aim is to identify AD, for which there are now some potential specific therapies.

Alzheimer's disease

AD represents over 70% of cases of dementia. The prevalence increases from 300 per 100 000 at age 60–69 years to 20% over age 85 years.

Pathology and aetiology

There is cerebral atrophy, usually starting in the temporal lobes with characteristic neurofibrillary tangles and senile plaques. An important constituent of the senile plaques is amyloid-β-protein, which is derived from amyloid-β-precursor protein (APP) and apolipoprotein E4. Studies support the importance of genetic abnormalities of both of these proteins in the aetiology of AD. The pathophysiology includes neurotransmitter defects, especially of cholinergic projection to the basal forebrain.

Clinical features

AD usually presents in three stages: (1) memory disturbance; (2) global cognitive decline with relatively intact personality; and (3) severe global decline with disorders of social behaviour, failure of self-care, incontinence and dependence.

The first symptom is commonly forgetfulness, which may be reported by family members or may cause failure at work. On formal testing there is evidence of more global impairment of cognitive function. As the disease evolves, depression (30%) and personality change (75%) commonly develop, especially apathy. Behavioural changes such as verbal and physical aggression, inappropriate sexual

Table 1	**Dementias associated with prominent physical abnormalities**	
Clinical feature	**Condition**	**Associated features**
Apraxic gait disorder or Parkinsonism	Frontal lobe tumour	Frontal lobe syndrome
	Hydrocephalus	Headache, incontinence
	Cerebral arteriosclerosis	
	Parkinson's disease/ cortical Lewy body disease	Prominent hallucinations
	Wilson's disease	Psychiatric disease/corneal Kayser–Fleischer rings
Myoclonus	Creutzfeldt–Jakob disease	Rapid progression
	Subacute sclerosing panencephalitis	Rapid progression
Chorea	Huntington's disease	Autosmal dominant
	Systemic lupus erythematosus	Systemic vasculitis, seizures and depression
Ataxia	Wernicke–Korsakoff syndrome	See above
Supranuclear gaze palsy	Hydrocephalus	See above
	Whipple's disease	Rare but treatable (p. 99)
	Multiple sclerosis	See pages 84–87
	Progressive supranuclear palsy	See page 89
Neuropathy/spinal cord syndrome	Vitamin B12 and folic acid deficiency	Usually raised mean red blood cell volume
Weakness and fasciculation	MND dementia	Evolves to MND with dementia (p. 108)

behaviour and eating disorders occur later in 30–85% of cases. Hallucinations and psychotic disturbance are less common. Seizures occur in 10–20% of cases.

An examination may reveal a gegenhalten pattern of increased tone (p. 22), release of primitive reflexes (pout, palmo-mental and grasp) but any major physical neurological deficits suggest a different or additional disease. The hippocampus may show extreme atrophy in AD on MRI but there is no diagnostic test.

Other dementias

Diffuse Lewy body disease
A characteristic dementia is associated with the development of the Lewy body, the pathological hallmark of Parkinson's disease (PD), in the cerebral cortex. There are marked fluctuations in cognition, mimicking reversible acute confusional states, visual hallucinations, usually faces or animals, and behavioural disturbances and agitation are prominent. There are usually some signs of Parkinsonism, which can be subtle or severe. The disease progresses more rapidly than AD but the hallucinations respond particularly well to cholinesterase inhibitors, e.g. rivastigmine.

Familial dementia
About 5% of Alzheimer's disease is familial (autosomal dominant). The age at presentation is usually in the 40s or 50s and the disease is more rapidly progressive than the sporadic form. Seizures are also more common. Huntington's disease is the other common autosomal dominant dementia, presenting with associated movement disorder (p. 93). Other inherited dementias are rare; they usually present at a younger age than Alzheimer's disease and are usually associated with physical neurological deficits. Wilson's disease is an important treatable cause (p. 92).

Infections
In younger patients, infections may cause dementia that is usually rapidly progressive. Examples include AIDS dementia, syphilis, subacute sclerosing panencephalitis (SSPE) and Creutzfeldt–Jakob disease (CJD) (p. 99). Syphilis is nowadays only very rare, though as it is treatable syphilis serology should be checked.

Other dementias
Structural brain disease, for example frontal tumours or hydrocephalus, can produce a dementia. Normal pressure hydrocephalus (NPH) is a syndrome where there is a loss of higher function, a gait apraxia (p. 62) and urinary incontinence. This is associated with an enlargement of the lateral ventricles, but not the cerebral sulci, without obstruction. Some patients improve after shunting. Diagnosis is difficult.

Occasionally dementia can be caused by metabolic or nutritional disturbance, e.g. hypothyroidism, vitamin B12/folic acid or thiamine deficiency. Thiamine deficiency is common (up to 7% of dementia) and is seen in alcoholics, the malnourished and occasionally in hyperemesis of pregnancy. It causes a characteristic picture of memory disturbance (Korsakoff's syndrome) with an inability to retain new information and variable retrograde amnesia associated with confabulation. In acute deficiency there may be Wernicke's encephalopathy with confusion and eye movement disorders, mixed with acute alcohol withdrawal.

Vascular disease, usually recurrent infarction (arteriosclerosis or rarely vasculitis) or occasionally recurrent haemorrhage (amyloid angiopathy, arteriovenous malformations) may cause a stepwise decline over months or years. There are usually other focal signs such as hemianopia. Cerebrovascular disease may occur in patients with senile dementia of Alzheimer's type.

Epilepsy may present with recurrent subtle seizures that mimic cognitive decline. Usually there is a history of more obvious seizures and of more clear-cut fluctuations in the patient's condition, with episodes of confusion early in the illness.

Focal cognitive decline
A progressive focal deficit suggests a focal lesion, e.g. a tumour. However, if no other structural abnormality is found then the likely diagnosis is a focal dementia. These are usually described in descriptive terms, for example progressive aphasia, semantic dementia or fronto-temporal dementia. These have focal, usually lobar, atrophy and their pathology is of Pick's disease.

Depressive pseudodementia
Depression may present with a 'pseudodementia' without the obvious mood changes usually associated with depression. Patients are usually more concerned about their memory problems than are their relatives. The reverse is true in dementia. Usually patients are able to give a clearer account of their illness. If there is any suggestion of depression, there is little to be lost by a trial of antidepressant therapy. Patients with early dementia may also be depressed.

Treatment
No medication influences the pathological changes of the common dementias but central cholinesterase inhibitors, such as donepezil, galantamine and rivastigmine, and the NMDA-receptor antagonist memantine, may improve cognitive function in AD. Medical management is directed at:

- Excluding or treating other treatable causes of dementia.
- Treatment of associated phenomena of mood disturbance and behavioural change. Antidepressants may be required. Neuroleptic agents may be needed to treat hallucinations or psychotic symptoms and can be used as mild sedatives.
- Provision of appropriate social support and help for the patient and carers.

Table 2 **Diagnostic assessment for dementia patients**
Blood count and erythrocyte sedimentation rate
Liver and renal function tests
Thyroid function test
Vitamin B12 and folic acid
Syphilis serology
MRI or CT brain scan*
Neuropsychological assessment
Electroencephalogram

* The purpose of the brain scan is to exclude treatable diseases. In most elderly demented patients it shows some cerebral atrophic change and ischaemic lesions, which may be no more severe than in cognitively normal individuals of the same age

---

> **Dementia**
>
> - Dementia is most commonly caused by Alzheimer's disease.
> - Features suggesting non-Alzheimer dementia are: young age, rapid progression and focal neurological or cognitive deficits.
> - Some rarer causes and associated mood or psychiatric disturbances are treatable.

Disturbances of vision

Common visual symptoms are loss of vision, blurring of vision or loss of part of the visual field. Occasionally more complex disturbances such as hallucinations or inattention may occur. Loss of vision may affect one eye or one visual field and patients may misinterpret this, for example mistaking a right homonymous hemianopia for a defect of vision in the right eye. It is important to establish which they mean, in order to decide which part of the visual pathway is affected (Fig. 1). The timing, evolution and duration of visual loss are crucial in diagnosis.

Monocular visual loss

Monocular visual loss may be due to a lesion affecting one eye or the optic nerve anterior to the optic chiasm. The pupil response is usually normal in disease of the eye itself but is usually impaired in optic nerve disease, either as a complete or relative afferent pupillary defect (p. 14).

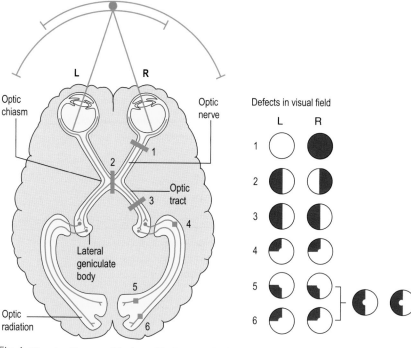

Fig. 1 **Visual pathways with sites of lesions marked.**

Acute reversible monocular visual loss

Amaurosis fugax causes sudden, reversible loss, lasting up to 30 min with complete and rapid recovery. It is usually due to embolism from the ipsilateral carotid artery to the retinal artery but may be associated with other causes of a transient ischaemic attack (TIA, p. 70). The patient describes a curtain coming down over their vision and episodes often recur. Typically the patient has no ocular signs at the time of being seen, but there may be cholesterol plaques from fragmented emboli in the retinal arterioles or carotid bruits to support the diagnosis. This should be investigated as a carotid artery TIA because there is a risk of subsequent middle cerebral artery infarction.

Retinal migraine occasionally occurs in younger patients. The episodes usually have a more gradual onset and last longer. There may also be a typical migraine headache.

Acute (closed angle) glaucoma can produce transient visual loss, occasionally without pain, although there will often be a typical history of coloured halos in vision preceding loss. Diagnosis requires ophthalmological assessment.

Optic neuritis usually occurs in young adults. It causes a visual loss that commonly evolves over 3–10 days then gradually improves over days to weeks. There may be pain behind the eye and flashing lights on eye movement. In the acute phase the optic disc may look pink, but then it becomes pale and atrophic with reduced colour vision and visual acuity, and a relatively afferent pupillary defect. It may be an isolated inflammatory lesion, but over half go on to develop multiple sclerosis.

Acute onset, persistent monocular visual loss

Anterior ischaemic optic neuropathy evolves over minutes to days. An altitudinal field defect, where the upper or lower half of the visual field is lost, is characteristic; the patient feels as if they are looking over a wall. There is often optic nerve head swelling with some fundal haemorrhages. In patients under the age of 55 years, this is likely to be due to atheromatous disease but in older patients it may be due to giant cell arteritis (GCA). In both types the condition may spread rapidly to affect both eyes but it is especially urgent to diagnose GCA because it is treatable with high dose corticosteroids. There is usually associated headache and weight loss and an elevated blood erythrocyte sedimentation rate (ESR) or plasma viscosity. An urgent temporal artery biopsy confirms the diagnosis in 60–80% of cases but treatment should not wait for results of the biopsy (p. 40).

Ocular causes of sudden onset visual loss include retinal detachment, vitreous haemorrhage and retinal vein thrombosis (p. 17).

Progressive monocular visual loss

This is commonly due to diseases of the eye, including senile macular degeneration in the elderly, diabetic retinopathy and chronic (open angle) glaucoma with a typical arcuate field defect.

Optic nerve disease occasionally causes progressive visual loss, most commonly from compression by meningiomas or gliomas of the optic nerve. There is progressive reduction in acuity and typical signs of optic nerve disease (Table 1).

Binocular visual loss

Almost any process that causes unilateral visual loss may affect both eyes or optic nerves. Some patients may not notice disease of one eye while the other remains normal and it is only when the remaining eye deteriorates that they become aware of a defect, especially with chronic processes such as glaucoma.

Table 1 **Types of visual loss**

Diagnosis	Age	Additional symptoms	Field defect	Acuity	Pupils	Other signs	Investigations
Amaurosis fugax	Middle-age to elderly	Other types of TIA	None between episodes		Normal between episodes	Carotid bruits, retinal cholesterol plaques	FBC, glucose, lipids, ESR, Doppler carotids
Acute ischaemic optic neuropathy	Middle-age to elderly	Headache, malaise	Altitudinal defect	Reduced	RAPD	Swollen optic disc with haemorrhages, later optic atrophy	ESR, glucose, lipids, temporal artery biopsy
Closed angle glaucoma	Young to middle-age	Eye pain, coloured halos	None between episodes		Dilated during episode	Hypermetropia raised intraocular pressure	Ocular pressure
Optic neuritis	Young adult	Pain and flashing lights on eye movement		Reduced	RAPD	Optic atrophy	Visual evoked potentials, MRI, CSF
Optic nerve tumour	Any age	None		Reduced	RAPD	Optic atrophy or papilloedema	MRI orbits
Open angle glaucoma	Middle-age to elderly	None		Normal early	Normal	Cupped optic disc	Ocular pressure
Pituitary tumour	Middle-age to elderly	Possible endocrine malfunction or extraocular nerve palsies	Bitemporal hemianopia (2)*	Initially normal	Usually normal	Optic atrophy or papilloedema sometimes	MRI pituitary fossa, serum prolactin
Optic radiation infarct	Middle-age to elderly	May have: ■ hemiparesis ■ hemisensory loss ■ dysphasia	Hemianopia or quadrantanopia (4, 5 or 6)*	Normal	Normal	Possible hemiparesis	CT or MRI brain
Bilateral occipital infarct	Middle-age to elderly	Brain stem disturbance		Blind	Normal	Possible brain stem signs	MRI brain and angiography

RAPD = relative afferent pupillary defect (p. 14)
* Numbers as in Figure 1

In these patients the defect is usually asymmetrical. Bilateral optic nerve lesions cause optic atrophy, reduced acuity, incongruous field defects with central scotomas that cross the midline, colour desaturation and abnormal pupil responses. Common neurological causes are optic neuritis and idiopathic intracranial hypertension (p. 40).

Unilateral retrochiasmal lesions produce field defects in both eyes that are homonymous (usually hemianopias or quadrantanopias) and respect the midline, with preserved visual acuity and usually normal pupil responses.

Acute bilateral visual loss

Causes of acute bilateral visual loss include pituitary lesions, temporal arteritis or other ischaemic optic neuropathy, acute demyelination, Leber's optic atrophy, bilateral intraocular disease (e.g. anterior uveitis) and bilateral occipital infarction (cortical blindness), sometimes as part of basilar artery thrombosis. Because pupillary responses are preserved in cortical blindness, these cases are sometimes misdiagnosed as hysteria.

Slowly progressive binocular visual loss

Chiasmal lesions commonly cause a bitemporal hemianopia, but if the lesion is not exactly central, the involvement of one eye may be greater than of the other. The field defect is often clearest on testing the central field to red pin. There is frequently reduced acuity and

there may be optic atrophy. The most common cause is a benign pituitary adenoma and there may be associated endocrine disturbance (p. 96).

Symmetrical anterior visual pathway disturbance occurs in toxic or metabolic causes of optic atrophy such as vitamin B12 or folate deficiency and tobacco-alcohol amblyopia and in some degenerative conditions, e.g. retinitis pigmentosa. Because of the symmetry, an RAPD may not be demonstrable.

Slowly progressive hemianopic defects usually reflect tumours of the retrochiasmal visual pathways.

Other visual disturbances

Inattention to the contralateral visual field without a field defect. This occurs in lesions of the parietal lobe, especially on the right. Patients tend to ignore stimuli presented to the left visual field, especially with simultaneous right-sided stimuli. When asked to draw a clock, they typically miss the numbers from 6–12, or squash all the numbers into the right half.

Agnosia. This is the inability to recognize or categorize objects presented visually in the presence of normal acuity. The objects may be identified immediately if palpated. Inability to recognize faces (prosopagnosia) is commonly part of the condition. It is usually due to bilateral visual cortex disease.

Visual hallucinations. These may be due to lesions in any part of the visual system. They may be simple patches of

colour or light, or complex images. They are most commonly seen in migraine or epilepsy but may occur in any visual disturbance, usually being restricted to the abnormal visual field. They may also be part of an encephalopathy (p. 52).

Some investigations of visual disturbance

■ Neuroimaging. MRI is the best modality for imaging the optic chiasm or optic nerve; views are as indicated.
■ The visual fields can be charted using several techniques, both manual and computerized.
■ Visual evoked potentials can give information about optic pathway function, especially optic nerve demyelination.

Disturbances of vision

■ The pattern of visual field loss usually gives the anatomical location of the lesion and the timing gives a clue to the pathology.

■ Pupillary responses to light and visual acuity are normal with lesions posterior to the optic chiasm.

■ Lesions of the optic nerve cause reduced visual acuity, central scotomas, reduced colour vision and abnormal pupillary responses.

■ Lesions of the chiasm may be best detected on testing fields to red pin.

■ Neuroimaging investigation needs to be tailored to the region of interest.

Weakness

Weakness is a common symptom and a commonly elicited sign on neurological examination. Weakness arises from lesions at every level of the nervous system. This produces:

- different types of weakness reflecting the element of the nervous system that is impaired (Fig. 1).
- different distributions of weakness reflecting the way in which the nervous system is organized.

As with all neurology, the time course of the development of the weakness, which comes from the history, is most important in understanding its aetiology. Sometimes patients complain of weakness when they mean something else, for example fatigue. Similarly, other abnormalities can be mistaken for weakness on examination (Box 1).

Table 1 Types of weakness and possible causes

Weakness	Possible causes
Hemiplegia	Stroke
	Multiple sclerosis
	Tumour
	Subdural haematoma
	Trauma
Brain stem syndrome	Stroke
	Multiple sclerosis
	Tumour
	Trauma
Spinal cord syndrome	Spondylosis
	Tumour
	Haematoma
	Trauma
	Multiple sclerosis
Cauda equina syndrome	Spondylosis
	Tumour
	Inflammatory lesion
Neuropathy	See pages 102–105

Type and distribution of weakness
(Table 1)

Upper motor neurone weakness
Lesions to the brain, brain stem and spinal cord produce upper motor neurone signs:

- increased tone (spasticity)
- brisk reflexes
- extensor plantars.

They produce a pyramidal distribution of weakness which particularly affects the extensors in the arms and flexors in the legs. With severe pyramidal weakness, the position assumed is flexed arms and extended legs.

It may not be possible to elicit the plantar response with a severe weakness. Muscles can thin in longstanding upper motor neurone lesions reflecting inactivity.

The distribution of the weakness reflects the site of the lesion (Fig. 2). Broadly speaking, hemisphere or brain stem lesions produce contralateral weakness affecting a combination of face, arm or leg depending on the site. There are usually other signs, either with disturbance of higher function speech or cranial nerve signs or sensory signs, to help locate the lesion.

Spinal cord lesions either produce unilateral or, more commonly, bilateral lesions below the level of other lesions. There are usually sensory signs to help in localization.

Lower motor neurone lesions
Lesions of the lower motor neurone, anterior horn cell nerve root or peripheral nerve produce lower motor neurone signs:

- wasting – this takes weeks to develop
- reduced tone
- loss of reflexes
- muscles that are wasting may develop fasciculations – spontaneous discharge of motor units.

The distribution reflects the pattern of lower motor neurone involvement. A generalized neuropathy can produce generalized weakness, though a distal weakness is more common (p. 102). Nerve root lesions and peripheral nerve lesions produce changes within the distribution of the nerve or root (pp. 82, 106). Usually there are associated sensory signs.

One important pattern of lower motor neurone weakness is the weakness of both legs, particularly of recent onset. This reflects a cauda

---

Box 1

Weakness that is not there
Patients may appear weak when they are not, if:

- they do not understand what you want them to do (altered higher function)
- they are slow to initiate movements (bradykinesia as in Parkinson's disease)
- they are not sure where their affected limb is (with marked loss of proprioception)
- the movement produces pain (arthritis).

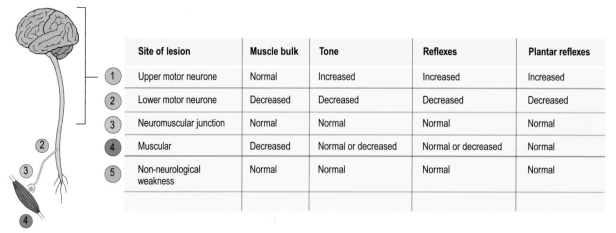

Site of lesion	Muscle bulk	Tone	Reflexes	Plantar reflexes
Upper motor neurone	Normal	Increased	Increased	Increased
Lower motor neurone	Decreased	Decreased	Decreased	Decreased
Neuromuscular junction	Normal	Normal	Normal	Normal
Muscular	Decreased	Normal or decreased	Normal or decreased	Normal
Non-neurological weakness	Normal	Normal	Normal	Normal

Fig. 1 **Sites of lesions and resulting weakness.**

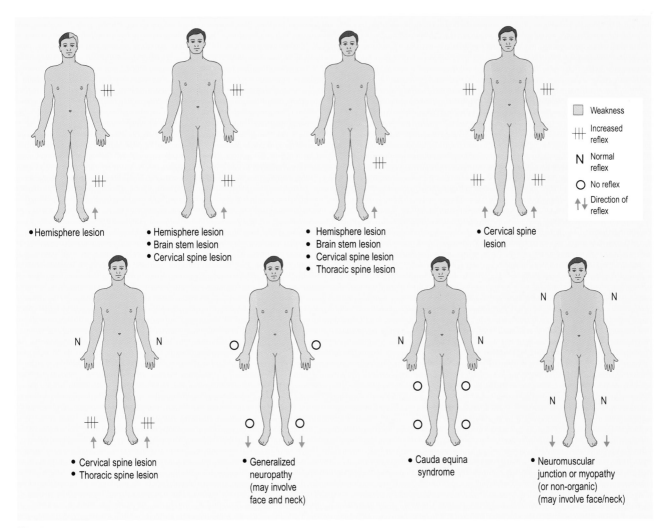

Fig. 2 **Distribution of weakness.**

equina lesion. This is usually associated with sensory and sphincter signs (p. 83).

Anterior horn cell disease produces prominent wasting and fasciculation with normal sensation. Some conditions produce upper and lower motor neurone signs. These include cervical and spine disease where spinal cord compression produces upper motor neurone signs, and where root compression produces lower motor neurone signs. There are usually associated sensory signs (pp. 80–84). Motor neurone disease (ALS) produces a mixture of upper motor and lower motor neurone signs without sensory loss (p. 108).

Neuromuscular junction weakness (p. 110)
This is uncommon and is usually due to myasthenia gravis. It is characterized by prominent, variable and fatiguable weakness. Muscle bulk, tone and reflexes are normal. Ocular muscles, bulbar muscles and the small muscles of the hand are particularly affected. There are no sensory impairments.

Muscle weakness
This can usually be distinguished from lower motor neurone weakness as there is less muscle wasting, with preserved reflexes until there is severe weakness. Sensation is normal.

Muscle disease produces weakness in several distributions. Indeed, this pattern of distribution has founded the basis of clinical classification (p. 112). However, most commonly it produces proximal limb weakness.

Non-neurologically determined weakness
This is the most difficult type of weakness to assess. This can reflect limitation because of pain, for example arthritis. However, with encouragement, full power can usually be sustained, even if only briefly.

Non-neurologically determined weakness usually has a collapsing quality where the patient gives way suddenly. The distribution is very variable and does not conform to anatomical boundaries. The difficulty is greatest with elaborated weakness, where there is neurologically determined weakness but its assessment is distorted by superadded non-organic weakness. Muscle bulk, tone, reflexes and plantar responses are all normal in non-organic weakness.

> ### Weakness
>
> - The pattern of weakness, the muscle tone and reflex changes allow the level of the nervous system producing the weakness to be identified.
>
> - There are five types of weakness: upper motor neurone, lower motor neurone, neuromuscular junction, muscle and non-organic.
>
> - Altered proprioception, inattention or bradykinesia in extrapyramidal disease can all masquerade as weakness.
>
> - The time course of the onset suggests the likely pathology.

Numbness and sensory disturbance

Sensory symptoms are very common, occurring in about 8% of the general population. Sensory symptoms and signs alone may lead to a diagnosis. They can also be very helpful in clarifying the diagnosis in patients with other symptoms and signs. However, sensory symptoms and signs are 'softer' than many other neurological symptoms and can occur without an established underlying cause.

Sensory symptoms and signs do not occur in diseases that solely affect muscle, neuromuscular junction or anterior horn cell. Their presence therefore excludes these diagnoses (unless another incidental reason can be found for them).

Clinical features

Numbness, tingling or pins and needles are the commonest sensory symptoms. The terms mean different things to different patients: you need to establish what the patient means, the distribution of sensory loss and the time course of the problem.

- What is it?
- Where is it?
- How did it come on?

What is it?

Sensory symptoms can be broadly divided into:

- **Positive symptoms**: an intrusive feeling of altered sensation, often referred to as numbness, tingling, pins and needles, though sensations may include pain.
- **Negative symptoms**: the realization that sensation is lost, usually noticed when the patient inadvertently touches the affected part.

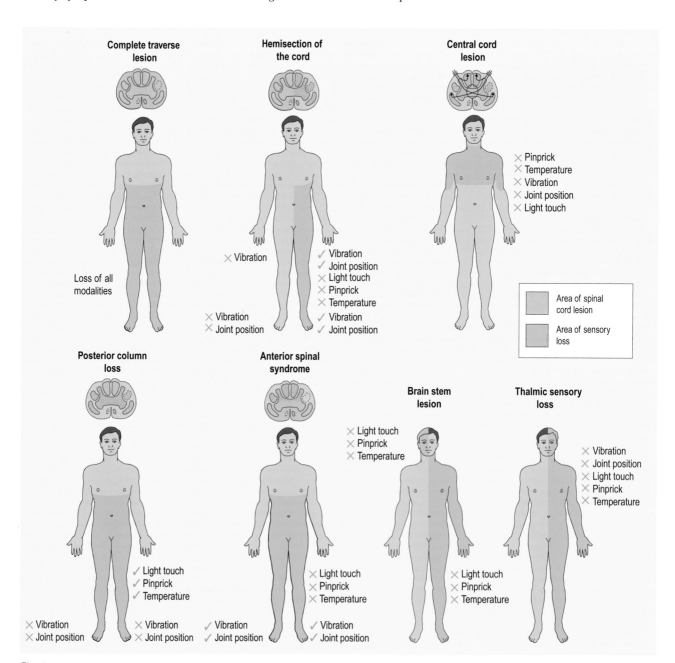

Fig. 1 **Sensory loss and associated conditions.**

Patients will often describe sensory disturbance as 'numbness' and this term alone can be used to mean:

- loss of sensation – a negative symptom
- a positive feeling of altered sensation – 'like the sensation as a local anaesthetic wears off'
- pain
- a limb may be described as numb when it is in fact weak, or vice-versa.

Tingling or pins and needles can usually be readily recognized as a distinct sensory symptom. Usually this can be localized more accurately than other positive symptoms, which can be very helpful for localization.

Loss of joint position sense (proprioception) is more likely to be described as clumsiness or unsteadiness or like having a tight bandage on rather than numbness. Cortical sensory loss is usually noticed because of the disturbance in function, with clumsiness or incoordination more prominent than sensory symptoms.

Negative sensory symptoms, or the finding of sensory loss without associated symptoms discovered on examination, occur particularly in the following situations:

- if the sensory loss is very longstanding or of slow onset, for example hereditary neuropathies
- when a cortical lesion also causes inattention so the area is ignored
- if in an area that is not functionally important, for example the thoracic dermatomes.

Where is it?

The distribution of the sensory symptoms and signs is important in determining the cause of the symptoms (Fig. 1). The common patterns of sensory symptoms follow the patterns of sensory loss illustrated. However this can be imprecise. For example, patients with carpal tunnel syndrome commonly feel their whole hand is numb, sometimes even the arm. Their feelings of tingling are usually more clearly localized to the hand, though they may be uncertain which fingers are affected. Patients with cervical root compression often describe numbness affecting the whole arm, their tingling however normally is more clearly related to a single root dermatome. In other circumstances even relatively minor symptoms can be very helpful. For example, a patient with numbness and weakness in both legs with upper motor neurone signs could have a problem at any level of the spinal cord, or possibly brain stem. If they have sensory symptoms or signs in the arms this indicates the level to be in the cervical cord or above.

How did it come on?

Important clinical features are the timing of the onset and pattern of sensory disturbance.

Transient sensory disturbance

Transient disturbances of sensation can arise from any level in the nervous system:

- Cerebral hemisphere and brain: include migraine, epilepsy and transient ischaemic attacks, CNS demyelination.
- Nerve roots and peripheral nerves: compressive radiculopathy and peripheral nerve compression.

- These types of symptoms are also often unexplained or may be psychogenic.

The timing of the onset and its duration, as well as the distribution, helps clarify this (Table 1).

Persistent sensory disturbance

The distribution of sensory disturbance and any associated motor or other signs are helpful in localizing the lesion. The timing and evolution gives additional information regarding aetiology in this group as well. In addition, sensory deficits can be progressive, reflecting progressive disease. The nature of this will depend on the affected level of the nervous system; some examples include:

- brain – space occupying lesions such as tumours, subdural haematoma
- spinal cord – demyelination, cervical spondylitic myelopathy
- nerve root – spondylitic radiculopathy
- peripheral nerve – peripheral neuropathy, common cause diabetes mellitus (pp. 102–105).

When there are persisting sensory symptoms more information can be obtained from examination. When examining for sensory loss, ignore equivocal findings, concentrate on definite abnormalities and map out their boundaries. The area may need to be re-examined to confirm the findings. This may allow a more definite pattern of sensory loss.

Sometimes sensory examination can be normal or minimally abnormal despite quite marked persisting symptoms. This can either reflect a central lesion or a non-organic sensory disturbance.

Understanding sensory loss will depend on the integration of sensory and motor signs.

Table 1 **Causes of numbness and of sensory disturbance**	
Condition	**Quality and distribution of numbness**
Focal epileptic seizure	Tingling, spreads down one side of the body in seconds as with the motor 'Jacksonian march'. There may be other epilepsy symptoms, such as altered awareness and limb jerking
Migraine aura	Tingling, builds up over minutes and is unilateral. The area of sensory loss reflects the cortical representation, spreading from one area of cortex to an adjacent area (e.g. lip to arm, to thigh, to foot). There are often other migraine symptoms; visual, headache/nausea
Transient ischaemic attack (TIA)	Sudden onset loss of sensation may be focal or unilateral. It may be associated with other deficits: visual, motor or speech
Stroke	Onset as TIA but slower recovery, may have residual signs
CNS demyelination	These usually come on over 2–3 days and last 4–5 weeks. In established MS, symptoms may last days, or be brought out by exercise or heat. Commonly in feet or hands but may have any distribution, and may have other symptoms: weakness, sphincter disturbance, with CNS signs
Peripheral nerve or root entrapment	A common problem. Symptoms within distribution of nerve or root may fluctuate; may be brought on by specific actions or in particular situations
Psychogenic	Fluctuating with variable quality. Other symptoms of anxiety, depression and hyperventilation

---

Numbness and sensory disturbance

- Sensory examination is an imprecise art. The subjective description of the cutaneous sensory abnormality is of limited value in diagnosis.

- The timing of the onset of paroxysmal sensory symptoms is important in diagnosis.

- The distribution of sensory loss is important in localizing the causative lesion

- Sensory symptoms and signs need to be integrated with other findings when trying to make a diagnosis.

Walking difficulties and clumsiness

Walking is very important to the way we live. The impact of losing this ability on a patient's lifestyle can be readily appreciated. It is not surprising that the ability to walk independently is a prominent factor in all the scales of neurological disability.

Walking on two legs is a complicated process. It requires:

- intact skeletal system
- muscular strength
- proprioception
- balance
- complicated central system for coordination and integration of these elements.

Any of the elements can malfunction. This section will consider the patterns of gait disturbance and a few problems associated with it, in particular syndromes of gait abnormality.

History

In taking the history of a patient with walking difficulties, consider particularly:

- the duration of progression of the gait disturbance documented by independent measures, such as aids used in walking and the distance that the patient is able to walk
- the current walking capacity in terms of distance or speed
- any falls
- pain in either the legs or low back, either continuous or brought on by walking.

Frequently the history will clarify the walking difficulty, especially where there is pain: for example, in a joint or calf pain brought on by distribution of vascular intermittent claudication. The onset of pain on walking can be neurogenic, usually arising from lumbar canal stenosis. This pain is usually radicular and is often associated with sensory symptoms. In some patients the deterioration in walking can be entirely due to unilateral symptoms, for example the dragging of one or other leg.

Gait analysis

On watching a patient walk, the disturbance can be broadly subdivided into symmetrical and asymmetrical gait disturbances (Fig. 1).

Asymmetrical gait disturbances

Non-neurological gait disturbances are usually asymmetrical. Any underlying orthopaedic problem, e.g. fixed hip joint or shortened limbs, are usually evident on closer inspection. The limp of someone in pain can usually be seen and corroborated by asking the patient about pain.

The basis of an asymmetrical gait caused by neurological abnormalities can usually be established by conventional neurological examination. These usually reflect unilateral abnormal tone or weakness. Three common patterns are:

- *Hemi-parkinsonian gait.* The arm swing is reduced on one side, the posture is slightly stiff and the gait can be slightly hesitant.
- *Hemiplegic gait.* One leg is stiff and is swung out and around, often catching the toe.

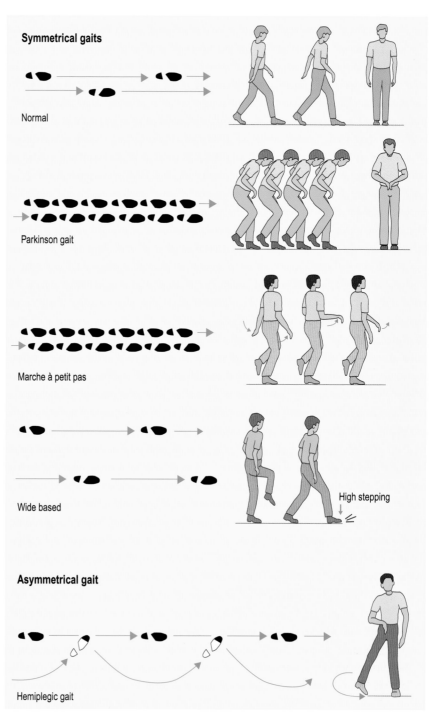

Symmetrical gaits

Normal

Parkinson gait

Marche à petit pas

Wide based

High stepping

Asymmetrical gait

Hemiplegic gait

Fig. 1 **Gait analysis.**

- *Foot drop*. This is a high stepping gait where the heel is brought up high to avoid catching the toe. This is noisy and there is usually a slap as the foot is brought down. This usually reflects unilateral lower motor neurone abnormalities.

Symmetrical gait disturbances

In some patients there may be a symmetrical gait disturbance. These can be broadly divided into:

- Broad-based gait, where the feet are widely spaced.
- Normally based gaits, with the feet a normal distance apart.
- Crossing or scissoring gait, where the feet cross. These indicate spasticity in both legs.

Heel/toe walking can bring out an imbalance. A patient with a broad-based gait will be unable to walk heel/toe.

Broad-based gait

The feet are separated to try and help balance, hence the inability to walk heel/toe. This usually reflects:

- a loss of proprioception (sensory ataxia)
- loss of coordination (ataxia).

Patients with impaired proprioception have a positive Romberg's test.

Ataxia with normal sensation indicates a midline cerebellar disturbance. There may also be limb incoordination which produces a clumsy ataxic gait with more widespread cerebellar disease.

Narrow-based gaits

Patients with narrow-based gaits usually have abnormalities of either:

- stride length
- stride pattern
- posture
- arm swings.

Specific conditions

Patients usually have the following gait abnormalities (Table 1).

Small steps

- Parkinsonism – short paced, stooped, poor arm swing. May have difficulty starting and stopping. When walking they appear to be falling forward, often trying to catch up with themselves (festinant gait).

- Marche à petit pas – small steps, upright posture, good arm swings. This usually reflects cerebrovascular disease.

Abnormal gait patterns

- Apraxic – great difficulty in starting with broken-up gait pattern. Almost seems to have forgotten how to walk. This usually reflects normal pressure hydrocephalus or diffuse cerebral disease.
- High stepping – bilateral foot drop produces high knee lift and slapping on walking. This can occur with a sensory ataxia, e.g. a patient with a peripheral neuropathy. Classically this is the pattern of gait seen in tabes dorsalis.
- Waddling – a patient with marked hip movement abnormalities will waddle in gait with prominent hip rotation. This can either reflect proximal pelvic weakness so that the pelvic position is not held normally, or bilateral hip disease.

Crossing-over gait – scissoring gait

Patients with bilateral leg spasticity with circumduction from both legs produce a scissoring gait.

Bizarre gait

When you see a patient who has a very bizarre gait, there are several factors to consider:

- chorea – patients with severe chorea often have bizarre gaits (e.g. Huntington's disease, Parkinson's disease on treatment)
- multiple diseases – patients with an orthopaedic problem and a neurological problem, e.g. a fixed hip and a contralateral hemiplegia
- non-organically determined gait – this should also be considered in a patient who seems to use a walking aid quite inappropriately, e.g. carrying a zimmer frame.

Clumsiness

Clumsiness is a symptom patients use to describe:

- weakness
- the effect of sensory loss, particularly posterior column loss
- bradykinesia
- incoordination.

These can usually be readily distinguished in the history or on examination. Examination needs to pay attention especially to the limb movements, including formal testing of coordination and any particular movement the patient has noticed provokes the problem, for example writing or holding a plate.

Cerebellar syndromes

Clumsiness, incoordination and ataxia are the major symptoms and signs found in cerebellar disease. Cerebellar syndromes occur in different diseases (Table 2). The clinical pattern can be divided into two broad categories: asymmetric syndromes due to focal lesions and symmetrical syndromes due to toxic, metabolic and degenerative causes. The most common causes are MS in younger patients, stroke in older patients and toxins including alcohol and some anticonvulsants. There are a number of rarer degenerative conditions, both inherited, such as the spinocerebellar ataxias (there are now seven genes identified for these conditions) and sporadic, such as multiple system atrophy. Paraneoplastic cerebellar syndromes can be associated with small cell lung and ovarian cancers, and antineuronal antibodies against the Purkinje cells can be found.

Table 1 **Causes of gait disturbance**	
Parkinsonism	See pages 88–89
Marche à petit pas	Diffuse cerebrovascular disease
Apraxic gait	Normal-pressure hydrocephalus
	Other diffuse cerebral diseases
Waddling gait	Muscle disease
	Hip disease
Crossing-over gait	Spinal cord disease
	Bilateral hemisphere disease
Ataxic gait	Cerebellar syndrome (see Table 2)

Table 2 **Causes of cerebellar syndromes**
■ Multiple sclerosis
■ Stroke
■ Tumour
■ Trauma
■ Degeneration
■ Metabolic – hypothyroidism
■ Paraneoplastic
■ Toxic – anticonvulsants and alcohol

Walking difficulties and clumsiness

- Walking is a very important function. Walking difficulties are a major cause of disability.
- Always examine a patient's walking as it may be the only abnormality.
- There are relatively few readily recognizable patterns of gait abnormality.

Stroke I

Stroke refers to damage of the brain caused by abnormalities of blood supply. This presents with a rapidly developing focal neurological deficit, which may lead to coma or death. If this deficit lasts less than 24 h it is referred to as a transient ischaemic attack (TIA) (p. 70).

Stroke is the third most common cause of death in developed countries. The incidence of first stroke is 2 per 1000 per year. The incidence increases with age. It is rare below 45 years of age and increases from 2 per 1000 per year for people aged 45–54 years to 10 per 1000 per year for those aged 65–74 years and to about 30 per 1000 per year in those aged over 80 years. About a quarter of these patients will be dead within 6 months (the majority of these within 1 month). Stroke is a major cause of disability; after their first stroke 40% of surviving patients will be dependent at 6 months.

Stroke is not a single diagnosis. Strokes differ in terms of their aetiology and pathogenesis, the area of the brain affected and the resulting clinical deficit. These differences have implications for investigation, treatment and prognosis.

Pathogenesis

Cerebral infarction accounts for 80% of strokes, 15% are primary intracerebral haemorrhages and 5% are due to subarachnoid haemorrhages (p. 72).

Cerebral infarction

Cerebral infarction results from an interruption in blood supply to an area of the brain. This can be due to (Fig. 1):

- emboli (30% of all strokes)
- thrombosis (30%)
- small vessel disease (20%).

Atheroma

Atheroma is an important factor in both embolic and thrombotic strokes. A similar pathological process, occurring in patients with the same risk factors, produces intracerebral small vessel disease.

The risk factors for atheroma, and other disease resulting from it, are given in Table 1. The most important risk factor is hypertension, with the risk increasing with the blood pressure.

Atheroma commonly arises at the junctions of arteries, for example the carotid bifurcation and the point where the two vertebral arteries join to form the basilar artery (Fig. 2).

The build up of atheroma may lead to narrowing of the arteries. This is usually a gradual process and anastomotic channels can develop, either around the circle of Willis (Fig. 2) or with enlargement of meningeal anastomoses. Stenosis can develop and proceed to occlusion of a vessel without resulting in cerebral ischaemia. However, the atheromatous plaque can lead to cerebral ischaemia in several ways:

- It can produce a stenosis that is not compensated for by anastomoses.
- The plaque may ulcerate and fragments can act as emboli.
- The base of an ulcerated plaque is irregular and may act as a focus for propagation of thrombus.
- Haemorrhage into an ulcerated plaque can produce a rapidly developing stenosis or occlusion.

Embolic strokes

An embolus is an abnormal particle within the bloodstream that can lodge in, and block, blood vessels. Emboli commonly arise from either the heart or the proximal arteries in the neck. The most common sources of emboli from the heart include thrombus from atrial fibrillation, mural thrombus following myocardial infarction and left ventricular dilatation.

Table 1 Risk factors for atheroma and relative risk of stroke	
Risk factors for atheroma	**Relative risk of stroke**
Hypertension	5
Diabetes	2
Smoking	3
Family history	
Cholesterol	
Excess alcohol intake	1–4

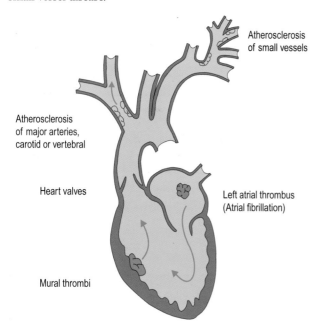

Fig. 1 **Pathophysiology of common causes of cerebral infarction.**

Atherosclerosis of small vessels

Atherosclerosis of major arteries, carotid or vertebral

Heart valves

Left atrial thrombus (Atrial fibrillation)

Mural thrombi

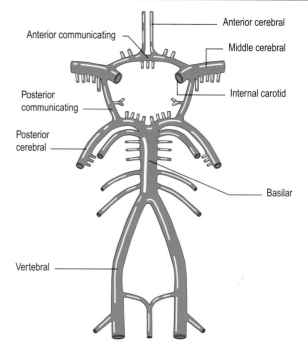

Fig. 2 **Circle of Willis.**

Anterior communicating

Anterior cerebral

Middle cerebral

Internal carotid

Posterior communicating

Posterior cerebral

Basilar

Vertebral

Rare embolic sources include bacterial vegetations in subacute bacterial endocarditis, calcium from heart valves or fragments from an atrial myxoma. Emboli from the heart account for about 10% of all strokes.

Emboli can come from the proximal neck vessels (artery to artery emboli) and these usually relate to atheromatous disease. The emboli consist of plaque debris, cholesterol crystals or platelet emboli, which arise from ulcerated atheromatous plaque. Other types include fat (from trauma) and air (from surgery).

Thrombotic strokes

Thrombosis arises in three main circumstances.

Abnormality in the vessel wall. Thrombosis usually occurs in the context of atheroma, which produces stenosis and irregularities in the vessel wall from which thrombosis can propagate. More rarely, thrombosis can occur in inflammatory arterial diseases, such as temporal arteritis, systemic lupus erythematosus, rheumatoid arthritis and other rarer diseases.

Abnormal tendency of the blood to thrombose. Thrombosis can also occur when there is a predisposition to clotting, for example polycythaemia, thrombocythaemia, sickle cell disease and coagulation disorders that result in thrombophilia (e.g. protein C and S deficiencies and antiphospholipid syndrome).

Stasis of the blood flow. Stasis usually occurs in association with severe atheromatous stenosis. An arterial dissection can arise if the intimal lining of an artery is torn, then blood can track beneath this layer in the wall. This produces a stenosis of the vessel and potential stasis and may lead to thrombosis. This is the commonest identifiable cause of stroke in young adults.

Small vessel disease

Intracerebral small vessel disease refers to the process of lipohyalinosis (or microatheroma) that occurs in penetrating and branch arteries, resulting in their occlusion. Patients with small vessel disease usually have a predisposition to atheroma.

Intracerebral haemorrhage

Intracerebral haemorrhage is usually due to hypertension (primary intracerebral haemorrhage). This occurs when small penetrating arteries within the brain rupture at sites of weakness, as a result of lipohyalinosis and microaneurysms (Charcot–Bouchard aneurysms). Intracerebral haemorrhages occur most frequently in the basal ganglia (50%) (Fig. 3), lobar white matter (20%), pons (10%) and cerebellum (10%).

Ruptured saccular aneurysms produce subarachnoid haemorrhage (p. 72). However, sometimes the direction of rupture of an aneurysm can result in most of the haemorrhage being intracerebral rather than subarachnoid. Arteriovenous malformations can rupture and produce intracerebral haemorrhage. Patients with bleeding disorders, particularly related to drugs (anticoagulants and thrombolytics such as streptokinase), can develop intracerebral haemorrhages.

Development of an ischaemic stroke

Cerebral infarction occurs after a few minutes of ischaemia. The consequence of ischaemia depends on its duration and severity. This will vary within the affected area of brain, with areas on the edge of the vascular territory of the affected vessel being relatively less affected, sometimes called the ischaemic penumbra. Severe ischaemia will lead to cell death while less-affected cells may have the potential to survive. There is increasing evidence that excitotoxic amino acids may be involved in the pathogenesis of the cell death. Other biochemical factors, such as the blood glucose, will also affect cell survival.

Areas of necrosis will then swell, so-called cytotoxic oedema, which may interfere with the perfusion of areas in the penumbra. This swelling increases over 5 days and then gradually clears. If large areas of brain are affected (e.g. a middle cerebral artery occlusion, p. 66), this may produce significant mass effect causing a further deterioration due to cerebral herniation. This is also seen in intracerebral haemorrhage where the haematoma increases the mass effect.

By 3 weeks the haemodynamic changes that led to the stroke are stable and the recovery phase of the stroke is dependent on recovery of the ischaemic penumbra and remodelling of brain function. The area of infarction shrinks, undergoing the process of gliosis. In patients who have had strokes affecting small deep perforating vessels, this process of gliosis leads to the formation of small lakes of fluid, so-called 'lacunes'.

Some rarer types of stroke

Hypotensive/watershed strokes. A period of systemic hypotension, for example during a cardiac arrest, can result in ischaemia in areas on the edge of two vascular territories (e.g. between middle and posterior cerebral arteries). This can produce strokes sometimes referred to as watershed infarcts.

Intracranial venous thrombosis. This occurs when there is an abnormality in haemostasis or when there is some irritation of the venous sinuses (e.g. surgery, infection, inflammation or tumour). These usually result in headaches, seizures and confusion, sometimes with focal signs. It may also present with raised intracranial pressure.

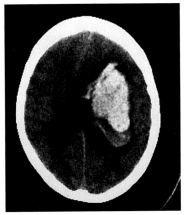

Fig. 3 **CT scan showing massive intracerebral haemorrhage.**

> ## Stroke I
> - Stroke is a common cause of death and disability.
> - Stroke is caused by cerebral infarction (80%), intracranial haemorrhage (15%) and subarachnoid haemorrhage (5%).
> - Atheroma is the most important cause of ischaemic stroke.
> - Ischaemic stroke can result from thrombosis or embolism.

Stroke II

Clinical features

A common feature of all strokes is the onset. The neurological deficit comes on over a short time, from seconds to a progression over hours. This contrasts with space-occupying lesions, which develop over weeks or months, and inflammatory lesions (such as plaques of demyelination in multiple sclerosis), which usually come on over days or weeks.

The clinical manifestations of stroke depend on the area of the brain affected, which in turn depends on which blood vessel is affected. The anatomy of the blood vessels supplying the brain can be subdivided according to vessel size (large or small) and vessel site (anterior or posterior) (Fig. 1):

- Anterior circulation
  - large vessels: the internal carotid artery (ICA) and its main branches the middle (MCA) and anterior (ACA) cerebral arteries
  - small vessels: branches from the MCA and ACA
- Posterior circulation
  - large vessels: the vertebral arteries, which join to form the basilar artery and its main branches, the posterior cerebral arteries
  - small vessels: branches from all these vessels.

The anterior circulation supplies the anterior two-thirds of the cerebrum, while the posterior circulation provides the supply for the occipital lobes of the cerebrum and the brain stem and cerebellum (Fig. 1).

A simple syndromic classification divides strokes into the following categories, which have important differences in terms of pathogenesis, treatment and prognosis:

- total anterior circulation stroke
- partial anterior circulation stroke
- posterior circulation stroke
- lacunar stroke.

Anterior circulation large vessel strokes

The MCA supplies most of the motor and sensory cortex, including that controlling the contralateral arm and face, both Wernicke's and Broca's areas in the dominant hemisphere, the internal capsule and optic radiation. The ACA supplies the motor cortex controlling the leg, the frontal lobe and the corpus callosum.

Total anterior circulation stroke

This can arise from a complete MCA infarct, from internal carotid disease or massive intracerebral haemorrhage.

Complete infarction of the area produces a devastating deficit. There is a dense flaccid hemiparesis, affecting the arm, face and leg. There is a homonymous hemianopia. The patient may be drowsy initially with eyes averted away from the hemiparetic side. There is a complete aphasia if the dominant hemisphere is affected and a marked inattention or neglect if the non-dominant side is involved. There may be a transient dysarthria and swallowing may be impaired. The patient may be incontinent. These strokes carry a high mortality and severe long-term morbidity.

Partial anterior circulation stroke

Infarction in the territory of one of the branches of the MCA produces different combinations of deficits depending on the

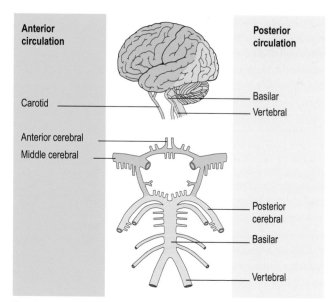

Fig. 1 **Anterior and posterior arterial circulation.**

affected hemisphere (Fig. 2). Some of the common ones are: inferior branch hemianopia – Wernicke's aphasia if dominant, or constructional apraxia if non-dominant; superior branch hemiparesis – Broca's aphasia if dominant or neglect if non-dominant. Distal branches lead to cortical infarcts with weakness only of one limb or isolated higher function deficits.

An ACA infarct produces á hemiparesis, of the leg more than the arm, with apathy and incontinence, and mixed aphasia if dominant or dyspraxia if non-dominant.

Lobar haemorrhage can produce a similar clinical syndrome.

Posterior circulation strokes (Fig. 3)

Large vessel syndromes

Posterior cerebral artery infarcts result in contralateral homonymous hemianopia and contralateral hemisensory loss. There may be some disturbance of higher function, such as altered memory or speech or cortical blindness. Occlusion of the basilar artery produces lesions of both posterior cerebral arteries and high brain stem lesions that may lead to 'a locked in' state – where the upper brain stem lesion prevents the conscious brain having any control over bulbar function or the limbs, though some control of eye movements can remain. Vertebral artery occlusion may leave no deficit or may produce one of the syndromes described below.

Other posterior circulation strokes

A large number of clinical syndromes (often eponymous) have been described arising from posterior circulation strokes. Cerebellar signs are commonly seen, indicating damage to the cerebellum or its connections. Nystagmus, dysarthria and diplopia are features that point to a brain stem lesion. A feature in this, and other brain stem diseases, is the crossed cranial nerve and long tract sensory or motor deficit. For example, the lateral medullary syndrome (the site of the lesion is the lateral medulla) comprises: lesions to the brain stem nuclei and cerebellar connections which produce ipsilateral facial sensory loss, Horner's syndrome, vocal cord paralysis and cerebellar ataxia, and damage to the spinothalamic tract which results in contralateral loss of pinprick and temperature sensation in the limbs.

In addition, brain stem events can result in lacunar syndromes.

Small vessel lacunar strokes

Lacunar strokes arise from occlusion of small branches of both the anterior and posterior circulation vessels. The lacunar syndromes are helpful in identifying the disease process but are often less helpful in identifying the exact site of the lesion. The lacunar syndromes are:

- Pure motor hemiparesis: face, arm and leg weakness with no other deficits. Usually an internal capsule lesion.
- Ataxic hemiparesis: motor hemiparesis with cerebellar type ataxia on that side. Lesion site is variable: posterior internal capsule, midbrain or pons.
- Dysarthria/clumsy hand syndrome: marked dysarthria with tongue and face weakness with hand clumsiness on the same side.
- Pure sensory stroke: hemisensory loss of superficial sensation. Usually thalamic lesions.
- Sensorimotor stroke is a combination of sensory and motor strokes.

Intracerebral haemorrhage

Distinguishing clinically between infarction and haemorrhage is unreliable. This can only be done with confidence by a CT scan performed within a week of onset. The occurrence of a severe headache or coma at onset makes haemorrhage more likely but it can be seen in infarction.

Other symptoms and signs

Headache is common though usually not a prominent symptom in ischaemic stroke: 10% have headache preceding the stroke and about 20% at stroke onset. About 50% of patients with intracerebral haemorrhage have headache at onset, which is usually more severe.

Horner's syndrome can result from carotid dissection due to damage of the associated sympathetic plexus. It is therefore an additional clue to aetiology when associated with signs of an ipsilateral anterior circulation event. (NB. This needs to be distinguished from Horner's syndrome related to brain stem lesions.)

The blood pressure may be increased, which may reflect previously

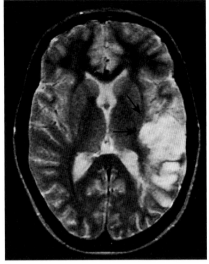

Fig. 2 **Partial anterior circulation infarct.**

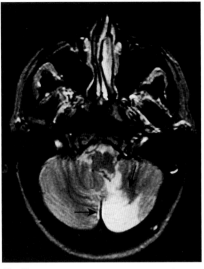

Fig. 3 **Posterior circulation infarct: right cerebellar.**

undiagnosed hypertension, though it is commonly observed in the early stages of stroke.

Symptoms and signs of associated and predisposing diseases

There may be symptoms and signs of associated diseases: for example, symptoms of angina, intermittent claudication, or signs of diabetic or hypertensive retinopathy or peripheral neuropathy.

Differential diagnosis

The diagnosis of stroke is usually straightforward (Table 1). Space-occupying lesions (SOL) are usually more insidious in onset than stroke, though some tumours can present with a 'vascular' onset, particularly if there is bleeding into a tumour. Cerebral abscesses have a more rapid progression than most SOL but the patient is usually unwell and septic. Chronic subdural haematoma is a very important diagnosis to consider because of the need for neurosurgical intervention. The onset is usually slower and very often the patient is mentally slower, as well as exhibiting focal deficits, and there may be signs of raised intracranial pressure.

In younger patients the onset of multiple sclerosis can be mistaken for a stroke and vice versa. Head injury is usually easily diagnosed but sometimes it can be difficult to tell whether the stroke caused the fall or the head injury resulted in the neurological deficit, particularly in elderly patients. Hypoglycaemia can produce focal deficits and this needs to be considered early in the assessment of diabetics with neurological deficits. A Todd's paralysis,

weakness in a limb after seizure, may mimic a stroke. In addition, patients with critical ischaemia, for example due to severe carotid stenosis, can present with focal seizures.

Special situations

Patients with multiple small deep infarcts may present with dementia (multi-infarct dementia). These patients often also have a gait disturbance, walking with small steps but a good arm swing. They may have focal neurological signs relevant to some of their strokes, such as hemianopias. There is considerable overlap with other dementing illnesses such as Alzheimer's disease because both conditions occur in the same age group, so there is some controversy as to whether 'vascular dementia' exists as an independent entity.

Table 1 **Differential diagnosis of stroke**

- Intracranial space-occupying lesion
  - tumour
  - bleed into tumour
  - abscess
- Subdural haematoma
- Multiple sclerosis
- Head injury
- Hypoglycaemia
- Seizures with Todd's paralysis

Stroke II

- The onset of the neurological deficit is important in the diagnosis of stroke.
- Strokes can be classified clinically as total anterior circulation strokes, partial anterior circulation strokes, and posterior circulation and lacunar strokes.
- Cerebral infarction cannot reliably be distinguished from haemorrhage on clinical grounds.

Stroke III

Investigations

Investigations are directed at answering the following questions:

- Is it a stroke?
- What kind of stroke is it?
- Why did the stroke occur?
- Are there any factors that could make it worse?

Is it a stroke? What kind of stroke is it?

Making the diagnosis of stroke on the basis of the history, either from the patient or a relative, and the examination is usually straightforward. The differential diagnosis that needs to be considered has been discussed previously (Table 1, p. 67). The clinical classification is considered on page 66. Haemorrhagic and ischaemic strokes cannot be reliably distinguished clinically.

The diagnosis of stroke can be confirmed by CT or MRI scanning, which will indicate whether the stroke is haemorrhagic. Early CT scans can be normal, indicating that the stroke is ischaemic and not haemorrhagic. The distribution of any abnormality will indicate the affected vascular territory (Fig. 1).

CT and MRI scans are recommended though are not yet performed in all patients.

Why did the stroke occur?

The likely aetiology of an ischaemic stroke can usually be determined from the history and examination. The range of investigations that may be used is given in Table 1.

Which of these investigations are used in a particular patient will depend on the clinical picture. For example a younger patient will be investigated more aggressively than an older patient; a patient with a history suggesting a possible cardiac source (e.g. previous rheumatic fever) will require full cardiac investigation. A patient without risk factors for atheroma would have a wider range of investigations. The investigation of the cause of a complete anterior circulation dominant hemisphere stroke is going to be tempered by the clinical condition of the patient.

In any patient with a small completed stroke in the anterior circulation, or one that could have come from the anterior

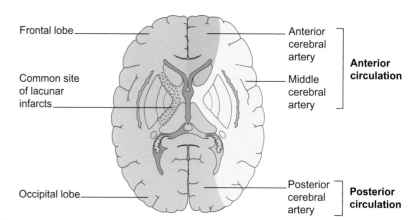

Fig. 1 **Vascular supply of the brain in the projection commonly used for scanning.**

circulation, a carotid Doppler scan should be performed to look for operable stenosis (see later).

A patient with a haemorrhagic stroke will usually be hypertensive and often have other risk factors for atheroma. In addition, consider whether there is a bleeding tendency (usually warfarin or thrombolytics). In younger patients who are not hypertensive, there may be a vascular abnormality that caused the haemorrhage, and cerebral angiography may be helpful.

Table 1 **Investigation of an ischaemic stroke**
Risk factors for atheroma
Blood pressure*
Blood tests
glucose*
cholesterol*
thyroid function*
liver function tests (?alcohol consumption)
Sources of embolism
Heart
ECG*
echocardiogram
blood cultures
24-h tape
Neck and intracranial vessels
carotid Doppler
angiogram or magnetic resonance angiography
Causes of tendency to thrombosis
Blood tests
full blood count*
thrombophilia screen (proteins C and S, lupus anticoagulant)
sickle cell screen
Causes of inflammatory vascular disease
Blood tests
plasma viscosity or erythrocyte sedimentation rate*
antinuclear factor, anticardiolipin antibodies
syphilis serology
temporal artery biopsy
The investigation needs to be directed by the clinical picture * Indicates tests performed in every patient with a stroke

Are there any factors that could make it worse?

Systemic metabolic disturbances, especially hypoxia and hyperglycaemia, will affect the function of the ischaemic brain and worsen the stroke. Stroke patients will frequently require hydration, either enterally or parenterally. Inappropriate fluid balance, particularly overhydration, may be detrimental and it is often helpful to monitor urea and electrolytes.

Treatment and prognosis

Treatment

The treatment of patients with strokes aims to:

- give general medical support of the patient
- minimize stroke size
- prevent complications of stroke
- optimize recovery
- prevent recurrence of stroke.

Much of the advice given below is based on clinical trial data. However, there are still many areas where current practice has not been formally proven to be of benefit. There are ongoing trials trying to find the best management strategies for many of these, for example feeding policy.

General medical support of the patient

Initially the patient with a large stroke may need to be resuscitated with protection of the airway, making them nil by mouth and giving nasogastric or parenteral fluids. Most patients will need assessment of their swallowing to determine whether it is safe for them to have oral fluids. In managing the fluid balance it is best to keep the patient slightly underhydrated for the first week to minimize cerebral oedema.

The blood pressure is elevated in over 80% of patients with strokes. Most should be managed conservatively as a reduction in blood pressure can further compromise the cerebral circulation. However, if there is more severe hypertension (diastolic > 120) a gentle introduction of antihypertensive therapy is appropriate. More severe hypertension associated with hypertensive encephalopathy needs aggressive management.

Hypoxia, hyperglycaemia and hypoglycaemia should be treated.

Minimize stroke size

There is increasing evidence that thrombolysis with recombinant tissue plasminogen activator (rTPA) decreases ischaemic stroke size and improves outcome if given within 3 and possibly 6 hours of stroke onset. Prior to treatment a CT scan needs to be performed to exclude haemorrhage or significant cerebral damage, which could be transformed into fatal haemorrhage by rTPA. This is only possible for a small number of patients and treatment is currently restricted to specialist centres. Aspirin may also reduce 30 day stroke mortality by 1% but heparin is unhelpful and neuroprotective agents have proved disappointing.

Prevent complications (Table 2)

Raised intracranial pressure may lead to fatal brain herniation and, when it occurs after a large anterior circulation infarct, it is usually unresponsive to treatment. However, a large intracranial haematoma can be surgically drained and large cerebellar strokes can cause brain stem compression and hydrocephalus and may need posterior fossa decompression to control intracranial pressure.

The complications of immobility are not unique to stroke. These require active nursing care with 2-hourly turns and appropriate positioning to prevent bedsores. Appropriate feeding, which may include using a nasogastric tube or percutaneous gastrostomy if more long term, positioning and physiotherapy to prevent pneumonia are required. Physiotherapy is initially used to maintain passive movements and prevent contractures.

Graded pressure stockings can be used as prophylaxis for deep vein thrombosis. Heparin should probably be avoided in the early phase of recovery from a haemorrhagic stroke and its use in ischaemic stroke is being evaluated.

Urinary catheterization should be avoided, if possible, as it increases the risk of infection. Laxatives and suppositories and enemas may be needed for bowel control.

The later complications are more difficult to prevent. Psychological support for the patient and the family from the doctors, nurses and therapists concerned can help a patient come to terms with the stroke. Social difficulties may sometimes be anticipated and minimized. However, it is important to recognize when a patient becomes depressed because this is treatable. Depression affects up to 50% of patients after stroke.

About 5% of patients will have a seizure within 1 year of their stroke. Anticonvulsants may be required.

Thalamic pain is a deep gnawing pain that can follow stroke, typically with some sensory involvement. This may respond to pain-modulating drugs such as amitriptyline and carbamazepine and can be difficult to treat.

Optimize recovery (p. 120)

The treatment of a patient with a stroke depends on a multidisciplinary team of: nurses, physiotherapists, occupational therapists, speech therapists, dietician, psychologists and social worker. This team aims to assist the patient in functional recovery and to help adapt the patient's environment to minimize the impact of the physical disability. The patient's family needs to be closely involved. After the patient leaves hospital there may be other agencies that can provide assistance, e.g. district nurses, day hospital or day centres.

There is evidence that care of stroke patients within a stroke unit, where there is a closely integrated team of therapists, reduces mortality by about 25% and improves functional recovery.

Prevent recurrence of stroke

The options available are the same as for transient ischaemic attacks (TIA) and are discussed on pages 70–71.

Prognosis

The outcome after a stroke depends primarily on the type of stroke and the clinical stroke syndrome. Primary intracranial haemorrhage carries a 50% mortality, with 50% of survivors dependent at 6 months. Total anterior circulation ischaemic strokes have a similar mortality but a higher (90%) level of dependent patients at 6 months. Partial anterior circulation strokes, lacunar strokes (Fig. 2) and posterior circulation strokes have a 10–15% mortality with 20–40% of survivors dependent at 6 months. Ischaemic heart disease is the most common cause of death following a stroke or TIA.

Table 2 **Complications of stroke**
Acute complications
Raised intracranial pressure and herniation
Aspiration and pneumonia
Complications of immobility
Pneumonia
Contractures
Deep vein thrombosis
Bedsores
Urinary tract infections
Constipation
Later complications
Depression
Epilepsy
Thalmic pain
Social problems

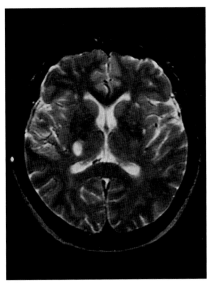
Fig. 2 **Lacunar Infarct.**

Stroke III

- Investigation of a stroke aims to confirm diagnosis, define the stroke type and pathogenesis and uncover any factors that could make it worse.

- Acute treatment of stroke aims to protect the patient from complications of stroke, minimize stroke size and optimize recovery.

Transient ischaemic attacks and prevention of strokes

A transient ischaemic attack (TIA) is an acute loss of neurological function or monocular vision caused by ischaemia with symptoms lasting less than 24 h. This occurs in 10% of patients prior to the development of a stroke. The annual incidence is 30 per 100 000.

A TIA is caused by artery-to-artery emboli or cardiac emboli. The pathogenesis is the same as for embolic stroke and is discussed on page 65. The investigation and management of TIAs and small strokes from which a good recovery has been made is the same because both provide a potential opportunity to prevent a more major stroke.

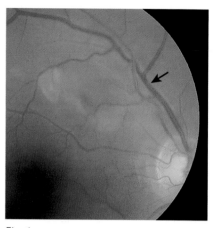

Fig. 1 **Cholesterol embolus on fundoscopy.**

Clinical features

These episodes are transient and therefore the diagnosis is made on the basis of the history. The onset is usually rapid over seconds or minutes. The resolution is more variable, with complete recovery in minutes to the full 24 h. A wide range of different clinical disturbances can occur. In considering them it is important to distinguish whether they arise from the anterior circulation (the carotids) or the posterior circulation (the vertebral and basilar arteries).

Anterior circulation TIAs include:

- amaurosis fugax (fleeting blindness) – loss of vision in one eye, 'like a shutter coming down'
- aphasia, or other language problems such as dyslexia or dysgraphia.

Posterior circulation TIAs include:

- homonymous visual field loss
- dysarthria
- combined brain stem symptoms: vertigo, diplopia, dysphagia; these are rarely TIAs if they occur in isolation
- bilateral weakness or sensory loss.

Anterior *or* posterior circulation TIAs include:

- unilateral weakness affecting the face, arm or leg in isolation or combination
- unilateral sensory loss affecting the face, arm or leg in isolation or combination.

TIAs rarely lead to blackouts or alteration of consciousness. If this occurs, alternative diagnoses should be considered.

Because TIAs are transient and alarming it is often difficult for the patient to characterize them exactly. It is therefore common not to be certain whether visual loss was monocular, indicating amaurosis fugax, or hemianopic, indicating a posterior circulation TIA. If in any doubt the investigations should be directed as for an anterior circulation event.

A history of risk factors for atheroma is important (Table 1, p. 64). In young women the type of oral contraceptive is important: the combined oestrogen–progestogen pill increases their risk by two to three times, but there is no increased risk with progesterone only.

Examination of a patient following a TIA usually reveals no neurological abnormalities. Occasionally a cholesterol embolus is seen on fundoscopy (Fig. 1). The cardiovascular system is more likely to reveal relevant abnormalities such as hypertension, hypertensive retinal changes, arrhythmias, heart murmur, signs of cardiac failure suggesting left ventricular dysfunction, loss of peripheral pulses and bruits.

Differential diagnosis

Most TIAs are sufficiently clear-cut for a confident clinical diagnosis to be made. The conditions that produce similar presentations include:

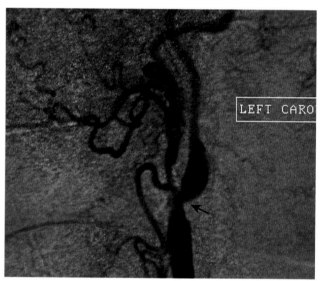

Fig. 2 **Angiogram showing carotid stenosis.**

- *Migraine.* There is usually a slower progression of the neurological deficit, taking 15–30 min to develop; there are usually positive symptoms such as flashing lights or marked tingling associated with this. There is usually an associated migrainous headache.
- *Partial seizures.* These are usually much shorter-lived, lasting seconds to a few minutes; when they recur they are very stereotyped.
- *Intracranial lesions.* These usually produce progressive deficits, occasionally they may produce intermittent symptoms.
- *Metabolic changes.* Hypoglycaemia can produce transient neurological deficits.
- *Peripheral nerve lesions.* For example, carpal tunnel syndrome produces intermittent sensory loss in the hands.

Investigation

Investigation is directed at looking for risk factors for vascular disease, potential sources of embolism in either the carotid arteries or in the heart, causes of tendency to thrombosis and causes of inflammatory vascular disease (Table 1, p. 64). The investigations need to be tailored to the patient. Younger patients will require more aggressive investigation, particularly if there are no risk factors for atheroma. In these patients careful evaluation of the heart and screening for thrombophilia and possible vasculitic processes are needed. Screening for sickle cell disease is indicated in all patients at risk.

In patients where the differential diagnosis is thought to include an intracranial lesion or partial seizures brain imaging with either CT or MRI is indicated. An EEG may prove helpful in the diagnosis of patients with partial seizures.

Secondary prevention of stroke and transient ischaemic attacks

Control of risk factors
Treatment of hypertension, control of diabetes, cessation of smoking and moderation in alcohol intake, and control of hypercholesterolaemia all combine to reduce the progression of atheroma. Recent trials have shown that even if a patient's serum cholesterol and blood pressure are 'normal', reducing them further will reduce the risk of another stroke. Most patients end up on a cocktail of a diuretic, an ACE inhibitor and a statin. These measures also reduce the risk of ischaemic heart disease, the commonest cause of death following TIA.

Postmenopausal oestrogen therapy (hormone replacement therapy) may increase the risk of stroke.

Aspirin
Aspirin reduces the recurrence of ischaemic stroke or TIA from 10% to 8% per year. A wide range of doses have been shown to be effective and an optimum dose has not been established. However the adverse effects are directly related to dosage. A typical dose is 150–300 mg per day. This is also useful in the prevention of other vascular complications.

Other antiplatelet agents
Dipyridamole has recently been demonstrated to be helpful when used in combination with aspirin. Clopidogrel, another antiplatelet agent, has been assessed in one large trial and has similar benefit to aspirin. The role of these newer agents is not entirely clear; they are useful in aspirin-intolerant patients.

Anticoagulation
There are several situations when anticoagulation has been demonstrated to reduce the risk of stroke. In patients with TIA or stroke in atrial fibrillation the risk of stroke is reduced from 12% per year to 4% by anticoagulation to an INR of 2–3, and the vascular mortality is reduced from 17% to 8%. The exact reduction in risk for patients with mural thrombosis and left ventricular dilatation has not been established in population studies but these are clinical situations where anticoagulation would be considered. The risk of recurrent stroke needs to be estimated in each patient and balanced against the risk of anticoagulation, including the risk of falls, difficulties taking the tablets or in monitoring treatment, etc.

Carotid stenosis
The North American Symptomatic Carotid Endarterectomy study and the European Carotid Surgery trials are landmark studies that evaluated the usefulness of this surgical procedure in a range of degrees of carotid stenosis (Fig. 2). Both studies found a reduced risk of recurrent stroke in patients with a greater than 70% stenosis in the surgical group and especially those with stenosis greater than 80% (Fig. 3). The benefit of surgery depends on achieving a low surgical morbidity and mortality (7% or less). The risk of stroke is greater with a tighter stenosis and if the plaque is ulcerated, so the benefit is greater for these patients. An occluded carotid artery poses no further risk of stroke.

Initial studies have found angioplasty to have similar effectiveness to endarterectomy, though further studies are ongoing. This technique has proved useful in the treatment of other peripheral and coronary artery stenoses.

Primary prevention of stroke
This revolves around the control of risk factors for atheroma in the general population, in particular the control of hypertension. Control of hypertension reduces the stroke rate by 40%, regardless of age.

There is dispute about the best management of asymptomatic carotid stenosis. Trials found that the stroke risk was about 2% per year in unoperated patients compared with 1% in the operated group, suggesting a very small benefit compared with a 2% operative risk. Put another way, 86 patients need to have the operation to prevent one stroke.

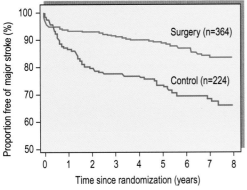

Fig. 3 **Kaplan–Maier survival curves to show survival time free of stroke in patients with 80–99% carotid stenosis following endarterectomy (surgery) and in controls.** (By kind permission of the Lancet: European carotid surgery trialists' collaborative group 1998. Randomised trial of endarterectomy for recently symptomatic carotid stenosis; final results of the MRC European carotid surgery trial (ECST). Lancet 351: 1379–87.)

> *Transient ischaemic attacks and prevention of strokes*
>
> ■ Diagnosis of TIAs depends on the history.
>
> ■ 10% of patients have a TIA prior to having a stroke.
>
> ■ Management relies on understanding the pathophysiology of the TIA.
>
> ■ Management includes control of vascular risk factors and use of aspirin, and in selected patients anticoagulation or carotid endarterectomy.

Subarachnoid haemorrhage

Subarachnoid haemorrhage (SAH) is an important and potentially preventable cause of death and neurological disability. SAH is uncommon, with an incidence of 6–20 per 100 000 per year. It is rare below the age of 20 years and most frequent between 40 and 60 years of age.

Pathology

SAH usually results from rupture of an intracranial aneurysm into the subarachnoid space, the space between the pia mater covering the brain and the dura mater lining the skull (Fig. 1a). These aneurysms, usually found on the circle of Willis (Fig. 1b), are usually saccular but may be fusiform. About 5% of SAH is caused by bleeding from an arteriovenous malformation (AVM).

The pathogenesis of intracranial aneurysms is uncertain. Proposed mechanisms include congenital defects in the muscular layer or acquired degenerative changes in the internal elastic lamina. Rarely they occur after trauma or infective emboli. Asymptomatic aneurysms occur in 2–5% of the population.

Aneurysmal rupture may lead to an intracerebral haemorrhage as well as subarachnoid haemorrhage and this intracerebral haemorrhage can produce focal neurological deficits depending on its site. Large subarachnoid bleeds can interfere with CSF reabsorption and produce hydrocephalus.

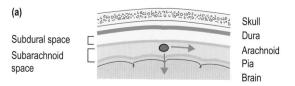

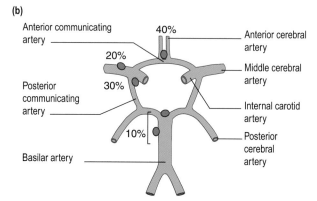

Fig. 1 **Pathology of subarachnoid haemorrhage. (a)** Aneurysms occur in the subarachnoid space, deep to the arachnoid mater and dura mater. The arrows indicate the direction of a bleed: may be intracerebral as well as subarachnoid. **(b)** Most aneurysms occur in the circle of Willis.

Clinical features

The classical presentation of SAH is:

- a sudden severe headache
  - 'as if hit by a bat'
- transient loss of consciousness
- vomiting
- neck stiffness and sometimes focal neurological signs.

It is important to realize that, while this is the classical presentation of SAH, not every patient has all these features. Sometimes the diagnosis of SAH is more difficult and up to 50% of patients are incorrectly diagnosed initially.

About a sixth of patients with SAH will die before reaching hospital. On arrival in hospital about a third are drowsy and 20% are stuporous or in coma. In those who can give a history almost all have had sudden severe headaches; rarely, it can come on slightly more slowly. Most patients have generalized headaches and occasionally it is localized. Fifty per cent of patients have had some loss of consciousness. Neck stiffness is found in about two-thirds of patients and localizing signs in 40% (motor deficits 15%, aphasia 15%, hemianopia 10%, sensory disturbances 5%).

A third nerve palsy with pupillary involvement is occasionally seen and is of particular significance, indicating enlargement or rupture of a posterior communicating artery aneurysm. Such patients need urgent referral to a neurosurgical unit and investigation to try to prevent aneurysmal rupture. In an unconscious patient, a third nerve palsy can also occur with uncal herniation due to raised intracranial pressure. A 6th nerve palsy can occur as a false localizing sign due to hydrocephalus. Ophthalmoscopy can occasionally reveal subhyaloid haemorrhage.

Hypertension occurs in about 50% of patients. About a third of patients who present with SAH have had another sudden severe headache in the weeks prior to their presentation. This probably represents a smaller bleed from which they have recovered.

Differential diagnosis

This depends on the presentation. If a patient presents with a sudden severe headache, without loss of consciousness or focal neurological signs, the most common differential diagnosis is 'thunderclap headache'. This diagnosis is only made once investigations for SAH are completed and are all negative. This occasionally recurs and is thought to be a migraine variant. Sometimes this type of headache is situation dependent, for example occurring during sexual intercourse or on exercise.

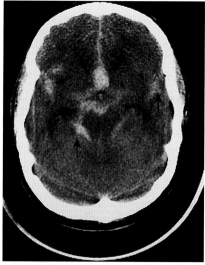

Fig. 2 **CT scan showing subarachnoid haemorrhage.** The subarachnoid blood appears white and fills the space around the brain that would normally contain CSF and would appear dark.

In a patient with headache, vomiting and a stiff neck who is a little confused and unable to give a reliable history, meningitis is the major differential diagnosis.

If the patient is found unconscious the differential diagnosis is that of coma (p. 50).

Investigations

Investigations are in two phases:

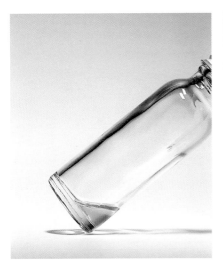

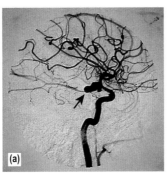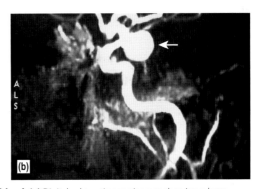

Fig. 4 **Discovering the source of the bleed. (a)** Digital subtraction angiogram showing a large multiloculated aneurysm arising from the middle cerebral artery (arrow), **(b)** MR angiogram showing an aneurysm on the middle cerebral artery (arrow).

Fig. 3 **Xanthochromic CSF.**

- *To prove that the patient has had an SAH.* A CT brain scan is positive (Fig. 2) in 95% of cases within the first 24 h after onset of headache but in only 67% by 3 days. If this is negative then a lumbar puncture should be performed, at least 6 h after the onset, when diffusely blood-stained CSF with xanthochromic (yellow) supernatant (Fig. 3) is found. This needs to be confirmed with spectrophotometry.
- *To discover the source of the bleed.* A four-vessel cerebral angiogram locates the aneurysm (Fig. 4a). About 1 in 10 patients with definite SAH will have no source of bleeding found and have a low risk of recurrence. Magnetic resonance angiography is increasingly used to locate aneurysms without the risks of angiography (Fig. 4b).

Complications

The main complications are:

- rebleeding from the ruptured aneurysm
- cerebral ischaemia because of vasospasm of the cerebral arteries; it is not clear how SAH causes vasospasm
- hydrocephalus.

These present with a deterioration in the level of consciousness or development of focal signs. They can only reliably be distinguished on repeat CT scanning.

Occasionally patients may develop hyponatraemia, neurogenic pulmonary oedema and cardiac arrhythmias. Patients may also develop complications from bedrest and impaired consciousness: deep vein thromboses and aspiration and basal pneumonia.

Treatment and prognosis

The objective of treatment is to prevent further rebleeding whilst minimizing the risk of complications.

Patients should be transferred to a neurosurgical centre. They require frequent neurological observations, including pulse, blood pressure and Glasgow Coma Scale, to monitor for deterioration. Appropriate nursing care should be provided for confused and unconscious patients (p. 51).

Rebleeding can be prevented either by endovascular occlusion of the aneurysm with a coil or by surgically clipping the aneurysm. Recent trials have found that, where technically possible, the endovascular procedure has a better outcome; however, some aneurysms are not amenable to this approach and are treated surgically.

The risk of ischaemic complications, thought to be due to vasospasm, can be reduced by sustained hypervolaemia (3 litres of normal saline per day) and a calcium antagonist (nimodipine). Aggressive control of blood pressure increases ischaemic complications, and antihypertensives should be avoided. Fludrocortisone or hypertonic saline can be used to treat hyponatraemia.

Hydrocephalus should be treated with an appropriate drainage procedure.

Patients who are alert on arrival at hospital have the best prognosis; three-quarters make a full recovery and there is a 10% mortality rate. In patients who are comatose on arrival, three-quarters die, 10% are severely disabled or in a persistent vegetative state and only 10% make a good recovery. Patients who are in a coma are therefore usually managed medically until their conscious level improves, when they would be considered for aneurysmal clipping.

Special situations

Unruptured aneurysms

Occasionally patients will be discovered to have unruptured intracranial aneurysms in addition to a ruptured aneurysm or if they are having angiograms for other reasons. Unruptured aneurysms have a risk of bleeding of 0.5% per year if over 10 mm and 0.05% per year if smaller. The decision whether to clip therefore depends on the life expectancy of the patient, the risk of the operation and the attitude of the patient to those risks.

Giant aneurysms

Giant aneurysms present in the same way as other space-occupying lesions, either by producing neurological deficits appropriate to their site or by acting as triggers for seizures. They are characteristically rounded lesions often with calcification at their edges. Neurosurgical treatment is difficult because these aneurysms often do not have a clear-cut neck to clip. Endovascular techniques, for example the introduction of coils into the aneurysmal sac, are proving a useful aid by causing thrombosis within the aneurysm.

Subarachnoid haemorrhage

- Classical presentation is with sudden severe headache and neck stiffness, frequently with loss of consciousness and focal signs.
- Sudden severe headaches need to be investigated as potential subarachnoid haemorrhages.
- 10% of patients with subarachnoid haemorrhage present in coma.
- 3rd nerve palsies that involve the pupil are due to posterior communicating artery aneurysms until proved otherwise.
- CT scanning and CSF examination are used to determine if a subarachnoid haemorrhage has occurred.
- Ischaemia, rebleeding and hydrocephalus are the main complications of subarachnoid haemorrhage.
- Intravenous fluids, calcium antagonists and aneurysmal clipping are the main treatments.

Epilepsy I: diagnosis

A seizure is a paroxysmal neurological event caused by the abnormal discharge of neurones. Epilepsy is defined as a tendency to recurrent seizures, i.e. two or more seizures. Epilepsy is not a single disease but it is a symptom of congenital or acquired CNS disease in the same way as weakness is a symptom in a range of different disorders. Different types of epilepsy can be classified according to different features, including seizure type, age of onset, prognosis and cause, and are more appropriately called the *epilepsies*.

The epilepsies are the most common serious neurological diseases; 5% of the population will experience an epileptic seizure at some point in their life. Their prevalence is 0.5%; 370 000 people in the UK are affected. Males and females are similarly affected. Peaks of onset occur in childhood/adolescence in relation to congenital causes and in the elderly are presumed to be secondary to cerebrovascular and degenerative diseases.

Seizures cause unpredictable loss of control, which makes epilepsy one of the most stigmatizing and socially disabling of all diseases, adversely affecting many aspects of life, such as increasing divorce rates, and adversely affecting employment opportunities. Epilepsy is associated with depression and psychiatric illness.

Diagnosis

The diagnosis of epilepsy is clinical, depending on the history from the patient and, critically, from any witnesses of the attacks. This can be supported by investigations such as an electroencephalogram (EEG), but the main contribution of the EEG is in syndrome classification. The differential diagnosis of blackouts is discussed on page 44.

Classification of seizures and epilepsy syndromes

Much of the confusion about the classifications in epilepsy arise because of a failure to appreciate that there are two inter-related classifications: a classification of seizure type (Fig. 1) and a classification of epilepsy syndromes (Table 1). Patients will often have several different types of seizure. The epilepsy syndrome includes diagnosis of seizure type and additional information, mostly relating to aetiology, including age, EEG and neuroimaging results. Where possible, patients' epilepsy should be classified by epilepsy syndrome rather than seizure type, which takes into account these other factors. The old terms 'petit mal' and 'grand mal' do not fit easily into this classification and should not be used.

There are three broad categories of epilepsy syndromes:

- *generalized epilepsies* – associated with a diffuse hyperexcitability of membranes that leads to synchronized generalized abnormal discharge of neurones.
- *focal epilepsies* (localization related) – discharges arise from a specific cortical region that can either remain localized or spread more generally.
- *provoked seizures* due to acute abnormalities, e.g. trauma, metabolic abnormalities, drugs or alcohol.

Patients who have had only a few attacks may not be classifiable into an epileptic syndrome.

Generalized epilepsies

These usually start in childhood or adolescence and have typical clusters of seizure types, including tonic-clonic seizures, absences and myoclonic jerks, combined with a characteristic

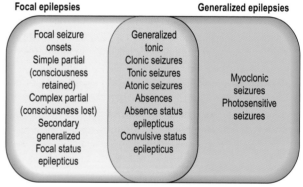

Fig. 1 **Seizure types in focal and generalized epilepsies.** Some seizure types occur only in focal or in generalized epilepsies but many can occur in both types and cannot easily be classified purely on the basis of clinical seizure type.

Table 1	**Some of the more common epilepsy syndromes (all generalized, except BECT)**				
Syndrome	Age of onset	Clinical features	EEG	Prognosis	Treatment
Childhood absence epilepsy (CAE)	3–12 years	Commonly in girls with many absences each day, mimicking daydreaming, rare convulsions	3 Hz spike and wave, often photosensitive	Usually remits in teens	Ethosuximide or sodium valproate
Juvenile absence epilepsy	7–17 years	Absences less frequent than CAE. Convulsions common	3 Hz spike and wave, rarely photosensitive	Good response to treatment, but may persist	Sodium valproate, ethosuximide, lamotrigine
Juvenile myoclonic epilepsy	10–20 years	Myoclonic jerks within first few minutes of waking and GTCS also in morning. Occasional absences	Polyspike and wave, sometimes photosensitive	Often persists but responds to treatment; worsens with carbamazepine	Sodium valproate, clonazepam, lamotrigine
West syndrome	3–7 months	Flexor spasms, tonic and atonic seizures with half of development. Mental retardation usual	'Hypsarrhythmia'; mountains on EEG	Poor, especially secondary cases with, for example, tuberous sclerosis. Very severe epilepsy	Adrenocorticotrophic hormone and vigabatrin
Lennox–Gastaut syndrome	2–9 years	Tonic and atonic seizures and atypical absences	Slow spike and wave at 2–2.5 Hz	Persistent epilepsy and mental retardation common	Carbamazepine, sodium valproate, lamotrigine
Benign partial epilepsy with centrotemporal spikes (BECT)	3–13 years	Occasional, motor seizures affecting one side of face, sometimes spreading. Usually nocturnal	Centrotemporal spikes, especially in sleep, shift between sides	Remits by age 20 years	Carbamazepine, often no treatment required

Table 2 **Symptoms of focal and generalized seizures**	
Seizure symptom	**Clinical significance**
Focal	
Focal limb jerking	Motor cortex onset
Focal tingling	Somatosensory cortex onset
Olfactory or gustatory hallucination	Temporal lobe onset
Visual hallucination	Occipital lobe onset
Limb posturing	Supplementary motor area onset
Swallowing/chewing movements	Temporal lobe
Generalized	
Generalized stiffening (tonic)	
Repeated generalized jerking (clonic)	
Intermittent symmetrical jerks (myoclonic)	
Absence with no focal symptoms	
Atonic drop attacks	

generalized EEG 'signature'. The most common forms are the idiopathic generalized epilepsies (IGE), which represent well-defined clinical syndromes (Table 2) and are not associated with structural brain disease. They generally have a good prognosis. There is a constitutional component with a significantly increased risk of epilepsy amongst family members.

West syndrome and Lennox–Gastaut syndrome are rarer generalized epilepsies of early childhood; they have a much poorer prognosis and may be associated with mental handicap and structural brain disease such as tuberous sclerosis.

Focal epilepsy

Focal epilepsy occurs at any age. The abnormal discharge appears to start in one part of the brain and may become generalized. The focal onset may be reflected in focal symptoms at the onset of the seizure, indicating the abnormal region of cortex (Table 2). The spread may be so rapid that the seizure appears to be a generalized convulsion from the outset and there are no early focal symptoms. There may be a post-ictal confusional state, during which the patient may wander and undertake stereotyped actions that appear purposeful ('automatisms'). These may include plucking at objects, or sometimes more sophisticated behaviours such as bedmaking or undressing. Without an EEG during the episode, this can be difficult to differentiate from complex partial status epilepticus (see below). An interictal EEG (between seizures) may show localized spikes or sharp waves. This helps to support the diagnosis but their location does not always accord with the region of seizure onset.

Focal epilepsy may be associated with focal structural brain disease. In younger patients this is usually hippocampal sclerosis or developmental abnormalities of the cerebral cortex. Trauma, cerebrovascular disease and tumours are also common causes, especially in older patients. The prognosis for seizure remission and mortality is worse than in generalized epilepsies.

The benign focal epilepsies of childhood, e.g. BECT (Table 1), are relatively common focal epilepsies that usually remit in adolescence and are not associated with focal structural abnormalities.

Status epilepticus

Status epilepticus is defined as seizures occurring for 30 min, either continuously or intermittently, without recovery. It is a medical emergency (see below). The seizures may be:

■ generalized convulsions (convulsive status epilepticus)
■ simple, partial or focal, e.g. jerking of one side of the body (non-convulsive status)
■ a confusional state, with or without abnormal motor activity (non-convulsive or complex partial status).

Investigation

An EEG is required to characterize the epilepsy but may be normal and this does not exclude a diagnosis of epilepsy. Repeating the EEG, especially with sleep deprivation, increases the diagnostic yield (p. 32). In some cases a prolonged, ambulatory EEG recording can 'catch' an attack, in which case it is helpful in diagnosis.

Adults presenting over the age of 20 years should undergo a CT or MRI scan to exclude a focal structural lesion. The sensitivity of MRI is much greater for subtle developmental abnormalities but CT is adequate to exclude larger lesions, e.g. most tumours. Younger patients should be scanned if there is clinical or EEG evidence of focal seizure onset.

Single seizures

It is not uncommon to see patients who have had only a single seizure or cluster of seizures over a few hours or an unwitnessed blackout that was probably a seizure. A potential structural trigger should be sought by a CT or MRI brain scan in all patients with focal onset seizures or in those over the age of 20 years. The advice following a single seizure is the same as for recurrent attacks (see below).

The prognosis for recurrence varies according to the seizure type, cause and associated clinical features. Most that recur do so within the first year. Focal seizures recur more frequently, especially if associated with congenital lesions or tumours. Sixty per cent of convulsions recur by 1 year. However, if there has been an acute precipitant ('provoked attack'), for example acute alcohol withdrawal or a metabolic disturbance such as liver or renal failure, which is successfully treated, the recurrence rate is lower. The EEG is relatively unhelpful in determining the risk of recurrence. If the EEG is very abnormal, recurrence is somewhat more likely than if it is normal. Most clinicians do not treat a single seizure.

Advice following one or more seizures

Epilepsy usually causes a frightening and unpredictable loss of consciousness. The patient needs to understand the nature of the problem and the clinician needs to try to encourage the patient to live a normal life, at the same time understanding that there will have to be some restrictions for the patient's own safety and the safety of others. For example, the patient can continue to go swimming, but should be accompanied by a competent adult. Family members, employers and schools need to understand the diagnosis and how to deal with seizures. It is also the duty of the doctor to tell the patient that the driving and vehicle licensing authority (DVLA) must be informed of the condition. This is the case for all types of seizures, including single seizures and single provoked seizures. Current regulations are that a patient should be seizure-free for 12 months – from all types of seizures including partial, complex partial or myoclonic seizures. In provoked seizures the DVLA may be more lenient but they must still be informed.

> *Epilepsy I: diagnosis*
>
> ■ Epilepsy is a symptom rather than a diagnosis in itself.
> ■ There are different sorts of seizures and more than one type of seizure can occur in a patient.
> ■ Epilepsy syndromes can be divided into generalized or focal onset disorders.

Epilepsy II: treatment and management

When to treat?

Most physicians would recommend treatment when a person has suffered two or more seizures within a 2-year period. The risk of recurrence after a first seizure varies according to the aetiology and seizure syndrome and may influence the decision on when to treat.

Principles of medical treatment

Which treatment to use depends on the epilepsy syndrome, seizure types and adverse effect profile. One drug should be used, where possible, and the dose titrated against response and adverse effects. Seventy per cent of patients will respond to first-line therapy, becoming seizure-free for at least 2 years. Monotherapy carries the lowest risk of adverse effects, which increase substantially with increasing numbers of drugs. For most drugs, the correct dose is the lowest effective dose that does not cause side-effects. A drug should not be considered ineffective until it has been tried to the maximum dose that does not cause adverse effects, which varies between patients. For refractory cases, more than one drug may be required and some will remain refractory to all agents. Using more than three drugs concurrently should be avoided.

Some refractory cases, on re-evaluation, prove to have non-epileptic (psychogenic) seizures, also referred to as pseudoseizures (p. 116). In others, poor compliance contributes to poor control.

In refractory cases where these factors have been excluded, if there is evidence of focal seizure onset, surgery may be considered (see below).

Choice of medication

The major divisions into generalized and focal onset epilepsies are important in the choice of drug (Fig. 1). Medications can be broadly divided into those useful in focal epilepsy, those with a broad spectrum of action and those for specific seizure types. Carbamazepine, lamotrigine and valproate are the commonest first-line drugs in the UK. The choice is also influenced heavily by the age of the patient because this affects their susceptibility to the side-effects of different drugs. For example, focal onset epilepsy in a young woman is often treated with carbamazepine or lamotrigine as first line because of its lower risk of teratogenicity, but sodium valproate is favoured in the elderly because of a lower risk of ataxia and falls. Lamotrigine is emerging as a broad-spectrum drug, well tolerated in many patient groups.

Measurement of drug levels in blood

This is of benefit in limited situations:

- in patients on polytherapy
- optimizing the dose of phenytoin and carbamazepine
- in the assessment of compliance.

In judging drug dosage, blood levels are most useful for patients on phenytoin therapy. The saturation kinetics of this drug give it a particularly narrow therapeutic window. There is substantial variability between patients. There is some value in measuring drug levels in patients receiving carbamazepine or barbiturates but little benefit for other drugs apart from finding out whether the patient is taking them (e.g. unconscious patient).

Adverse effects

The adverse effects of antiepileptic drugs are common and are listed in Table 1. Sedation can occur with all drugs and is the most common complaint, especially with polytherapy. Another concern is teratogenicity, which rises with the number of drugs taken. Women of childbearing age on antiepileptic medication should be counselled of the risk and their medication minimized prior to conception. Although not proven to be of benefit, folic acid supplements (5 mg daily) are generally prescribed to women of childbearing age taking antiepileptic drugs as it may help to prevent neural tube defects, a particular worry with sodium valproate.

Drug interactions

Carbamazepine, phenytoin and phenobarbital are potent liver enzyme inducers. They increase the rate of elimination of the contraceptive pill so that a higher-dose pill needs to be taken to compensate. They also increase the metabolism of other drugs eliminated via the liver, including other antiepileptic drugs. Sodium valproate inhibits liver metabolism of some drugs. The drug most sensitive to these effects is lamotrigine; its half-life varies from 12 h (with concurrent enzyme inducer) to 70 h with concurrent sodium valproate. The new drugs gabapentin, topiramate and levetiracetam are principally renally excreted so interaction is less of a problem.

When to stop treatment

In general, the same factors that predict seizure recurrence are also associated with relapse on cessation of treatment. If medication is withdrawn after 2 years of being seizure-free, there is a risk of recurrence of 25–40%. There is no absolute predictive test, and seizure recurrence is always less if patients continue with treatment than if they stop. For this reason, the decision to stop treatment is largely a personal one. For

Focal epilepsy	Either	Generalized epilepsy
Carbamazepine[1,2]	Lamotrigine[1,2]	Ethosuximide (absences)
Gabapentin[2]	Valproate[1,2]	
	Topiramate[2]	Clonazepam (myoclonus)
Phenytoin[1,2]	Levetiracetam	
Tiagabine	Clobazam	Piracetam (myoclonus)
Vigabatrin	Phenobarbital[2]	

Fig. 1 Drugs used in focal and generalized epilepsies.
[1] Drugs widely used as first line in the UK.
[2] Drugs licensed for monotherapy.

Table 1 Adverse effects of anticonvulsant drugs

Adverse effect	Drugs
Sedation	All drugs, especially phenobarbital and benzodiazepines Substantial individual variation
Diplopia and ataxia	Phenobarbital, phenytoin, carbamazepine, lamotrigine
Rash	Carbamazepine, lamotrigine, phenytoin
Gastrointestinal effects	Carbamazepine, sodium valproate
Weight gain	Sodium valproate, vigabatrin, gabapentin, others infrequently
Weight loss	Topiramate
Reversible hair loss	Sodium valproate, vigabatrin
Teratogenic effects	Proven for carbamazepine (safest), phenytoin, phenobarbital, clobazam, sodium valproate, topiramate. Unknown for other new drugs
Visual field loss	Vigabatrin (rarely used as a result)

example, a woman who wants to start a family may accept a recurrence of partial seizures if it means that her baby is not exposed to the teratogenic effects of drugs *in utero*, but a travelling salesman may wish to continue with medication indefinitely, rather than increase the risk of losing his driving licence.

Surgical treatment of epilepsy

Patients with focal onset seizures not controlled by drugs should be considered for neurosurgical treatment. Before undertaking surgery, the epilepsy must be demonstrated to come from a single part of the brain that could be removed, without leaving any major neurological deficit. It requires detailed MRI studies, EEG recordings, including recordings of seizure onset (sometimes with intracranial electrodes), and neuropsychological assessment to establish the risks of surgery for cognitive function. The forms of epilepsy most amenable to surgical treatment are temporal lobe epilepsy due to mesial temporal sclerosis and epilepsy due to foreign tissue lesions.

Prognosis of established epilepsy

The natural history of epilepsy is poorly understood. The prognosis for remission depends on the epilepsy syndrome and is generally good. Most generalized epilepsies remit in adolescence or early adult life, except juvenile myoclonic epilepsy which usually persists. Partial epilepsy syndromes, especially those with a congenital cause, are usually more persistent, but 80% of these also achieve a 3-year remission by 9 years after onset. The EEG is of little value in determining prognosis in most cases.

Epilepsy mortality

The mortality of patients with epilepsy is up to three times that of age-matched controls. The increase is seen mostly in focal epilepsies. Some of this excess is due to the underlying cause of the epilepsy, e.g. tumours, and some is clearly due to seizure-related events, e.g. status epilepticus or drowning. There remain patients who die suddenly probably following a seizure. This is called sudden death in epilepsy and may affect up to 0.5% of

epilepsy sufferers per year. The likely causes are apnoea or fatal cardiac dysrhythmias due to unwitnessed seizures.

Management of status epilepticus

Status epilepticus is a medical emergency and convulsive status epilepticus (CSE) is life-threatening. CSE causes a variety of secondary manifestations, including hypoxia, acidosis, myoglobinuria, renal failure, disseminated intravascular coagulation and hyperthermia. Most of these complications reverse rapidly on cessation of seizures but, untreated, the mortality is high.

Treatment is directed to:

- general resuscitation
- stopping the seizures
- treating the underlying cause.

Patients fall into two general categories: those with a previous diagnosis of epilepsy and those presenting for the first time, in whom serious new disease underlying the seizures is likely (Fig. 2). The cause may be metabolic dysfunction, drugs, intracranial mass lesions, haemorrhage or infection. These patients need to be investigated for metabolic disturbance, undergo urgent neuroimaging and, if this is normal, CSF analysis, especially to look for encephalitis. An EEG may also help with this diagnosis.

Treatment should be initiated immediately to stop the seizures and to prevent further seizures. In general, if the seizures stop, most of the secondary metabolic abnormalities will correct rapidly. First-line treatment is a benzodiazepine (lorazepam or diazepam intravenously or rectal diazepam) then a loading dose of 10–15 mg/kg of phenytoin given by intravenous infusion.

In patients with a known history of epilepsy, drug withdrawal seizures should be considered and urgent anticonvulsant blood levels obtained. If there is drug withdrawal, the same drug should be restored if possible, otherwise treatment should be along the same lines as with *de novo* cases. If patients with known epilepsy respond rapidly to treatment, such intensive investigation may not be required, but if they do not respond, investigation should proceed as above.

If patients do not respond rapidly to treatment, the diagnosis should be reconsidered. If seizures are not controlled the patient should be entubated and ventilated and given thiopentone. EEG monitoring is needed to monitor control of seizures. Many cases of 'refractory status' turn out to have psychogenic seizures, rather than epilepsy, but this is a difficult diagnosis and requires specialist advice.

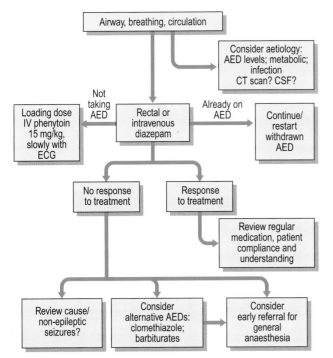

Fig. 2 **Management of convulsive status epilepticus. (AED, anti-epilepsy drug.)**

> ### Box 1
>
> **Instructions for carers witnessing a convulsive seizure**
> - Remove any objects on which the individual may harm themselves.
> - Put the patient into the recovery position.
> - Call an ambulance if convulsion lasts longer than 10 min.
> - Do not try to put anything into the patient's mouth.
> - Do not try to restrain the convulsion.
> - If the person wanders after the convulsion, gently guide them to safety, do not try to exercise restraint.

> ### Epilepsy II: treatment and management
> - Choice of drug depends on the epilepsy syndrome and adverse effects.
> - Monotherapy should be used if possible.
> - Some drugs interfere with the oral contraceptive pill or are teratogenic.
> - Status epilepticus is a medical emergency.

Head injury

Head injury is an important cause of disability and death. In western countries, trauma is the most common cause of death in patients aged under 45 years. Half of these patients die as a result of head injury. Overall there is a mortality rate of 20–30 per 100 000 per year. The survivors are often disabled with a prevalence of disabled survivors of up to 400 per 100 000.

The causes of head injury are falls, assaults and road traffic accidents (RTAs). The relative frequency varies from country to country and according to age. About a quarter of head injuries are due to RTAs in all age groups. In those aged under 15 years and over 65 years, falls are the most common cause; in those between the ages of 15 and 65 years, assaults are the most common cause.

Patients with acute head injuries are looked after by neurosurgeons or orthopaedic surgeons. Neurologists can be involved in their care, particularly in the recognition and management of the sequelae of head injury.

Pathology and pathogenesis

Cerebral injury

Head injury may lead to a brief loss of consciousness without associated pathological changes in the brain. The mechanism for the loss of consciousness is not clear.

With more severe head injury, brain damage can occur because of the direct trauma to the brain. This arises from direct disruption of the brain, shearing of axons and intracerebral haemorrhage. These injuries occur at the site of trauma and opposite the site of injury, so-called contre-coup injury. Contre-coup injury results from acceleration/deceleration forces moving the brain within the skull.

There may be secondary brain injury (Fig. 1) due to brain oedema, which causes raised intracranial pressure and can lead to cerebral herniation (p. 48). The raised intracranial pressure, usually associated with hypotension, leads to hypoperfusion of the brain and therefore cerebral ischaemia. Infratentorial lesions can obstruct CSF flow and lead to hydrocephalus.

Intracranial haematomas

Extradural haematomas occur when the middle meningeal artery bleeds into the extradural space (Fig. 2). This can occur

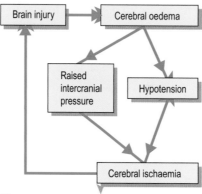

Fig. 1 **Mechanisms of secondary head injury.**

some time after the head injury and should be considered in any patient with deterioration following an apparently good recovery from a head injury.

Subdural haematomas occur either acutely, usually with some intracerebral bleeding, or chronically (Fig. 3). The latter occurs when damaged cortical veins ooze into the subdural space.

Intracerebral haematomas (Fig. 2) are the most common, occurring both at the site of direct trauma and at the contre-coup site.

The mass effect of any of these bleeds may lead to cerebral herniation.

Skull fractures

These can be divided into simple and depressed fractures and basal skull fractures. The latter are difficult to see on skull X-rays but are associated with particular physical signs such as periorbital bruising or Battle's sign (Fig. 4). These may also be associated with cranial nerve damage, especially facial and auditory nerves. Basal fractures also produce bleeding into the middle ear, seen as either blood behind the ear drum or coming from the external ear, or CSF rhinorrhoea. CSF rhinorrhoea is seen as clear fluid coming from the nose – fluid which, unlike mucus, contains glucose, which is easily tested for. (A more specific test is isotransferrin.) The presence of a skull fracture substantially increases the risk of significant intracranial haemorrhage.

Basal and compound fractures can produce a dural leak, which provides a potential route of entry of infection into the CNS.

Clinical features

The clinical features of head injury are varied and depend on the severity of the

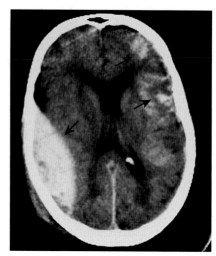

Fig. 2 **CT scan showing an extradural haematoma on the right (arrow) and intracranial haemorrhage on the left (double arrow).**

injury and the part of the brain affected. This can be complicated by delayed events such as intracranial haemorrhage. The clinical setting alters the evaluation. For example, in patients with multiple injuries there can be trauma elsewhere, with multiple fractures and abdominal and chest trauma. In these and other patients there may be associated cervical spine trauma.

The severity of a head injury can be assessed in several ways:

- The level of consciousness, reliably and easily measured using the Glasgow Coma Scale (p. 122), is an important clinical measure.
- Signs indicative of a basal skull fracture (see above).
- The pupil reactions, an important indicator of herniation.
- The finding of focal neurological signs.

These measures can be monitored and any change is particularly important in the management of these patients. The vital signs need to be monitored.

Fortunately, most patients will have less severe head injuries. The same measurements need to be made but a history may be obtainable from the patient. From the history of the episode, perhaps from witnesses, some estimate of the potential forces involved can be made. The occurrence and duration of loss of consciousness is an important indicator. The amount of memory lost by the patient, before the injury (retrograde amnesia) or after the injury

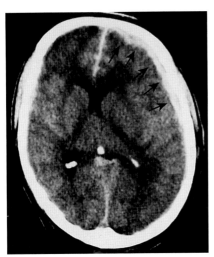

Fig. 3 **CT scan showing a subdural haematoma (arrow) producing some mass effect with displacement of the midline structures.**

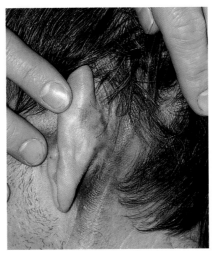

Fig. 4 **Signs of basal skull fracture: Battle's sign.**

(anterograde amnesia), is an important indicator of severity of injury.

One group of patients of particular concern are those who have made an initial recovery from their head injury but then later deteriorate again after a 'lucid interval'. This is the classical history of patients with extradural haemorrhage, though it can occur with subdural haemorrhage. It can also occur because of neck trauma resulting in carotid dissection. These complications are rare in patients who have not fractured their skull (1 in 1000).

Differential diagnoses

The differential diagnosis of head injury will depend on the clinical presentation. In patients who present unconscious or confused the differential diagnosis is wide and is discussed on page 50. In patients who have had a head injury with a period of anterograde and retrograde amnesia there may be uncertainty as to whether the head injury was the primary event or the result of a blackout.

Investigation and management

The investigation and management depends on the severity of the head injury. Patients with mild head injuries without loss of consciousness or with loss of consciousness of less than 5 min, with a normal examination and no skull fracture, can be allowed home in the care of a responsible adult with a warning card outlining the possible types of deterioration. Patients at risk from developing complications are those with longer than 5–10 minutes (min) unconsciousness, a seizure at onset, altered consciousness or focal signs on

examination and evidence of a skull fracture. These patients need to be admitted and monitored. CT or MRI of the brain is needed in most of these patients. These are optimally managed in a neurosurgical centre.

The aim of treatment is to prevent secondary brain damage. This focuses on avoiding hypotension, maintaining oxygenation and avoiding raised intracranial pressure. Intracranial pressure may be reduced by surgical procedures to evacuate intracranial haematomas and shunt for hydrocephalus, and medical interventions with mannitol, mechanical ventilation and forced hyperventilation; this may need monitoring with intracranial pressure monitors. Cytotoxic oedema is maximal about 3–4 days after the injury. This specific treatment needs to be combined with general medical care as for any unconscious patient.

Once the patient is stable and improving there are many aspects that will require rehabilitation. This will involve physiotherapy and occupational therapy, and may require speech therapy. There are frequently psychological and behavioural difficulties with personality change, frontal disinhibition and memory loss. These latter problems make the rehabilitation of patients following severe head injuries somewhat different from patients with other brain injuries such as stroke and are often most effectively managed at a specialist unit.

Other complications

In addition to the consequences of brain damage there are other complications.

Post-traumatic syndromes

Even after a mild head injury, patients can become anxious, have difficulty concentrating and sleep poorly. This may be associated with particular recollections of the accident and a change in behaviour, e.g. avoiding driving. This is a post-traumatic stress disorder. There is uncertainty about whether this is affected by compensation claims relating to any accident. Patients may develop a migraine-like headache following head injury, which usually spontaneously improves over 2 years.

Anosmia (loss of sense of smell) can occur as a result of damage to the fibres passing through the cribriform plate. This is permanent. Patients may still appreciate tastes and chemical irritation such as ammonia.

Post-traumatic vertigo can occur and is most commonly benign positional vertigo (p. 46).

The frequency of post-traumatic epilepsy depends on the severity and type of the head injury. Severe head injuries with intracranial haematomas or post-traumatic amnesia (PTA) over 24 hours have a 12% risk of epilepsy in 5 years. More moderate injury with skull fracture or PTA over 30 min has a 1.6% risk at 5 years. Milder head injuries have the same rate as the background population of 0.5%.

Prognosis

The outcome of head injury depends on the severity of the injury and age of the patient, with younger patients doing better. Most head injuries are mild or moderate and there is a good recovery: if PTA is less than 1 hour, 90% of patients are back at work in 2 months; if PTA is longer than 24 hours then 80% of patients return to work in 6 months. Patients with more severe head injuries are often left with some disability. They do, however, continue to improve for longer, over 2 years, than patients with other brain injuries such as stroke.

> ### Head injury
>
> - Head injury is a common cause of death and neurological disability.
>
> - Brain injury results from a combination of direct trauma, haemorrhage, hypoxia and raised intracranial pressure.
>
> - Acute management of head injuries aims to control the secondary mechanisms of brain injury: haemorrhage, hypoxia and raised intracranial pressure.

Spinal cord syndromes

Spinal cord disease and injury account for major long-term morbidity. The most common causes in young people are spinal cord trauma, which has a prevalence of 50 per 100 000, and multiple sclerosis affecting the spinal cord (60 per 100 000). The spinal cord terminates at the lower border of L1; most lumbar spine diseases cause radiculopathy and not spinal cord syndromes (p. 82).

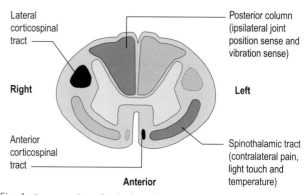

Fig. 1 **Cross-section of spinal cord.** Note the sensory input (red) from, and motor output (black) to, the right side.

Clinical presentation

The clinical presentation of spinal cord disease depends on:

- the level of the lesion
- the parts of the spinal cord affected
- the pathological process.

The level of the lesion

A spinal lesion can only affect function below the level of the lesion. In assessing a patient there will be a motor level (the highest myotome affected), a reflex level (the reflex with the highest segmental supply affected) and a sensory level. The lesion must be at or above the highest level. Pain at the level of the lesion may radiate along a nerve root level – myeloradiculopathy (p. 82) – and the spine may be tender at this level. Structural spine abnormalities, e.g. tumour, cause pain exacerbated by coughing, straining or sneezing. At the level of the lesion, reflexes may be lost from associated root or anterior horn cell involvement.

The parts of the spinal cord affected

The clinical picture will vary depending on which spinal tracts are affected. There are four main tracts involved (Fig. 1):

- *Corticospinal tract*. Symptoms: weakness and unsteadiness and stiffness in walking, sometimes with spontaneous spasms of the legs. Signs: increased tone and reflexes, and extensor plantar responses.
- *Dorsal column (sensory)*. Symptoms: ataxia and clumsiness in the hands. Signs: loss of joint position and vibration senses.
- *Spinothalamic tract (sensory)*. Symptoms: lost or altered cutaneous sensation or pain. Painless injuries and secondary deformity may occur, leading to neuropathic or 'Charcot joints'. Signs: loss of pain and temperature sensation, injuries, burns and deformity.
- *Lateral columns (sphincter disturbance)*. Altered sphincter function implies abnormalities of its supply bilaterally in the lateral columns, often indicating extensive, spinal disease, requiring urgent investigation.

Patterns of spinal cord lesion

There are five main patterns of spinal cord lesion:

- Total spinal transection causes loss of all function below the level of the lesion (paraplegia or tetraplegia), with urinary retention and constipation. NB. In acute cases, 'spinal shock' may cause flaccidity and areflexia.
- Hemicord 'Brown–Séquard' syndrome causes ipsilateral spasticity and posterior column sensory loss, and contralateral spinothalamic loss (which may be asymptomatic).
- Central cord lesions cause early sphincter disturbance and spinothalamic loss, which may be bilateral. Loss of pain and temperature sensation may appear suspended (p. 60). Wasting, weakness and areflexia occur in the affected segments as a result of anterior horn cell loss, with spasticity below this.
- Dorsal column loss. Symptom: ataxia. Signs: loss of proprioception and vibration sense.
- Anterior cord syndrome. There is striking preservation of dorsal column sensation with loss of all other functions.

Pathological processes

Trauma

This is a common cause of spinal cord disease, especially in young men. Stabilizing the spine is important and the patient should be moved carefully. Other parts may also be injured, e.g. brain, chest, abdomen or limbs.

Neoplasms

These are usually extrinsic malignant metastases to the vertebrae and cause neurological compromise by expansion into the vertebral canal or by vertebral collapse (Fig. 2a). Common primary malignancies are bronchus, breast, myeloma, lymphoma and prostate. Primary extrinsic tumours are usually benign neurofibromas or meningiomas (Fig. 2b). Malignant lesions are painful and present acutely or subacutely. Benign lesions are usually painless and may develop very slowly.

Intrinsic (intramedullary) tumours are rare and are usually astrocytomas or ependymomas. They usually present gradually, sometimes over many years, and are often painless.

Inflammatory spinal cord disease

This is most commonly due to multiple sclerosis (p. 84) but may represent an isolated episode, sometimes after infection. Other causes include sarcoidosis or collagen vascular diseases, e.g. Sjögren's syndrome or systemic lupus erythematosus. They typically cause a neurological deficit evolving over a few days, but some slower syndromes occur.

Infection

This is a rare but important cause of acute, subacute or chronic syndromes. Paraspinal or epidural abscesses are painful and may present acutely (pyogenic) or more insidiously (tuberculous) with associated systemic symptoms (fever, sweats and weight loss). Brucellosis is an important cause of a subacute syndrome in parts of the world where unpasteurized milk is consumed. Myelopathy can develop chronically in infection with syphilis or HIV (p. 100). It is also seen in patients from the tropics with human T-cell lymphotropic virus I (HTLV-I) infection: 'tropical spastic paraparesis'.

Vascular

Infarction produces a sudden onset of symptoms that are usually painless.

Anterior spinal cord syndrome with a level at T8–T11 is the most common (relating to the artery of Adamkiewicz), but other patterns of spinal disturbance can occur. Vascular malformations of the spinal cord, e.g. dural arteriovenous fistulae, may produce a progressive deficit resembling a tumour. A characteristic feature is exacerbation of symptoms by exercise, which causes 'claudication' of the cord.

Degenerative cervical disc disease
This is the most common cause of spinal cord compression, especially in the neck (Fig. 3); its frequency increases with age. Cord compression can be due to:

- degeneration of interverterbral discs with extrusion of disc material into the spinal canal – acute disc
- formation of osteophytes, which impinge upon the spinal canal
- forward or backwards slip of vertebrae, introducing kinks into the vertebral canal and thickening
- calcification and protrusion of the ligamentum flavum and dentate ligaments.

Pain is variable and the rate of progression may be acute or chronic. There is often associated root disease (p. 82).

Vitamin B12 and folate deficiencies
These present with a subacute myelopathy, especially affecting the dorsal columns. There may be a megaloblastic anaemia and other neurological changes such as mental slowing, cerebellar ataxia and peripheral neuropathy.

Genetic
A myelopathy is a component in a large number of rare inherited diseases, especially the 'spinocerebellar degenerations' such as Friedreich's ataxia. This is an autosomal recessive condition due to a defect in frataxin. Ataxia begins between 8 and 15 years, with loss of reflexes (axonal neuropathy), optic atrophy and later cardiomyopathy; the patients are chairbound by their 40s. There is a slightly increased risk of diabetes. In familial spastic paraparesis, patients usually have severe spasticity of the legs with relative preservation of power and compensatory hypertrophy of the upper limb muscles.

Syringomyelia
This is a rare but classical disease. There is progressive expansion of a fluid cavity in the spinal cord, probably due to altered CSF dynamics. The cause may be a congenital abnormality such as a Chiari malformation (elongated cerebellar tonsils protrude through the foramen magnum, compressing the medulla at the craniocervical junction) or a tumour or trauma. The presentation is with a central cervical cord lesion (see above), which usually progresses slowly. The cavity may spread up to the medulla to give lower cranial nerve signs: 'syringobulbia'.

Investigations
Neuroimaging (usually MRI) should be undertaken as an emergency in progressive myelopathies, primarily to exclude a surgically treatable cause. The spine at the clinical level should be imaged. More indolent presentations, e.g. a patient with numb hands and stiff legs, evolving over a year, need less urgent investigation.

Occasionally bihemispheric disease can mimic spinal cord disease (classically a parasagittal meningioma), so a brain scan may be needed.

Other investigations depend on the clinical situation.

Treatment

Emergency treatment
In acute presentations, until spinal instability can be excluded, the patient should be moved with extreme caution, avoiding excessive flexion or extension of the neck, ideally with a hard collar. If an infective cause can be excluded, high doses of corticosteroids may protect the spinal cord from injury and temporarily reverse some of the deficit, especially in malignant compression. Spinal cord compression needs immediate neurosurgical referral and decompression.

Specific treatment
Specific treatment depends on the cause. Surgery is used in cases of extrinsic compression by a disc, spondylosis or benign tumour and selected cases of malignant tumour. Cervical spondylosis may be treated by posterior laminectomy, excision of disc material or anterior cervical decompression and fusion with grafts usually taken from the iliac crest. Osteophytes and ligamentous thickening may also require excision. There is uncertainty about the management of cervical spondylosis, who to treat surgically and when to manage conservatively.

Radiotherapy and chemotherapy are used for the treatment of malignant tumours. High-dose corticosteroids are used for non-infective inflammatory causes. Surgical decompression at the foramen magnum may help syringomyelia, if there is an associated Chiari malformation. Long-term rehabilitation is discussed on page 120.

Prognosis
The prognosis of myelopathy depends on the cause and the severity and duration of the deficit. The aim of treatment is to preserve function. Therapy, especially surgical treatment, often does not reverse existing deficits and this needs to be taken into account in deciding on the timing of treatment and in counselling the patient.

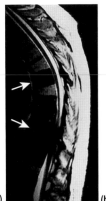
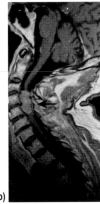

(a)　　　(b)

Fig. 2 **Spinal cord compression. (a)** Multiple vertebral metastases (arrows) causing spinal cord compression; **(b)** cervical spinal cord compression caused by a large meningioma (arrow).

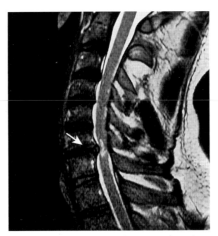

Fig. 3 **A T2-weighted sagittal MRI scan of the cervical spine showing a C6/7 disc compressing the spinal cord.** There is associated signal change within the cord.

> ### Spinal cord syndromes
> - Progressive spinal cord disease is a medical emergency.
> - Spinal cord syndromes are predictable from the anatomy of the spinal cord.
> - The lesion must be at or above the level of the highest neurological sign.
> - Common causes are trauma, spondylosis, multiple sclerosis and tumours.

Radiculopathy

Disease affecting the nerve roots is common. The most common sites of involvement are the lumbar spine (annual incidence of severe cases of 150 per 100 000) and cervical spine (annual incidence of 20 per 100 000).

Aetiology

The most common cause is compression by displaced intervertebral discs or degenerative spine disease. Disc protrusions are most common at C5, C6 in the neck, L5 and S1 in the lower back, although it occurs at other levels. There are several causes:

Acute disc

This occurs in young individuals in the absence of other major degenerative spine disease. In acute presentations there is often a history of recent injury or straining, e.g. lifting. This results from herniation of the nucleus pulposis through a rupture in the annulus fibrosis, a so-called 'soft disc' (Fig. 1).

Spondylosis

In older adults spondylotic disease may present with radiculopathy, usually at similar levels, but somewhat more frequently can affect other cervical and lumbar levels. The discs initially dehydrate, thus losing height and the disc annulus prolapses. This leads to osteophytic outgrowths on the vertebral bodies and instability of the apophyseal joints, which then hypertrophy. The osteophytes and hypertrophied facet joints may then compress the nerve roots, producing a radiculopathy, or the spinal cord, producing a myelopathy.

Other rarer causes

Tumours may cause radiculopathy at any level and may be primary nervous system tumours arising on the nerve root (e.g. neurofibroma or meningioma) or spinal bony metastases compressing the nerve root (Figs 2 and 3). Common sources of secondaries are tumours of breast, bronchus, prostate, kidney, thyroid and lymphoma. An apical lung tumour (Pancoast tumour) causes wasting of small muscles of the hand (T1) and a Horner's syndrome.

Inflammatory conditions may cause radiculopathy; the most common is shingles (Herpes varicella zoster virus) infection (p. 100). Rarely, radiculopathy can be due to inflammatory or malignant meningitis.

Symptoms and signs

Radiculopathy presents with pain, weakness, reflex changes and sensory loss; the pattern of loss for the most commonly affected roots is given in Figure 4.

- *Pain* radiates from the spine in the distribution of the affected nerve root. In disc prolapse the onset is often acute and may be related to physical exertion. With mechanical causes, the pain is made worse by manoeuvres that increase intraspinal pressure: coughing, sneezing or straining. Moving the limb to stretch the nerve root exacerbates the pain (Fig. 5). Spinal tenderness and restriction of movement are common but are non-specific as they occur in mechanical back pain without radiculopathy.
- *Weakness and reflex changes.* There may be loss of function in the distribution of the nerve root. This manifests as weakness of muscles innervated by that root and alteration or loss of sensation in a dermatomal distribution. There may be wasting or fasciculation of the muscles innervated by that root with loss of reflexes.
- *Sensory loss* in the distribution of the affected nerve root.

In addition, *upper motor neurone signs* or sensory signs below the level of the radiculopathy in the cervical spine imply compression of the spinal cord as well as the nerve roots: 'myeloradiculopathy' (p. 80).

Polyradiculopathy

Involvement of more than one nerve root cannot be caused by mechanical disease such as a disc protrusion at only one level, except where multiple roots travel together in the cauda equina (central disc prolapse, see below). Polyradiculopathy implies an inflammatory process, such as Guillain–Barré syndrome (p. 104), inflammatory meningitis, e.g. sarcoidosis, or a neoplastic process within the spinal fluid, a malignant meningitis, infiltrating the nerve roots with lesions at multiple levels.

Investigation and management

This is directed by the clinical presentation and the likely diagnosis. Polyradiculopathy is discussed on page 104.

The investigation of choice for a single-level radiculopathy is an MRI scan of the relevant spinal level. Electromyography

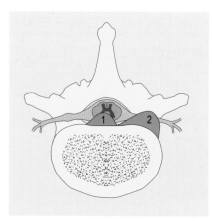

Fig. 1 **Acute herniation – the 'soft disc'.** This leads to (1) cord compression or (2) radicular compression.

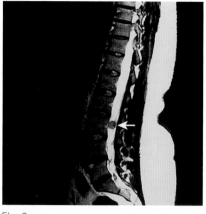

Fig. 2 **MRI showing a neurofibroma in the lumbosacral canal (arrow).**

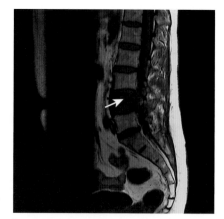

Fig. 3 **An MRI of the lumbosacral spine showing a vertebral secondary leading to collapse of vertebral body and compression of the cauda equina.**

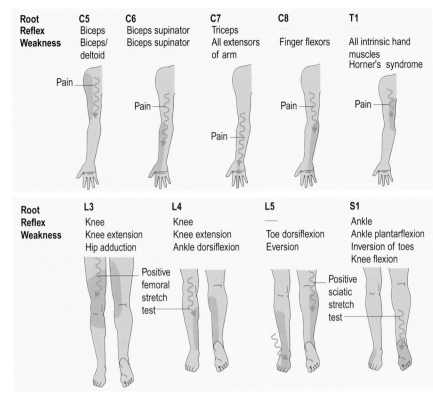

Root	C5	C6	C7	C8	T1
Reflex	Biceps	Biceps supinator	Triceps	Finger flexors	
Weakness	Biceps/deltoid	Biceps supinator	All extensors of arm		All intrinsic hand muscles Horner's syndrome

Root	L3	L4	L5	S1
Reflex	Knee	Knee	—	Ankle
Weakness	Knee extension Hip adduction	Knee extension Ankle dorsiflexion	Toe dorsiflexion Eversion	Ankle plantarflexion Inversion of toes Knee flexion

Fig. 4 **Pattern of loss for the most commonly affected nerve roots.** The right arm and back and front of the right leg are shown.

may help to show a radicular pattern of denervation and nerve conduction excludes a neuropathy but is unhelpful in identifying the cause of the radiculopathy.

CSF examination may be indicated in multiple radiculopathy or in cases with clinical evidence of systemic illness.

Treatment of radiculopathy depends on the cause and severity. Optimum treatment of the most common causes, lumbar and cervical disc prolapse, has not been established by randomized trials and remains an area of uncertainty. The following is common practice.

Lumbar disc disease

In initial presentations with pain and no neurological deficit, initial treatment is with a minimum period of rest, then mobilization and subsequent education to avoid back strain/injury. If the radicular pain (the pain in the leg, not the back) continues, surgical treatment may be considered. Where there is neurological deficit associated with acute disc protrusion, especially if severe or progressive, then surgery is considered at an earlier stage. The most common operations are removal of a protruding disc using a dissecting microscope: 'a microdiscectomy'; older procedures include resection of the vertebral lamina to decompress the root: laminectomy.

Cervical disc protrusions

Most of cervical radiculopathies are due to disc protrusions or spondylotic changes. Both tend to improve spontaneously or with conservative therapy, e.g. with physiotherapy, a soft collar or traction. Where pain persists or there is marked radicular weakness, surgery can be helpful. The approaches vary from single-level discectomy to anterior approaches with removal of the disc and bone grafting.

Other causes

Benign compressive tumours are treated by surgical decompression. Malignant lesions may respond to radiotherapy, chemotherapy or surgery.

Special situations

Lumbar central disc prolapse

This is an emergency akin to spinal cord compression. If a lumbar disc prolapses into the centre of the spinal canal ('central disc prolapse'), all the roots of the cauda equina may be affected at and below the level of the prolapse. The level is usually the same as unilateral prolapse – L5 or S1. It causes severe back pain radiating into both legs, usually in sciatic distribution, bilateral foot drop, weakness of flexors of both hips and knees and sphincter disturbance. Ankle jerks are lost and there is distal sensory loss in the feet with sacral anaesthesia and loss of the sacral reflex. Management is with urgent surgical decompression.

Lumbar canal stenosis

More chronic involvement of multiple roots is seen in lumbar canal stenosis in older patients. In these patients the complaint is of increasing leg weakness on walking, also referred to as neurogenic claudication. The patient often becomes stooped and paradoxically may find it easier to go up hill than on the flat. There are usually no neurological signs. Surgical decompression is usually helpful.

Spina bifida

This congenital neural tube defect may result in a paraparesis. Management is primarily supportive and helping to prevent complications resulting from the paraparesis, such as pressure sores and urinary infections. The frequency of this is decreasing.

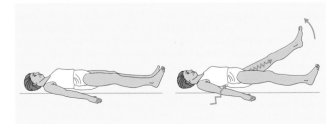

Fig. 5 **Sciatic stretch (straight leg raising).** With the patient supine, the examiner gently raises the leg straight up off the couch, causing back pain to radiate in the leg in a sciatic distribution, implying an L5 or S1 lesion.

Radiculopathy

- Radiculopathy presents with pain radiating into the distribution of the sensory nerve, lower motor neurone signs in the myotome or dermatomal sensory loss.

- The most common sites are at L5/S1 and C5/C6.

- Common causes are prolapsed intervertebral discs and spondylotic disease.

- Treatment depends on the cause and severity.

Multiple sclerosis I

Multiple sclerosis (MS, disseminated sclerosis) is a common disorder affecting about 1 in 1000 individuals in the UK. It is a major cause of disability in young adults. The diagnosis of MS requires two separate episodes of central nervous system demyelination separated in *space* and *time*.

Pathology

The pathological hallmark of MS is the plaque. This is an area of demyelination, with loss of myelin and relative preservation of axons (Fig. 1). Active lesions may have an associated inflammatory response and oedema. In more chronic lesions the oedema and inflammation have resolved and there is a demarcated area of gliotic scarring.

Plaques can be found in any part of the white matter of the brain and spinal cord. There is a predilection for the periventricular white matter, the corpus callosum and optic nerves.

Pathophysiology

The area of demyelination disrupts the conduction of a nerve impulse (Fig. 2). This initially blocks conduction, but with recovery conduction is slowed and the refractory period is prolonged. Conduction along such segments is particularly sensitive to temperature changes and may fail if the temperature rises (which leads to Uhtoff's phenomenon, see below).

Pathogenesis

The aetiology of MS is unknown. There is a minor genetic component (the relative risk of a first-degree relative developing MS is two to four times that of the general population) and there is a tendency for an association with HLA antigens DR2 and DW2.

There is some geographical and racial variation in disease prevalence: lower rates are found in tropical countries and migrants from low-prevalence areas remain at low risk if they move over the age of 15 years; if younger, they take on the risk of their new home. The significance of these observations is not clear.

Investigation of an immunological basis for MS or an underlying viral infection have so far proved fruitless.

Clinical features

The peak age of onset of MS is 25–35 years. It is rare below 15 years and over 60 years. It is more frequent in women than men (about 1.5:1). There are essentially two patterns of disease (Fig. 3):

- *Relapsing remitting* form, with clear relapses followed by recovery. The frequency of relapses and duration of remission vary considerably. This may go on to produce a *secondary progressive* form, where there is a progressive increase in disability.
- *Primary progressive* form that deteriorates from onset. This accounts for about 10% of patients.

Symptoms and signs

Sensory

Sensory symptoms are the most common presentation, occurring as the first symptom in up to 40% of patients. The feelings are described as numbness, coldness, pins and needles, swelling or tightness. They may be radicular, especially in the limbs and over the lower trunk. The onset is usually over a few days with resolution in weeks to months.

Signs may be absent or relatively subtle, usually affecting vibration sense and proprioception more than superficial modalities. Sometimes signs can be more prominent than the symptoms with a sensory level or occasionally a marked loss of proprioception in a hand (so-called deafferented hand).

Visual

Optic neuritis is a common initial manifestation of MS. A visual disturbance evolves over a few days with distortion of the central vision and impairment of colour perception. There may be pain on eye movement. Visual loss can be mild to severe. Patients have a relative afferent pupillary defect and a central scotoma. The optic disc usually appears normal (retrobulbar optic neuritis) though may be swollen with papillitis. Vision improves over months, though may be incomplete, particularly if visual loss was severe initially. Optic atrophy may develop following an episode of optic neuritis (Fig. 4).

Uhtoff's phenomenon is the decrease in visual acuity following a rise in temperature, due to exercise, a hot bath or a fever.

Motor

Weakness usually affects the legs. It can be an early symptom. Later in the disease it produces a paraplegia, which may have marked spasticity, increased reflexes and extensor plantars. Weakness of the arms is less frequently a problem. An evolving paraparesis is the usual pattern of primary progressive MS.

Spinal cord

Motor and sensory problems can be clearly localized to a single lesion in the spinal cord: myelitis. In MS this is usually incomplete, for example

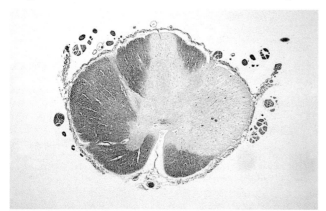

Fig. 1 **Myelin stain showing plaques.**

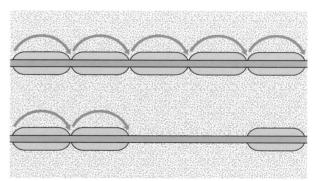

Fig. 2 **Effects of demyelination on an axon:** saltatory conduction is blocked.

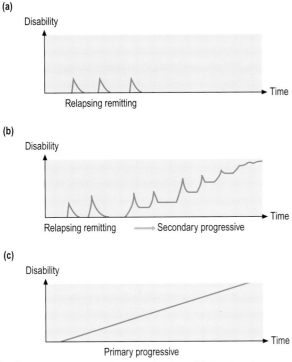

(a) Disability — Time
Relapsing remitting

(b) Disability — Time
Relapsing remitting ⟶ Secondary progressive

(c) Disability — Time
Primary progressive

Fig. 3 **Various patterns of progression in multiple sclerosis over time. (a)** Relapsing remitting; **(b)** relapsing remitting to secondary progressive; **(c)** primary progressive.

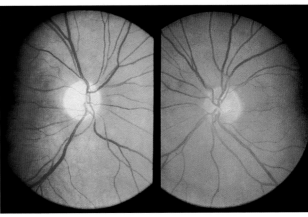

Fig. 4 **Optic atrophy.** Note pale discs.

Table 1 **Simplified Kurtzke expanded disability status scale**

0	Normal
1	Signs but no disability
2	Minimal disability*
3	Moderate disability* but able to walk
4	Relatively severe disability, but able to walk up to 500 m; up 12 h a day
5	Walking limited to 200 m; not able to do a full day's work without special help
6	Uses walking aid; limited to 100 m
7	Wheelchair bound; able to transfer in and out of chair
8	Bedbound, some arm function
9	Helpless and bedbound
10	Dead

* In other functions: motor, cerebellar, brain stem, sensory, bowel and bladder, visual

producing a hemicord lesion (called a Brown–Séquard syndrome), though it can be complete – transverse myelitis. Some patients have a progressive spinal cord involvement.

Brain stem and cerebellum
Double vision is a common early symptom. This can be associated with a range of eye movement abnormalities (6th, 3rd or occasionally 4th nerve palsies), skew deviation and lateral gaze palsies and, most characteristic, an internuclear ophthalmoplegia (INO) (p. 19).

Dizziness, usually with other brain stem symptoms (diplopia, facial numbness or dysarthria), may occur.

Nystagmus is a common finding. Ataxic nystagmus is found with an INO.

Gait and truncal ataxia are commonly found later in the disease. There may be marked limb incoordination with associated cerebellar tremor.

Higher function and mood
Minor cognitive deficits are found in patients with MS. Dementia is uncommon. Some of the cognitive deficit may reflect depression and anxiety related to the difficulties caused by this chronic disease.

Classical descriptions often refer to the euphoria seen in the disease. This can occur but is rare and is eclipsed by the large number of patients with depression.

Sphincter and sexual function
The development of urgency and frequency of micturition, and to a lesser extent defecation, usually parallels the motor weakness in the legs. The urinary symptoms reflect a small unstable upper motor neurone type bladder. Urinary symptoms can arise with detrusor sphincter dyssynergia – a loss of coordination of detrusor contraction and sphincter relaxation leading to retention and a bladder that empties incompletely. This can result in repeated infections and overflow incontinence.

Impotence is a common problem in men.

Others
Lhermitte's phenomenon is an electric shock feeling going down the back and into the arms and legs after bending the neck. It occurs in MS and to a lesser extent in patients with other cervical cord disease.

Epilepsy is slightly more common (3%) than in the general population.

Fatigue is often a very prominent syndrome in MS. This is often very debilitating and can occur in patients with otherwise relatively mild disease.

Precipitating factors
Relapses occur more commonly after infections. There is a slight increase after trauma, though evidence is less clear-cut. There is a relative reduction during pregnancy with a slight increase afterward – over the whole period the rate is stable.

Measuring disability
MS is a very variable disease. To try to assess treatment it is imperative to have a reliable and valid measure of disability. This is straightforward for single components of disability, e.g. acuity and field, in assessing visual recovery after optic neuritis. A scale to cover the multiple possible disabilities found in MS will inevitably be less reliable: the most frequently used scale is the Kurtzke disability status scale (Table 1). This uses mobility as the major determinant. The scale is not linear (a one-point change means different things at different points on the scale) and has limited reliability. It is, however, the scale used in all recent major trials.

> ### Multiple sclerosis I
>
> - MS is common, with a peak onset at 25–35 years of age.
> - MS is a disease of the CNS with multiple episodes of demyelination occurring at different times in different parts of the CNS.
> - The optic nerves, brain stem and spinal cord are the most commonly affected sites.

Multiple sclerosis II

Differential diagnosis

The diagnosis of MS depends on identification of multiple episodes of demyelination separated in space and time. The occurrence of a single episode does not lead to a diagnosis of MS. The differential diagnosis for the most characteristic episodes will be considered individually. The differential diagnosis of multiple episodes will then be considered.

Single episodes

Optic neuritis. The most important differential is with optic nerve compression. This is usually more insidious in onset and is progressive. This can be ruled out by MRI scan. Between 25 and 60% of patients first presenting with optic neuritis go on to develop MS.

Spinal cord syndromes. The most important differential diagnosis is spinal cord compression (Fig. 1a). In more insidious spinal cord syndromes the differential diagnosis includes rarer spinal cord disease such as vitamin B12 deficiency, HTLV-1 myelopathy and familial spastic paraparesis. In patients lacking sensory signs, consider amyotrophic lateral sclerosis; associated lower motor neurone signs allow a distinction. After first presentation with complete transverse myelitis, patients later develop MS; those with partial spinal cord syndromes more often progress (70%).

Brain stem syndromes. The differential diagnosis is wide, including tumours, brain stem encephalitis, cranial polyneuritis, an Arnold–Chiari malformation or vascular disease, the last being the most common alternative in older patients. MRI may clarify this differential; CSF examination and other investigations may be needed.

Multifocal CNS disease. The relapsing remitting form of MS can be mimicked by other inflammatory diseases such as systemic lupus erythematosus, sarcoid, Behçet's disease and polyarteritis nodosa, and infectious diseases such as Lyme disease and syphilis. These are all rare. A monophasic illness characterized by widespread multifocal demyelination can occur either in isolation (acute disseminated encephalomyelitis) or after an infection (post-infectious encephalomyelitis). In these conditions there are multiple areas of

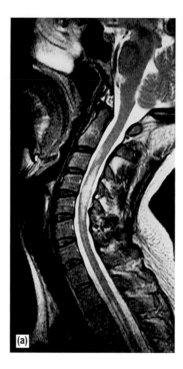

(a)

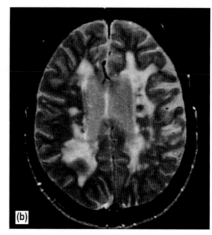

(b)

Fig. 1 **MRI in multiple sclerosis. (a)** A T2-weighted scan of the cervical spine showing intrinsic high-signal changes; **(b)** a proton-weighted axial scale scan showing periventricular high-signal changes.

demyelination separated in space *but not in time.*

Investigations

The investigation of a patient with suspected MS can be divided into:

- excluding other causes for the clinical syndrome
- finding abnormalities characteristic of MS.

Excluding other causes

Some of the most common presentations and their investigations are discussed above. The investigation of any first presentation is more intensive than the investigation of a relapse. However, even patients with an established diagnosis of MS can develop unrelated neurological complications.

Finding characteristic abnormalities

Demonstrating clinically silent lesions. MRI is particularly powerful at detecting clinically silent lesions in MS. These tend to occur in characteristic sites within the white matter: the periventricular region and corpus callosum (Fig. 1). Similar changes can be seen in the spinal cord, though these are more commonly found when symptomatic. If a scan is enhanced with gadolinium then active lesions can be seen; the enhancement persists for 6–8 weeks.

Abnormalities on the MRI scan of the brain are found in over 90% of patients with clinically definite MS. There is a loose correlation between the changes on MRI and disability; however, patients with severe disability can have almost normal MRI scans while patients who are clinically normal have marked abnormalities on MRI.

Not all patients with MRI abnormalities of this type have MS. Over 50 years, T2-weighted abnormalities are seen in a normal population. Similar lesions occur in cerebral ischaemia, sarcoidosis, Behçet's syndrome and other vasculitic illnesses. In patients who present with a single episode of demyelination, the finding of MRI abnormalities substantially increases the risk of developing MS.

Neurophysiological tests can also be used to show that there has been unrecognized demyelination. This is usually done in the visual pathways using visual evoked responses (VER), which will be delayed if there has been demyelination, or in the sensory pathways with somatosensory evoked responses. They are not diagnostic of MS and will be abnormal in the symptomatic eye if the optic nerve is being compressed. VERs are abnormal in about 80% of cases of clinically definite MS.

Finding characteristic changes. Examining the CSF for oligoclonal bands can be helpful in the diagnosis of MS. Routine analysis of the CSF usually produces a normal result: the white cell count may be slightly elevated (< 15 cells/ml). Protein electrophoresis, using isoelectric focusing, may find oligoclonal bands in the CSF but not in serum. This indicates intrathecal immunoglobulin synthesis. This is present in 95% of patients with clinically definite MS. It occurs in other diseases, infections (e.g. neurosyphilis, Lyme disease) and in inflammatory diseases (e.g. Behçet's syndrome and systemic lupus erythematosus).

Complications
The complications of MS have much in common with other disabling neurological conditions. Common medical problems seen in MS are summarized in Table 1. The social impact of the disease can include loss of job, divorce or social isolation. Depression is common and suicide can occur.

Prognosis
The prognosis is variable and any comments about long-term prognosis are complicated by the improved diagnostic methods that allow milder disease to be recognized. On the basis of currently available studies, life expectancy is reduced by between 5 and 10 years. Half the patients have moved into the progressive phase of the disease by 10 years and half require aids to walk by 17 years. About 15% have a very benign form of the disease with only a few relapses and minor, if any, disability. Where disease is mild after 5 years, severe disease develops infrequently. Several factors influence prognosis. Relapsing remitting disease has a better prognosis than primary progressive. Men tend to do worse than women. Sensory symptoms or optic neuritis at onset tend to indicate a better prognosis.

Management and treatment

Management
It is important for the patient to understand the nature of their condition. The popular conception of MS is that of a severely disabled patient in a wheelchair.

While this may occur, it is important that a newly diagnosed patient and their family appreciate that many patients can follow a more benign course. They need to be helped sympathetically to come to terms with the condition, particularly with the uncertainty of the future. The range of problems that may accompany the problem means that a range of help is required from the family doctor, physiotherapists and occupational therapists, making it important for there to be a team approach supporting the patients and carers.

Treatment
There is as yet no cure for MS. Treatment is aimed at alleviating symptoms. Some newer therapies may prove useful in reducing the frequency of relapses and slow progression of disability.

Symptomatic treatment
Steroids accelerate the recovery following a relapse. They are usually given intravenously (as methylprednisolone) over 3 days. Steroids can be used in patients with progressive MS but the response is usually more disappointing than in relapsing remitting disease.

Specific symptoms can be helped. The most common problems are summarized in Table 1. Pain may occur and usually responds to pain-modulating drugs such as amitriptyline or carbamazepine. Carbamazepine may also help some paroxysmal symptoms such as Lhermitte's or trigeminal neuralgia. Tremor is usually difficult to treat, occasionally stereotactic thalamotomy may be helpful. Depression is common and needs to be treated with appropriate support and antidepressants. Physiotherapy is helpful at optimizing the level of function of the patient and occupational therapy optimizes the patient's environment to minimize the impact of disabilities. Speech therapy may be helpful in some patients.

Disease-altering treatments
The variability of MS in terms of prognosis and its diverse clinical manifestations make it difficult to conduct therapeutic trials. Some immune-modulating drugs such as cyclophosphamide and azathioprine have been shown to have minor beneficial effects.

More recently, studies of beta-interferons and copolymer-1 (COP1) have found encouraging results. Two preparations of beta-interferon (1a and 1b) and COP1 have been studied in ambulant patients with relapsing remitting disease with two relapses in the past 2 years. All three studies have demonstrated a similar reduction in the frequency of relapses from about three to two in the 3-year follow-up; COP1 and beta-interferon 1a have demonstrated a small effect on disability. The studies of beta-interferon used MRI changes as a surrogate marker of disease activity and found this to be reduced. The introduction of these drugs was controversial, partly because of cost (about £8000 per patient per year).

Beta-interferon is given either subcutaneously or intramuscularly; side-effects include local irritation at the site of injection and flu-like symptoms. Some patients develop antibodies to beta-interferon though the significance of this is not clear. Longer-term follow-up data are limited. One study found slowing of progression in secondary progressive forms of the disease.

Other demyelinating diseases
Devic's disease. This consists of bilateral optic neuritis and myelitis. It occurs in children and is usually monophasic.

Cerebellitis. This acute ataxic syndrome follows viral infections, particularly chickenpox in children. It is benign and self-limiting.

Table 1 **Treatment of complications**

Problem	Treatments	Comment
Spasticity	Baclofen, dantrolene, tizanidine Physiotherapy	Reducing the tone with drugs must be balanced against the increased weakness
Fatigue	Amantadine, pemoline, modafinil	NB. Fatigue may be a symptom of depression
Ataxia	Isoniazid (with pyridoxine)	Usually there is little response
Bladder problems		
Unstable bladder	Oxybutynin	Consider urinary infection and treat
Uncoordinated bladder	Intermittent self-catheterization ± oxybutynin	
Erectile faliure	Intracorporeal injections of papaverine or alprostadil; sildenafil	
Constipation	Bulking agents and stool softeners May need manual evacuation	

Multiple sclerosis II
■ The investigations in MS aim to exclude alternative diagnoses and find changes consistent with MS.
■ MRI characteristically finds periventricular and corpus callosum white matter changes on T2-weighted images.
■ Symptomatic treatment can help spasticity, urinary frequency and complications such as depression.
■ Newer drugs have demonstrated some alteration in the course of the disease in relapsing remitting MS.

Parkinson's disease and other akinetic rigid syndromes I

In 1817 James Parkinson wrote 'Essay on the shaking palsy'. The clinical syndrome he described, with tremor, rigidity and slowness of movement, is referred to as Parkinsonism or an akinetic rigid syndrome. The most frequent pathological cause of this syndrome is Parkinson's disease.

Parkinson's disease is common, affecting 1 per 1000 of the population. The disease is quite rare below the age of 50 years, and increases in frequency with age, affecting 1.5% of patients aged between 70 and 79 years and 3.5% of patients over 80 years.

Clinical features

The classical features of Parkinson's disease are TRAP:

- **T**remor
- **R**igidity
- **A**kinesia or bradykinesia (a- = lack of, brady- = slow, kinesia = movement)
- **P**ostural instability.

Early symptoms are often subtle. The patient may describe stiffness, difficulty in fine movements, especially writing, fatigue and a feeling of slowing down. Some patients will first notice a tremor. The onset is usually unilateral or may be limited to one limb.

The tremor, occurring in 70% of untreated patients, typically occurs at rest but may occur on sustained posture and mainly affects the hands. It is coarse and slow. The rigidity is usually best appreciated at the elbow and wrist. The increase in tone is not sustained and repeatedly gives, producing the characteristic cogwheeling.

The face is immobile and the skin may appear greasy (Fig. 1). There may be a dysarthria, with a monotonous voice that tends to trail off. Fast repeated movements tend to slow up, so called bradykinesia. This can be tested by asking the patient to drum their fingers on a table or repeatedly bringing index finger and thumb together. Writing becomes small and spidery (Fig. 2). The posture tends to becomes stooped and the patient stands with slightly flexed elbows (Fig. 3). On walking there is a loss of arm swing, the steps become shorter and there may be difficulty starting or stopping. The patient may be unsteady or fall on turning. This reflects the loss of postural reflexes; these can be tested by standing behind the patient and gently pulling the patient backwards. This would normally lead to a minor adjustment in posture, but a patient with altered postural reflexes may take multiple steps backwards. In more severe disease there may be freezing – where the patient cannot start to walk – a form of akinesia. The gait may be festinant, where the patient cannot stop once started.

Later in the disease there may be some altered higher function, sometimes a slowness of thought (bradyphrenia); occasionally there may be a global dementia. The frequency is a matter of controversy. A significant alteration in higher function raises the possibility of alternative diagnoses (see below).

Drug treatment of Parkinson's disease produces a range of clinical responses and adverse effects. These are considered in the next section.

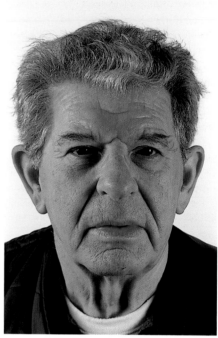

Fig. 1 **Parkinsonian facies.** Patient shows a fixed immobile expression and slightly greasy skin.

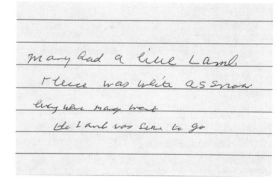

Fig. 2 **Writing of a patient with Parkinson's disease.**

Differential diagnosis

In many patients the diagnosis is straightforward. In other patients, particularly early in the disease, diagnosis can be difficult.

The differential diagnosis depends on the pattern of the presentation. Tremor is one of the most common early symptoms. The main differential diagnosis is with essential tremor (p. 92). Essential tremor is not present when the limb is relaxed and at rest and is usually most prominent on sustained posture or with movement. However, if a patient voluntarily holds the hand in a resting position, a postural tremor may look like a rest tremor. Essential tremor may produce a yes–yes head tremor or titubation, and a trombone tremor of the tongue, features not seen with Parkinson's disease.

The presentation with unilateral stiffness may be mistaken for a unilateral hemiparesis. The muscle stiffness may suggest muscular or rheumatic diagnoses. The fatigue and weight loss may be interpreted as features of malignancy or, combined with the slowness of thought and deed, as depression.

The gait patterns most commonly mistaken for Parkinson's disease are the 'marche à petit pas' of diffuse cerebrovascular disease and, less frequently, the apraxic gait of normal pressure hydrocephalus (p. 63).

A common, and usually easily identified, cause of Parkinsonism is drug-induced Parkinsonism. This is produced to varying degrees by different dopamine antagonists such as the phenothiazines and other antipsychotics.

In younger patients, Wilson's disease is a rare but important differential diagnosis (p. 92).

There are a range of syndromes that share several features with Parkinson's disease, but which have different pathological findings. These have been referred to as 'Parkinson's plus' syndromes. These are all relatively rare. However, together there are a significant number of affected patients; indeed, in a series of 100 postmortem examinations of patients considered to have Parkinson's disease, 20% were found to have other forms of Parkinsonism. The most common such syndromes are (1) multisystem atrophy, where there is autonomic failure, cerebellar signs and signs of upper motor neurone involvement, and (2) progressive supranuclear palsy (or Steele–Richardson syndrome), where there is a supranuclear palsy (an inability to look up voluntarily, while preserving upgaze on doll's head testing, p. 19), prominent loss of postural reflexes and dysarthria. Both these syndromes tend to respond poorly to treatment and have a worse prognosis than idiopathic Parkinson's disease. In initially assessing someone with suspected Parkinson's disease it is therefore worthwhile testing eye movements carefully and measuring standing and lying blood pressure. In patients with a significant loss of higher function and prominent hallucinations on low-dose therapy, diffuse Lewy body disease should be considered.

Pathology and pathogenesis

The characteristic pathological feature of Parkinson's disease is the loss of the pigmented dopaminergic cells of the zona compacta of the substantia nigra. In some of the remaining neurones there are eosinophilic cytoplasmic inclusions called Lewy bodies (Fig. 4). Similar changes are seen elsewhere in the brain stem, such as the locus ceruleus and the dorsal motor nucleus of the vagus.

The cause of Parkinson's disease is not known. There are a few clues.

In the early part of this century there was an epidemic of encephalitis lethargica (EL), thought to be a viral infection. Following recovery, patients developed Parkinsonism either directly or over 20 years later. In some modern cases of EL antibasal ganglia antibodies have been found. More recently, a designer drug – MPTP – has been found to cause Parkinsonism in humans and other primates. Pathologically, MPTP-induced Parkinsonism mimics idiopathic Parkinson's disease very closely, and even Lewy bodies are found. These observations suggest there may be an environmental factor in the aetiology of the disease.

There are suggestions that there may be genetic factors, particularly in the mitochondrial function, that make some individuals more likely to develop Parkinson's disease. There are several rare inherited forms, which usually have younger onset and sometimes subtle differences in clinical presentation, including defects of Parkin and α-synuclein.

Investigations

There are no specific diagnostic investigations for Parkinson's disease, which is a clinical diagnosis. A diagnostic test based on the response to apomorphine, a dopamine agonist, has been used with limited effectiveness.

Where diagnostic uncertainty exists, investigation is aimed at eliminating alternative diagnoses, e.g. CT or MRI scanning to look for normal-pressure hydrocephalus or small vessel disease. Some investigators have tried to use the response to certain drugs as a diagnostic test, with limited success (see next section). Positron emission tomography using radiolabelled levodopa is a research technique that may be useful. An isotope 'DAT' scan can show deficits of dopaminergic pathways and help distinguish between Parkinsonism and essential tremor but not differentiate between different causes of Parkinsonism.

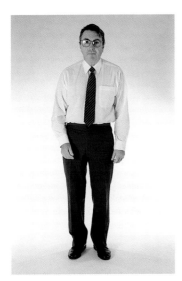

Fig. 3 **Posture in Parkinson's disease.** Note the slight stoop and the position of the right arm.

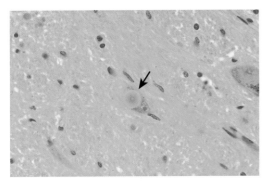

Fig. 4 **Lewy body in substantia nigra.**

> ### Parkinson's disease and other akinetic rigid syndromes I
>
> - Parkinsonism is the clinical syndrome of tremor, rigidity, bradykinesia and postural instability.
> - The most common cause of Parkinsonism is idiopathic Parkinson's disease.
> - The characteristic neuropathological feature of Parkinson's disease is a loss of pigmented dopaminergic cells from the substantia nigra.

Parkinson's disease and other akinetic rigid syndromes II

There is no cure for Parkinson's disease. The treatments available are directed at minimizing the symptoms and disabilities of the patient. Several agents have been tried to provide a neuroprotective effect and slow the deterioration of the disease, and a range of treatments such as transplantation may prove useful in the future.

The life expectancy of a patient with Parkinson's disease is only minimally reduced.

Pharmacology

In simple terms a reduction in dopamine and dopaminergic neurones underlies Parkinson's disease. This dopaminergic system is antagonized by a cholinergic system. There are several levels for possible pharmacological intervention (Fig. 1; Table 1).

Treatment

There is no standard treatment for Parkinson's disease. The therapies available are symptomatic treatments and therefore they need to be directed to the patient's symptoms. This therefore will involve a close involvement of the patient and carer in the planning of treatment.

Neuroprotection

There is no agent currently available that is proven to be neuroprotective. Some recent studies using functional imaging as a surrogate marker for disease progression suggest pramipexole and ropinirole may slow disease progression.

Symptomatic

There is much debate as to how to initiate treatment. Levodopa preparations are effective and, if they are not, an alternative diagnosis should be considered. However, it is suggested that early use of levodopa increases long-term complications (see below). Mild early symptoms are therefore usually best treated with other drugs such as selegiline, amantadine or anticholinergics.

In more severe disease, when these measures do not alleviate symptoms and when patients perceive themselves as limited in their activities, then dopamine agonists or levodopa preparations can be used. There is some evidence to suggest that dopamine agonists induce long-term complications less frequently; however, they provide effective symptomatic relief in less than half of the patients treated. There is some suggestion that the early use of a controlled-release preparation will minimize the fluctuation of dopamine levels and therefore prevent long-term complications of treatment; this is as yet unproven. Thus there is no definite evidence to

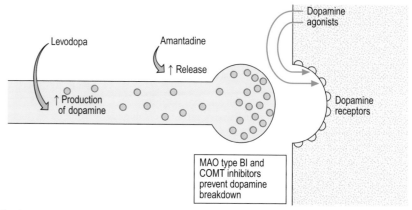

Fig. 1 **Sites of action of drugs used in the treatment of Parkinson's disease.**

Table 1 **Drugs used in the treatment of Parkinson's disease**

Groups of drugs	Examples	Comment
Levodopa preparations	Sinemet (levodopa plus carbidopa) Madopar (levodopa plus benserazide)	Precursor of dopamine combined with a dopa-decarboxylase inhibitor to prevent metabolism outside the brain
	Sinemet CR, Madopar CR	Controlled-release preparations
Dopamine agonists Ergot	Bromocriptine, lisuride Pergolide Cabergoline Apomorphine	Broad-spectrum dopamine agonists More specific agonist to D2 dopamine receptors Given subcutaneously by pump
Non-ergot	Ropinirole, pramipexole	
Dopamine-releasing agents	Amantadine	Weak symptomatic effect. May help dyskinesias
Monoamine oxidase B inhibitor	Selegiline	Mild symptomatic effect Smoothes delivery of levodopa
Co-methyl-transferase inhibitors (COMT)	Entacapone	Potentially augment the effect of levodopa
Anticholinergics	Procyclidine Benztropine	Limited efficacy Useful for tremor Prominent adverse effects

favour one strategy or another. Generally, younger patients (< 70) are started on dopamine agonists and older patients on levodopa preparations. The dose of whichever levodopa preparations or dopamine agonists are selected is then titrated against symptoms.

Complications of long-term treatment

After 5 years, 75% of patients will develop a complication of treatment. This occurs because of progression of the disease, a reduction in responsiveness to levodopa and a narrowing of the therapeutic window. These result in:

- fluctuations
- dyskinesias
- drug failure.

Fluctuations

As the therapeutic window narrows, patients notice a more dramatic change in their symptoms when the drug levels are above or below a critical threshold. Initially this occurs at the end of the dose, as the drug effect wears off. This can be helped by either increasing the frequency of doses, adding

(a) Early dopaminergic effect

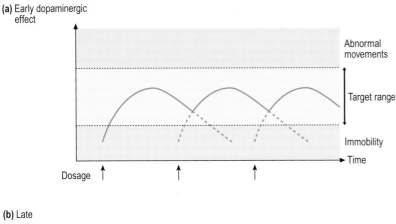

(b) Late

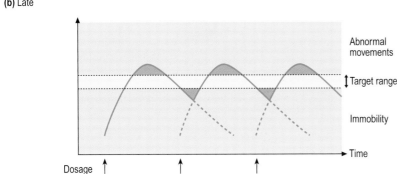

(c) Late treated

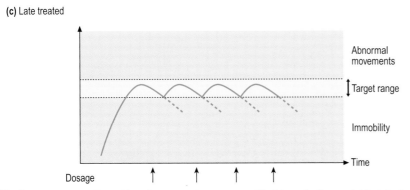

Fig. 2 **Therapeutic effect of levodopa at various stages of Parkinson's disease. (a)** Early in the disease; **(b)** later in the disease with the drug effect wearing off towards the end of the dose and with peak dose dyskinesias; **(c)** changes in therapy in the patient in (b) which improves response.

selegiline or a COMT inhibitor, adding a dopamine agonist or using a controlled-release form of levodopa (Fig. 2). In some patients the transitions seem to be more marked and random and the patient can swing violently from the rigid immobile 'off' state to an 'on' state where the patient has severe dyskinesias without any period of useful mobility. This is the 'on-off' effect. This is difficult to treat, but may be improved by using strategies to smooth levodopa levels (as above), by adding a dopamine agonist that has a longer half-life or by using apomorphine given subcutaneously by pump.

Dyskinesias

These are involuntary abnormal movements that can occur at the peak of a dose or when the dose is coming on or wearing off. They are usually irregular writhing movements (chorea or athetosis), though may involve painful dystonic movements (this is where agonist and antagonist muscles both contract and lock the limb in one position). These are managed by trying to smooth the dose of levodopa or by reducing the dose of levodopa and adding a dopamine agonist.

Drug failures

As the disease progresses, the response to treatment gradually declines. This is manifest by a decline in the best response to treatment. The loss of postural stability, which responds poorly to any drugs, gradually increases.

Other treatments

Some patients develop significant nausea on levodopa preparations or dopamine agonists. This type of nausea responds very well to domperidone. Other antiemetics should be avoided.

A significant number of patients with Parkinson's disease are depressed and may benefit from antidepressants.

Salivary drooling is a late symptom in some patients and improves with anticholinergics.

Hallucinations can occur, both from drug therapy or an underlying cognitive disturbance. An alteration in dopaminergic therapy may help; alternatively a small dose of quetiapine or olanzapine may help.

Neurosurgery was quite widely used in the past to treat tremor by thalamotomy. Pallidotomy and subthalamic stimulation are being reintroduced with some success. With the advent of accurate image-guided stereotaxic surgery, this is being used in very selected patients.

Transplantation of fetal substantia nigra is an experimental treatment that has been reported to show some benefits, though with significant side-effects.

Treatment of other akinetic rigid syndromes

While the response to treatment of the 'Parkinson's plus' syndromes is poor, patients will often get some useful benefit from levodopa preparations and dopamine agonists.

Drug-induced Parkinsonism improves when the precipitating drug is removed or the dose reduced.

Parkinson's disease and other akinetic rigid syndromes II

- A reduction in dopamine and dopaminergic neurones underlies Parkinson's disease.
- Drug treatment is symptomatic only.
- The principal treatments are levodopa preparations and dopamine agonists.
- Late complications of drug treatment include fluctuations, dyskinesias and drug failures.
- Failure to respond to levodopa suggests that the patient does not have idiopathic Parkinson's disease.

Other movement disorders

There is a wide range of movement disorders other than Parkinsonism. In most cases the diagnosis is based on the clinical description of the abnormal movement. The most important of these will be discussed.

Tremors

Essential tremor
Essential tremor is a common problem, with a prevalence of 3 in 1000. It is a slowly progressive 5–8 Hz tremor that is postural and worse on action. It is usually asymmetrical, involving the hands and affecting writing and fine movements (Fig. 1). It may affect the head (yes–yes head titubation). Patients usually present later in life but have generally been aware of the tremor for many years. About 60% of patients will notice a marked improvement with small amounts of alcohol. About half the patients have a family history when the inheritance is dominant.

The diagnosis is clinical. Most patients respond well to propranolol. Primidone, an anticonvulsant, may be useful if beta-blockers are contraindicated or ineffective. Very occasionally, in severely affected patients stereotactic thalamotomy may be needed.

Other tremors
- *Physiological tremor.* A tremor of 8–12 Hz that is normally present but can be enhanced by anxiety, hyperthyroidism, drugs (such as beta-

agonists or sympathomimetics) and alcohol withdrawal.
- *Cerebellar tremor.* A slower tremor (3 Hz) that increases as the limb is moved towards the target (intention tremor). There may be yes–yes head titubation.
- *Rest tremor.* See section on Parkinsonism.
- *Orthostatic tremor.* A rare tremor which appears in the legs on prolonged standing. It is treated with clonazepam and levodopa.

Focal dystonias
Dystonia is the involuntary co-contraction of agonist and antagonist muscles.

Cervical dystonia
This is a common condition. The involuntary contraction in the neck muscles results in:

- abnormal head movements
- abnormal head position
- neck pain.

The direction of movement and abnormal head position vary depending on which muscles are overactive. For example, if one sternocleidomastoid is overactive, the head will turn to the opposite side; if both splenius capitis are affected, the head will look up (retrocollis). Often the patient will be aware that a particular manoeuvre, for example touching the cheek in a certain position (referred to as a 'geste'), can stop an abnormal movement.

In most patients no cause is found. Sometimes this can be triggered by neuroleptics or, occasionally, structural lesions in the basal ganglion.

Patients can be treated symptomatically with botulinum toxin. This toxin weakens the affected muscle for 3–4 months, so relieving symptoms. Side-effects are infrequent, mostly producing weakness in the treated muscles or, rarely, adjacent muscles, e.g. muscles of speech and swallowing.

Writer's cramp and other task-specific dystonias
These conditions, of unknown aetiology, were previously considered to be psychiatric. During a specific activity an abnormal tension and posture develops in the hand. This most commonly occurs during writing, but has been associated with a range of skilled motor

tasks such as typing, playing the guitar or playing darts. In writer's cramp the way the pen is held often changes and the patient may complain of breaking pens and pressing very hard on the paper.

The response to treatment is poor. Patients do best if there are ways of avoiding the activity involved, e.g. move from hand writing to using a computer. Occasionally botulinum toxin can help.

Blepharospasm
This is an uncommon problem where the eyes close involuntarily. This can be sufficiently severe to render the patient effectively blind. It responds well to botulinum toxin injections.

Other focal dystonias
- *Spasmodic dysphonia.* This is rare. Speech is variable and often has a high-pitched strangled quality; it may be tremulous.
- *Oromandibular dystonia.* The mouth and tongue are affected and the jaw may close on the protruded tongue.

Both conditions respond to botulinum toxin.

Generalized dystonias
These are all rare and can occur following neonatal jaundice (kernicterus) or with athetoid cerebral palsy. A rare genetic disease called dystonia musculorum deformans produces a progressive generalized dystonia.

A rare but important condition is levodopa-responsive dystonia. This produces a fluctuating dystonia that develops in children and may mimic spastic diplegia (cerebral palsy). It responds well to a small dose of levodopa.

Wilson's disease
This is a rare (3 per 100 000) but very important disease because it requires specific treatment to prevent deterioration. This condition needs to be considered in all young patients with unusual neurological or psychiatric problems.

There is a defect in copper metabolism, which leads to an accumulation of copper in the liver and the basal ganglia. It has autosomal recessive inheritance.

The presentation is variable. Children may present with liver problems, psychiatric disturbances or a wide range of movement disorders, most notably tremor, Parkinsonism, dysarthria and

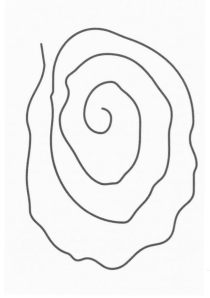

Fig. 1 **Writing in essential tremor.** Note the spiral has become larger (cf. Parkinsonism).

incoordination. The finding of Kayser–Fleischer rings, brown corneal deposits that can be seen with an slit lamp, is said to be pathognomonic. Diagnosis depends on a low blood copper and caeruloplasmin and an elevated 24 h urinary copper.

Treatment is with chelating agents such as D-penicillamine or oral zinc, which impairs copper absorption.

Chorea

Chorea is a term used to describe abnormal movements that are fidgety and twitchy with no position being sustained. If the movements are mild they can be made to look semipurposeful.

Huntington's chorea

This is a dominantly inherited condition that produces a progressive movement disorder and dementia. Most patients develop their symptoms between 30 and 60 years of age and can develop either psychiatric symptoms, particularly changes in personality, or the movement disorder initially. In addition to chorea, tongue protrusion and a very bizarre gait may be prominent.

The diagnosis can now be made genetically by finding an expanded trinucleotide CAG repeat on the short arm of chromosome 4.

The condition is progressive and treatment is symptomatic. Tetrabenazine or haloperidol may help the movements.

Patients with a family history of the disease can now be tested presymptomatically to discover whether they carry the gene. While practically this is easy, the implications of a positive result are such that this needs to be done only after a full and expert discussion with the patient and often other family members, who will also be affected by the result.

Others forms of chorea

Sydenham chorea (post-streptococcal chorea) occurs several months after the streptococcal illness, usually in teenagers. The chorea may affect only one side. It usually resolves spontaneously. Diagnosis of recent streptococcal infection can be demonstrated serologically.

Systemic lupus erythematosus can be associated with chorea, usually in patients with the lupus anticoagulant. Chorea can occur in pregnancy, with the oral contraceptive, hyperthyroidism and with neuroleptic drugs (see below).

Hemiballismus

This is a more dramatic movement of one side of the body, which is thrown around violently, sometimes injuring the patient. This usually arises from vascular lesions of the contralateral subthalamic nucleus. Hemiballismus usually resolves spontaneously.

Tic syndromes

Tics are stereotyped movements. They are voluntary movements undertaken to satisfy an inner urge. They can be suppressed temporarily. They can occur in the absence of other neurological problems, simple motor tics, or be associated with the utterence of obscenities (Gilles de la Tourette's syndrome), other neurological problems (previous head injury or stroke) or neuroleptic drug administration.

Myoclonus

Myoclonus is the occurrence of sudden, shock-like involuntary movements. It can occur in epilepsy as a form of seizure (p. 74) and normally in association with sleep. It can occur without other neurological deficits (essential myoclonus), when it usually responds to clonazepam or sodium valproate. It is a prominent feature in postanoxic encephalopathies and some neurodegenerative diseases.

Neuroleptic malignant syndrome

This is the onset of rigidity, fever, autonomic disturbance and impaired consciousness associated with an elevated creatine kinase. It can occur at any time in association with neuroleptics. Therapy involves withdrawal of the neuroleptics, antiparkinsonian drugs and dantrolene and appropriate support. Mortality can be as high as 25%.

Restless legs syndrome (Ekbom's syndrome)

This is an unpleasant sensory feeling occurring in the legs, particularly at night, that is relieved by moving the legs. It may occur with a peripheral neuropathy, iron deficiency, uraemia or lumbar spondylosis, but is usually idiopathic. Treatment is with clonazepam, levodopa or dopamine agonist.

Hemifacial spasm

This is an uncommon problem that usually occurs later in life. There are episodes where half the face briefly goes into spasm; these may almost appear rhythmical at times. This is usually due to compression of the facial nerve by an aberrant posterior fossa vessel: microvascular compression. The spasms may remit spontaneously. Treatment with botulinum toxin is effective. If symptoms are severe and the patient is otherwise well, a microvascular decompression of the nerve is effective.

Drug-induced movement disorders

Acute. Oculogyric crises occur in about 2% of patients given neuroleptics (including the antiemetics prochlorperazine and metoclopramide) and particularly occurs in young men. The effect is dramatic: the jaw clenches, the face grimaces, there is marked torticollis and retrocollis and there may be opisthotonus (back muscles going into spasm and hyperextending the back). Treatment is with intravenous anticholinergics, followed by oral anticholinergics, and is equally dramatic.

Parkinsonism. Neuroleptics can produce an akinetic rigid syndrome indistinguishable from idiopathic Parkinson's disease. Older patients are more likely to be affected. This may improve over months despite continued neuroleptic therapy. Anticholinergics and amantadine are the only therapies available.

Akathisia. This is a very common problem in patients on long-term neuroleptics. It consists of a motor restlessness manifested as stepping up and down on the spot, or leg swinging. This is usually resistant to treatment.

Tardive dyskinesias. Tardy means late and tardive dyskinesias are movements that occur either after prolonged therapy or some time after drug exposure. The most characteristic is the orolingual dyskinesia – a repetitive lipsmacking and chewing – but most movement disorders mentioned above have been described in association with neuroleptics. A detailed history of previous exposure to neuroleptics is essential in assessing anyone with a movement disorder.

> ## Other movement disorders
>
> - Essential tremor responds to beta-blockers.
> - Cervical dystonia, blepharospasm, hemifacial spasm and some focal dystonias are treated effectively with botulinum toxin.
> - Wilson's disease should be considered in all younger patients with movement disorders or psychiatric illnesses.
> - Neuroleptic drugs can provoke all types of abnormal movement.

CNS neoplasia I: intracranial tumours

In adults, primary intracranial tumours represent only 3% of tumour-related deaths, and have an annual incidence of 4–7 per 100 000. Intracranial metastases are more common. Intracranial tumours are the second most common tumour in childhood with an annual incidence of 2–3 per 100 000.

Pathology
Intracranial tumours can be divided into intrinsic and extrinsic (Table 1).

Intrinsic
Intrinsic tumours are within the substance of the brain, either primary or secondary. *Primary intracranial tumours* do not metastasize outside the CNS, and thus lack a central feature of malignant tumours elsewhere in the body. The concept of malignancy in primary intrinsic CNS tumours is therefore different from tumours elsewhere in the body. Malignancy in cerebral tumours is only a relative term and they are graded according to histopathological appearance (high = more malignant). They can arise from different cell lineages of neuroectodermal origin; gliomas arise from glial cells, and can be divided into specific cell types such as astrocytes (leading to astrocytomas and glioblastoma multiforme), oligodendrocytes (leading to oligodendrogliomas) and ependymal cells (leading to ependymomas). The histological type and grade are the primary determinants of prognosis. Different parts of a tumour may have different grades and a low-grade tumour may suddenly become more aggressive, in association with a change in histological characteristics.

The pattern of tumours differs in adults and children. In adults (Table 1), 70% of tumours are supratentorial; in children, 70% of tumours are infratentorial.

Secondary intracranial tumours (or intracerebral metastases) occur in up to 20% of patients with cancer at postmortem examination. In most of these patients the primary tumour is known. The difficulty arises when intracranial metastases is the presentation. These most commonly arise from carcinoma of the lung and breast, and melanoma.

Extrinsic
Extrinsic tumours arise from intracranial structures outside the brain substance, most commonly from the meninges, resulting in meningioma, the cranial nerve, producing a Schwannoma or neurofibroma, or the pituitary (p. 96).

Aetiology
The aetiology of most brain tumours is unknown. Hypotheses include the pathological activation of embryonic cell rests, e.g. in primitive tumours such as teratomas, or the dedifferentiation of mature cells to more primitive cells and neoplastic transformation. The importance of genetic changes is supported by the large number of inherited syndromes of CNS tumours, e.g. neurofibromatosis (p. 97). There are changes at specific sites of the genome in many tumours, including chromosome 22 loss in up to 70% of meningiomas,

P53 gene (involved in DNA repair) in up to 40% of astrocytomas and epidermal growth factor receptor gene amplification in up to 40% of glioblastoma multiforme (GBM). These changes represent an exciting development in understanding but their exact role is unclear; because none is seen in 100% of the appropriate tumour type, other factors must also be important. Endocrine factors are important in some tumours; meningiomas are more common in females, grow more rapidly in pregnancy and may express oestrogen receptors.

Clinical features
Intracranial tumours present with four types of symptoms.

Focal neurological deficit. This is the most common presentation. Tumours may interfere with the function of adjacent neural tissue. As the tumour enlarges this effect increases, resulting in a progressive focal neurological deficit, depending on the site of the lesion. More malignant tumours usually expand more rapidly and cause a more rapid progression of symptoms.

Raised intracranial pressure. This is the presenting feature in 20% of patients with intracranial tumours and occurs at some stage in 60% of cases. The typical headache of raised intracranial pressure is worse on lying down, bending down or straining and is associated with nausea and vomiting. Initially it may be present each morning and clears after rising. Many patients do not have the classical headache, but there are usually other features: unsteadiness, dulled mentation or drowsiness. Signs include gait ataxia, papilloedema (may be absent), failure of upgaze and false localizing signs: 3rd and 6th nerve palsies. Drowsiness is an ominous sign, suggesting a critically elevated intracranial pressure. Occasionally tumours within the ventricles may cause a sudden, intermittent obstruction to CSF outflow. This causes a sudden severe headache, sometimes with collapse or loss of consciousness.

Epileptic seizures. These occur in 20–50% of tumours affecting the cerebral hemispheres and are focal in onset (p. 74). Low-grade tumours, e.g. oligodendroglioma or meningioma, may cause seizures 10 or more years before other symptoms.

Endocrine disturbance. This may result from tumours in the region of the pituitary gland (p. 96).

Table 1 **Approximate frequency of different intracranial tumours**

Tumour	Percentage of total	Comments
Intrinsic		
Glioblastoma multiforme	20	High-grade glioma; poor prognosis
Astrocytoma	10 (48 in children)	Lower-grade glioma
Metastases	10*	Often multiple
Oligodendroglioma	5	Slow growing. Often frontal or temporal and calcifies
Ependymoma[†]	5 (10 in children)	Arise from ependymal lining, usually of 4th ventricle
Medulloblastoma[†]	5 (45 in children)	Arise from cerebellum. May metastasize within CNS
Primary CNS lymphoma	Rare except in AIDS	May be multifocal
Extrinsic		
Meningioma[†]	15	Arise from meninges and indent brain, may erode bone
Pituitary adenoma[†]	7	Chiasmatic visual disturbance and endocrine effects
Schwannoma, e.g. of acoustic nerve[†]	7	Benign
Other	16	Includes teratomas, pinealomas, etc.

Estimates are taken from a combination of series
[†] Potentially curable
* Metastases are much more common. This estimate is of those with solitary intracranial metastases

Differential diagnosis

The differential diagnosis depends on the presentation. Other space-occupying lesions can share all the characteristics described above and constitute the main differential diagnoses. These include chronic subdural haematomas, intracranial abscesses and giant aneurysms. Obstructive hydrocephalus from non-malignant causes can closely mimic an intracranial tumour. Other differential diagnoses are considered in the sections on headache and epilepsy.

Investigation

MRI shows over 95% of intracranial tumours. A CT scan may miss small lesions. Often, the differential diagnosis can be narrowed considerably by the site and appearance of the lesion. Multiple lesions suggest metastases and investigations for an extracranial primary source may establish the diagnosis. For single lesions, and sometimes with multiple lesions, intracranial biopsy will be required to achieve a histological diagnosis.

Management of intracranial tumours

Treatment differs depending on the clinical situation, site of the tumour, the eloquence of the related part of the brain and the type of tumour. The objective of treatment will vary, from curative resection of a meningioma (Fig. 1) to palliation in a glioma (Fig. 2). Some rarer tumours have different treatment objectives (p. 96).

The optimum management for most kinds of intracranial tumours has not been established by prospective randomized clinical trials. Especially difficult is the management of low-grade gliomas whose natural history is only being observed following the advent of improved brain imaging.

Presurgical management

The cerebral oedema related to the tumour may respond temporarily to steroid therapy: usually dexamethasone. Intravenous mannitol may achieve a rapid but transient reduction if the intracranial pressure is critically elevated. The arterial blood pressure should be maintained to overcome raised intracranial pressure and maintain cerebral perfusion. Adequate fluid balance and sometimes inotropes may be needed. Artificial ventilation with hyperventilation may produce hypocarbia, causing cerebral vasodilatation and increasing brain tissue perfusion.

Seizures are treated as focal epilepsy (p. 76). In the emergency situation a loading dose of intravenous phenytoin is often used.

Surgical treatment

Resective surgery. Certain tumour types may be cured by resection, especially extrinsic tumours, e.g. meningioma.

Palliative surgery. This may be undertaken where the tumour cannot be resected. Intrinsic tumours do not have a clear margin to allow resection and a purely surgical cure is not possible. There are two types of procedure:

- biopsy aiming to establish the diagnosis with minimum brain damage; image-guided techniques are helpful
- debulking procedures.

The success of any debulking procedure depends on the site. Tumours in 'silent' areas are more accessible to debulking than eloquent areas, such as the motor cortex. Debulking tumours has been shown to improve prognosis for GBM and astrocytoma. Removal of a large cystic component may be of particular benefit. Obstructive hydrocephalus may be treated by ventriculoperitoneal shunts or by ventriculostomy (opening a hole from the third ventricle to the basal cisterns). This may be undertaken as a palliative procedure or as an emergency, prior to more definitive tumour surgery.

Radiotherapy

Primary radiotherapy is the main mode of palliation for metastatic disease, including meningeal infiltration, and may be effective primary treatment in some rarer tumours, e.g. primary cerebral lymphoma or pineal region germinoma.

Adjunctive radiotherapy has been shown to improve the prognosis of GBM by an average of 5 months and the 10-year survival of astrocytoma from 11% to 40%. It is used to prevent seeding of tumour for medulloblastoma or ependymoma.

Chemotherapy

Chemotherapy for the more common tumours is unproved and under evaluation, but some benefit has been reported in the treatment of GBM and oligodendroglioma. Some tumours are more sensitive, e.g. medulloblastoma.

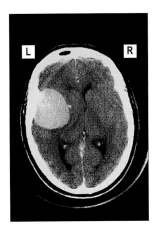

Fig. 1 **Meningioma.** Meningiomas arise from the meninges and have a component attached to the meninges, and may cause bony erosion. They typically have a smooth boundary and they may be calcified. They enhance diffusely with contrast. Common sites are parasagittal, attached to the falx cerebri, in the posterior fossa, attached to the tentorium and at the sphenoid ridge.

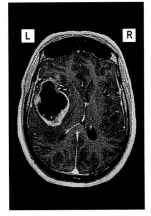

Fig. 2 **Glioblastoma multiforme.** An intrinsic lesion, often with a heterogeneous appearance due to necrosis and cyst formation and considerable oedema. They enhance patchily or may show ring enhancement. The main differential diagnoses are cerebral abscess and metastasis.

CNS neoplasia I: intracranial tumours

- In adults metastases are more common than primary intracranial tumours.
- Intracranial tumours commonly present with progressive focal neurological deficit, raised intracranial pressure or seizures.
- Emergency treatment is directed at reducing cerebral oedema and treating seizures.
- The operability of tumours depends on their location as well as their type.

CNS neoplasia II: special situations

This chapter deals with pituitary tumours, some less common tumour presentations and some inherited syndromes with a particular predisposition to developing CNS tumours.

Pituitary tumours (common)

Pathology

Nearly all tumours are benign pituitary adenomas. The incidence increases with age: 20% of 80-year-olds have small adenomas at postmortem examination. Prolactinomas represent 60–70%, growth hormone-secreting tumours 10%, non-secreting tumours 30% and tumours secreting thyroid-stimulating hormone or adrenocorticotrophic hormone are rare. Less common pituitary lesions are craniopharyngiomas, meningiomas, metastases and granulomatous diseases.

Clinical features

These include endocrine malfunction, visual disturbance and headache.

Endocrine disturbance may be due to abnormal excessive hormone secretion or impaired hormone secretion following damage to hormone-secreting cells. The most common features in adults are infertility, amenorrhoea, loss of libido and hypothyroidism. Acromegaly, gigantism, Cushing's syndrome, diabetes insipidus and hypoadrenalism occur less commonly.

Visual disturbance occurs because of compression of the optic chiasm and is typically chronic or subacute deterioration of vision in both eyes. The chiasmal lesion leads to a bitemporal hemianopia, especially to red pin, and may lead to reduced acuity. The fundi are usually normal but there may be papilloedema or optic atrophy. Eye movement abnormalities occur if the tumour has expanded into the cavernous sinus and compresses the 3rd, 4th or 6th nerves.

Headache is a late feature and may reflect bony erosion or hydrocephalus.

A rare but important presentation is with pituitary apoplexy, characterized by acute visual disturbance associated with headache, malaise and systemic collapse. This is due to infarction of a pituitary tumour causing swelling and acute adrenal failure. It may occur after postpartum haemorrhage in women with pituitary tumours.

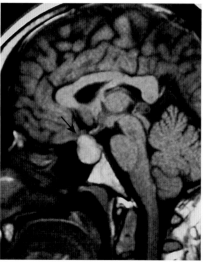

Fig. 1 **MRI scan of a pituitary tumour.**

Investigations

A highly elevated serum prolactin level (>4000 mU/l (normal < 400)) implies a prolactinoma. More moderate elevations may be seen with other pituitary tumours that block the inhibition of prolactin release by dopamine. The tumours and their relation to other structures, especially the optic chiasm, are best seen on MRI (Fig. 1) but may also be seen on a CT scan with dedicated pituitary views. Endocrine assessment may be required, e.g. thyroid function, adrenal function, follicle-stimulating hormone and luteinizing hormone.

Treatment

Pituitary tumours can be divided into two main categories: prolactin-secreting prolactinomas that can usually be treated with medication alone; and other tumours that require surgery. Prolactinomas respond to dopaminergic agonists such as bromocriptine or cabergoline. This treatment not only prevents secretion of the hormone but also causes tumour shrinkage, so surgery is not usually required unless vision is immediately threatened. Growth-hormone-secreting tumours may also respond to dopaminergic agonists or octreotide (an analogue of somatostatin) but other tumour types need surgery if there is any suggestion of neurological compromise. Radiotherapy may be of value in some inoperable cases. Endocrine failure requires appropriate treatment. The prognosis with modern treatment is good.

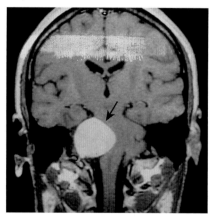

Fig. 2 **MRI scan of a cerebellopontine angle tumour.**

Craniopharyngiomas

These are rare and usually occur in children. They arise from embryonic cell rests of Rathke's pouch at the junction of the stem of the infundibulum and the pituitary. They usually present with a combination of pituitary, chiasmal and hypothalamic features, sometimes with hydrocephalus. The hypothalamic involvement causes mental dulling and disorders of autonomic control, including diabetes insipidus, eating disorders and disturbances of thermoregulation. Most cases are amenable to surgical cure.

Cerebellopontine angle tumours (rare)

Pathology. Most commonly acoustic nerve Schwannomas (often referred to as acoustic neuromas); see also neurofibromatosis type II. Also meningiomas of trigeminal, facial and acoustic nerves and cholesteatoma.

Clinical features. Seventy-five per cent of patients present with progressive deafness in one ear. Any patient with unilateral sensorineural hearing loss requires investigation to exclude this diagnosis. Less commonly, there may be ipsilateral facial weakness, facial sensory loss, ataxia and headache. Neurological deficits in the limbs occur later with brain stem compression.

Investigation. An MRI scan (Fig. 2) (a CT scan may miss early tumours) and audiometry to document hearing loss.

Treatment. Surgical resection can be undertaken via various routes. Suboccipital transmeatal microdissection minimizes risk to the facial nerve, which is immediately adjacent to the 8th nerve in the auditory

Table 1 Inherited central nervous system (CNS) tumour syndromes

Condition	CNS manifestations	Cutaneous manifestations	Comments
Neurofibromatosis I (peripheral)	Optic nerve glioma in children, cortical dysgenesis, mental retardation, seizures, syringomyelia, hydrocephalus	Peripheral nerve neurofibromas, epidermal molluscum fibrosum, café au lait patches, massive plexiform neurofibromas, axillary freckles	Pigmented Lisch nodules in the iris by age 5 years Bone cysts, precocious puberty, phaeochromocytoma. Defect of neurofibronin
Neurofibromatosis II (central)	Bilateral acoustic Schwannoma, multiple spinal neurofibroma, multiple meningioma, glioma	Few cutaneous lesions	Chromosome 22 abnormality
Tuberous sclerosis	Seizures, mental retardation Cortical dysplasia and tubers (often calcified)	Hypomelanotic regions, adenoma sebaceum, subungual fibromala, shagreen patches	Cardiac rhabdomyoma and dysrhythmias, angiomyolipoma of liver, kidneys, testes, thyroid, gastrointestinal tract. Defective Tuberin and Hamartin gene
Von Hippel–Lindau syndrome	CNS haemangioblastoma, especially cerebellum and spinal cord, syringomyelia	None	Retinal haemangioblastoma, renal carcinoma, phaeochromocytoma, benign renal, liver or pancreatic cysts

Table 2 Paraneoplastic central nervous system disorders

Syndrome	Clinical features	Comments
Cerebellar degeneration	Progressive cerebellar syndrome over weeks to months Sometimes myoclonus, diplopia, hearing loss	In 50% it is the presenting feature of the neoplasm. Anti-Purkinje cell antibodies present. Bronchus, breast, female genital tract, lymphoma
Encephalomyelitis (rare)	Anxiety, depression, hallucinations, Korsakoff amnesic state and brain stem signs	Anti-Hu antineuronal antibodies present; 80% bronchus, also prostate, breast, neuroblastoma
Sensory ganglionitis (rare)	Dysaesthesiae spread over weeks from feet to include all limbs and face. Sensory ataxia and autonomic disturbance common	CSF protein elevated, anti-Hu antibodies present. Differential diagnosis: Sjögren's syndrome and idiopathic cases
Opsoclonus–myoclonus syndrome (rare)	Acute onset of opsoclonus (dancing eyes) and myoclonus with ataxia	Usually due to neuroblastoma in children. Sometimes bronchial or breast. Breast carcinoma produces anti-Ri antibody

canal. Function can be monitored perioperatively by facial nerve electromyography and auditory evoked potentials. The prognosis is good, especially for early tumours.

Pineal region tumours (rare)

These tumours present with visual disturbance and headache and Parinaud's syndrome, characterized by failure of upgaze, eyelid retraction, dilated unreactive pupils, convergence–retraction nystagmus (on attempted convergence, all extraocular muscles contract, pulling the globe back into the orbit), hydrocephalus and papilloedema.

In addition to a CT or MRI scan, markers for germ cell tumours (α-fetoprotein and β-human chorionic gonadotrophin) may help.

Surgical resection is difficult. Germinomas are very radiosensitive and some authorities suggest radiotherapy without histological confirmation, if tumour markers are elevated. Chemotherapy may also be of benefit. Teratomas, astrocytomas and dermoids can occur.

Other tumours

Numerous eponymous syndromes are described for tumours at the skull base. They present with pain and associated cranial nerve deficits, depending on the location of the lesion. Neurofibromas and Schwannomas, meningiomas and bony metastases or direct invasion by adenocarcinoma of the nasopharynx can all present this way. The differential diagnosis is from chronic meningitis (p. 98), osteomyelitis and inflammatory processes, e.g. sarcoidosis or Tolosa–Hunt syndrome.

Special situations

Malignant meningitis. Malignant infiltration of the meninges may present with chronic meningitis, often with communicating hydrocephalus. Common features are headache, radicular pain, multiple cranial nerve palsies and polyradiculopathy in the limbs, usually evolving over a few weeks. Common causes are adenocarcinoma, lymphoma, leukaemia and melanoma. Diagnosis is made from the clinical picture and on CSF examination. In 25% of cases it may not be possible to identify malignant cells even with two lumbar punctures. MRI may help in identifying bulky meningeal masses and meningeal enhancement. Occasionally meningeal biopsy is indicated. The prognosis is very poor. Palliative intrathecal chemotherapy (methotrexate, cytarabine or thiotepa) may improve prognosis and prevent neurological deterioration.

Inherited tumour syndromes. A variety of inherited diseases present with nervous system tumours, some with typical skin abnormalities (Table 1). They are rare. Most are inherited as autosomal dominant traits. The genetic locus of some of these conditions has been characterized but the pathophysiology is not yet understood.

Paraneoplastic syndromes (Table 2). The nervous system is especially susceptible to non-metastatic manifestations of malignancy. In some cases, humoral factors have been demonstrated, especially antibodies to Purkinje cells of the cerebellum in paraneoplastic cerebellar disorders, which differ in nature according to the primary tumour and are in higher titre in CSF than in blood. Certain tumours are particularly prone to causing these syndromes, especially small cell bronchial carcinoma, breast and female genital tract carcinoma and lymphoma. Paraneoplastic syndromes affecting other parts of the nervous system include: subacute myelopathy, retinopathy, stiff person syndrome and Lambert–Eaton myasthenic syndrome.

> ## CNS neoplasia II: special situations
>
> - Pituitary tumours may present with neurological or endocrinological symptoms.
> - Prolactinomas can usually be treated without surgery.
> - The clinical presentation determines the site of the tumour and narrows pathological possibilities.
> - Systemic malignancy may present with CNS paraneoplastic syndromes or malignant meningitis.

Infections of the nervous system I

The central nervous system is protected by the blood–brain barrier and neurological infections are relatively rare in the western world. There are, however, many different infections that can occur. In this section the more common infections are discussed. Other infections, such as leprosy and HTLV-1 myelopathy, are dealt with elsewhere.

The infections affecting the immunocompetent host will be explored before discussing the immunocompromised states including acquired immune deficiency syndrome (AIDS).

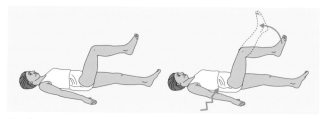

Fig. 1 Kernig's sign. Flex the leg at the hip and knee and try to extend the knee. Low back pain with this procedure indicates meningeal irritation.

Meningitis

Bacterial meningitis

This occurs in 5–10 per 100 000 per year in the developed world. The most common organisms are *Haemophilus influenzae*, *Neisseria meningitidis* and *Streptococcus pneumoniae*. *N. meningitidis* tends to occur in epidemics. Neonatal meningitis is usually due to *Escherichia coli* or group B streptococcus. In developing countries, tuberculous meningitis is also common but usually clinically distinct (see below).

Overcrowding and poverty have been shown to be risk factors.

Meningitis can occur with organisms crossing the blood–brain barrier during systemic infection or as a result of a breakdown in the barrier, for example after skull fracture or a neurosurgical procedure. In the latter cases a wider range of organisms is seen.

The clinical features of meningitis are:

- headache
- fever
- neck stiffness.

There may also be altered consciousness, seizures and focal signs in about 15% of patients. Patients may have a positive Kernig's sign (Fig. 1), another sign of meningism. Meningococcal meningitis may be associated with a purpuric rash (Fig. 2).

Bacterial meningitis is a medical emergency. Treatment should begin as soon as the diagnosis is suspected and should not await investigation results or on occasion investigation. Acute treatment is usually with systemic penicillin and a third generation cephalosporin, though alternatively ampicillin and chloramphenicol may be used.

Blood cultures should be taken immediately. Lumbar puncture is important to confirm the diagnosis and determine the organism. However, if the patient has focal signs, altered

Table 1 **Typical changes in the cerebrospinal fluid (CSF) in different types of meningitis**				
	Cell count	**Differential**	**CSF protein**	**CSF glucose**
Bacterial	> 200/µl	Polymorphs	> 1.5 g/l	< 40%
Viral	50–200/µl	Lymphocytes	< 1.0 g/l	Normal
Tuberculous	50–500/µl	Lymphocytes	> 1.0 g/l	< 40%
Partially treated bacterial	50–500/µl	Mainly lymphocytes	Variable	Normal or reduced
Normal	< 5/µl	Lymphocytes	< 0.45 g/l	> 60% of blood glucose

consciousness or has had a seizure, then a CT brain scan or MRI needs to be done prior to the lumbar puncture. In severely ill children, LP may lead to deterioration and should be avoided. The CSF findings are indicated in Table 1. The Gram stain and culture are usually diagnostic, and can be helped by newer tests for specific bacterial antigens.

The main differential diagnoses are subarachnoid haemorrhage and other meningitic illnesses.

There is a 10% mortality; 20% of patients have some sequelae, most commonly hearing loss, but also higher-function deficits and epilepsy.

Aseptic meningitis

Aseptic meningitis is a term used to cover those with a clinical and CSF picture of meningitis without bacterial culture from the CSF. This therefore covers a wide range of aetiologies, in particular viral infection, other non-bacterial infections and inflammatory processes such as sarcoid and malignancies. This can also reflect parameningeal inflammatory processes such as brain abscess. Partially treated bacterial meningitis will also present like this.

Viral infections are usually less severe than their bacterial counterparts, with less severe headache, neck stiffness and fever. This occurs in about 10 per 100 000 per year. A wide range of viruses has been found to cause meningitis, though the enteroviruses are the most common. The management is conservative and perhaps the most important contribution is to make as definite a diagnosis as possible so as not to miss other treatment

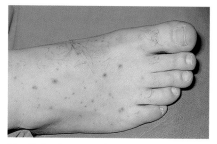

Fig. 2 Meningococcal rash.

opportunities. If in doubt, especially where the differential diagnosis is partially treated bacterial meningitis, treat as for bacterial meningitis.

Tuberculous meningitis

This is a more insidious onset meningitis. There is usually a general malaise associated with a progressive headache, which may be followed by development of multiple lower cranial nerve palsies and radiculopathies. The diagnosis may prove to be difficult. Investigations may find abnormalities such as an elevated viscosity, though this is variable. The CSF findings reflect the more chronic process with a lower level of lymphocyte pleocytosis, raised protein and low glucose. The differential diagnosis is wide and includes other infections such as fungal infections, brucella or spirochaetal disease and non-infectious diseases such as sarcoid and malignant meningitis, particularly lymphoma. Diagnosis can be difficult as culture of *Mycobacterium tuberculosis* takes 6 weeks. Newer techniques such as polymerase chain reaction (PCR) are proving to be helpful. Treatment is often

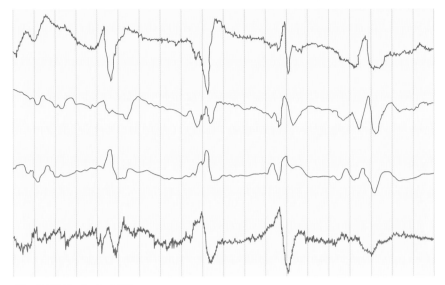

Fig. 3 **EEG in classical CJD.**

initiated on a suspected diagnosis having ruled out alternatives as far as possible. Triple therapy with isoniazid, ethambutol and rifampicin, plus pyrazinamide, which crosses the blood–brain barrier well, is used. Treatment is for 9 months.

Encephalitis

Infectious encephalopathies, either alone or with an associated meningitis (meningoenphalitis) present with altered behaviour, seizures, confusion or coma (p. 50). These patients often have a history of a prodromal infection and are febrile. Their CSF shows some abnormalities: a slightly lymphocytic pleocytosis (50–150 cells/µl) and an elevated protein level, usually with a normal glucose level. Brain imaging is usually normal. The EEG is slow, and cannot distinguish between infective and other encephalopathies.

Viral encephalitis occurs in about 10–15 per 100 000 per year. The syndrome can be caused by a range of different viruses; some are sporadic, such as herpes simplex virus (HSV), Epstein–Barr virus and adenovirus; others are epidemic, such as arbovirus infections (e.g. eastern equine encephalitis); and others such as rabies, are transmitted by animals. Virological diagnosis is often made after the acute illness, serologically or from viral culture. PCR is showing promise in the earlier diagnosis.

Outside epidemics, the major concern is whether the encephalitis is due to HSV, which is the proven cause in less than 10% of cases of viral encephalitis. The diagnosis is considered more frequently because specific antiviral therapy is available. The virus demonstrates a predilection to affect the temporal lobes. Clinically this is manifest as behavioural changes, speech disturbances, hemiplegia and seizures. The most common and disabling sequela, short-term memory loss, results from this. If the diagnosis is considered, the patient should be treated with aciclovir intravenously. Without treatment the mortality rises to 80%, but falls to 30% with antiviral treatment. Patients with other sporadic viral encephalitis usually have a more benign course, resolving spontaneously. Most of these patients now receive aciclovir to cover the possibility of HSV.

Cerebral abscess

Cerebral abscesses are now rare. They result from:

- direct spread into the brain from adjacent tissues (75%), such as paranasal sinus infection, or middle ear and mastoid infection
- haematogenous spread (25%), particularly from a proximal source of infection such as endocarditis.

The presentation is with progressive headache (75%), focal neurological symptoms or signs (50%), fever (50%) and seizures (30%). The brain scan shows one or more usually ring enhancing lesions with associated oedema. There may be features of the primary infection, ear or sinus, and markers of systemic infection. The main differential diagnosis is cerebral tumours (p. 94). Management is with a combination of antibiotics and surgical drainage. There is a high incidence of epilepsy following cerebral abscess.

Non-bacterial intracerebral abscesses can occur. They are seen in toxoplasmosis, fungal infections, cerebral amoebiasis, cysticercosis or echinococcus in restricted geographical areas or in the immunocompromised (see below).

Slow infections

There are several infections that present in a chronic or subacute manner and can simulate degenerative disease. Subacute sclerosing panencephalitis, a progressive intellectual deterioration with seizures, myoclonus and progressive tetraparesis, occurs in late childhood and adolescence as the sequela to measles. Whipple's disease is a rare infection with *Tropheryma whippelii* that can affect the bowel and, occasionally, the CNS. It is usually associated with supranuclear gaze disorder and sometimes with a bizarre rhythmical movement of the eyes and mouth. It is variable in its clinical manifestations.

The spongiform encephalopathies, Creutzfeldt–Jakob disease (CJD) and new-variant CJD, are rare but have been intensively studied recently. CJD occurs in about 1 per million per year; new variant CJD has had about 100 cases reported by 2004. They are caused by abnormalities in prion proteins. Some cases of CJD occur from transmission from using infected dural transplants or human pituitary extracted growth hormone. Most CJD is sporadic, but 5% of cases are familial and due to mutation of endogenous prion protein (chromsome 20), referred to as the Gerstmann–Straussler syndrome. The onset of the sporadic disease is usually between 50 and 70 years of age with dementia and subsequently myoclonus and typical EEG changes (Fig. 3); median survival is less than 1 year.

New-variant CJD presents in young adults with psychiatric disturbance, followed by dementia, ataxia and dystonia progressing over months. Myoclonus and typical EEG changes of classical CJD are absent. New-variant CJD is caused by transmission of bovine spongiform encephalopathy (BSE) from cattle to humans.

> ### Infections of the nervous system I
>
> - Bacterial meningitis is a medical emergency.
> - Bacterial meningitis presents with headache, fever and neck stiffness.
> - Encephalitis can present with headaches, confusion, behavioural changes and seizures.

Infections of the nervous system II

Spinal infections

Specific infections of the spinal cord are caused by viruses such as HTLV-1, polio, herpes zoster, herpes simplex and Epstein–Barr, bacterial and other infections including syphilis (see below) and Lyme disease. Infection can also spread from the spine. The spinal cord and cauda equina may also be affected by meningitic processes described previously and in association with meningoencephalitis.

HTLV-1 is a retrovirus. It is common in the West Indies, Africa and southern USA and in immigrants from these areas. Myelopathy occurs in a small proportion of sero-positive patients (2–5%) and presents as a slowly progressive weakness and stiffness in the legs with sensory symptoms and prominent bladder symptoms. The arms are rarely affected. Oligoclonal bands are positive in the CSF. The main differential diagnosis is with multiple sclerosis. Treatment is symptomatic.

Poliomyelitis is now extremely rare. It can lead to a myelitis and leave significant neurological deficit (p. 109).

Other viruses, particularly from the herpes group, can produce a transverse myelitis, though this is usually in the immunocompromised.

Pyogenic infection in the vertebral body or in the epidural space can lead to an epidural abscess (Fig. 1), producing back pain often associated with fever. This is followed by radicular pain and then symptoms and signs of spinal cord or cauda equina involvement. If this diagnosis is suspected then urgent investigation with spinal MRI is needed, as early drainage of the abscess and high-dose antibiotics is the only hope of reversing this process. A similar, if slower onset is associated with tuberculous epidural abscess. Treatment of this is primarily antituberculous therapy, though in some patients surgery is needed.

Peripheral nerve infections

The most common peripheral nerve infection is shingles (5 per 1000 per year), resulting from herpes zoster dorsal root ganglionitis. This is usually thoracic and can be managed conservatively. When it occurs in unusual sites or more than one dermatome, it is useful to consider whether there is an underlying cause for immunosuppression. When it occurs in the ophthalmic branch of the trigeminal nerve there is particular concern as this innervates the cornea and corneal

ulcers can occur. Neuralgic pain may develop following the infection, which usually settles spontaneously but sometimes persists. Oral aciclovir shortens the illness and reduces the frequency of postherpetic neuralgia. Aciclovir eye drops are used in ophthalmic zoster. Carbamazepine and amitriptyline are helpful in patients with postherpetic neuralgia.

Syphilis

Syphilis used to be the great mimic in neurology and syphilis serology was performed on all patients with neurological disease. Neurosyphilis is now rare. Pathologically, neurosyphilis occurs because of a chronic syphilitic meningitis and an endarteritis. These result in a large number of neurological abnormalities that can be categorized into four neurological syndromes, most of which occur years after the original infection.

- *Meningeal syphilis* – within 6–12 months of infection: it presents as a chronic meningitis with multiple cranial nerve palsies.
- *Meningovascular syphilis* – 5–10 years after onset it presents as young stroke.
- *Tabes dorsalis* – 15+ years after infection. This results from chronic damage to the cauda equina and dorsal root ganglia from chronic meningitis. It presents with lightening pain in the legs, loss of sensation in the legs, producing Charcot joints, and a wide-based high-stepping gait (originally called locomotor ataxia).
- *Paretic syphilis* (or general paralysis of the insane) – 15+ years after infection there is a progressive dementia, classically with prominent delusions, associated with personality change, weakness and gait disturbance.

The diagnosis of syphilis is in two phases. Blood serology (TPHA, VDRL and FTA) identifies patients with current or prior infection. CSF examination is used to determine the activity of infection, measuring cell count, protein and VDRL titre. Treatment is with prolonged (21 days) supervised courses of intramuscular penicillin.

Tropical neurology

Infections play a larger part in neurology in tropical countries. For example, cysticercosis, schistosomiasis and paragonimiasis

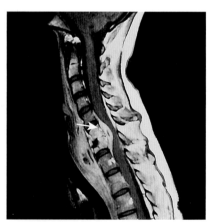

Fig. 1 **MRI showing epidural abscess associated with discitis leading to spinal cord compression.** The abscess is the ring enhancing lesion (arrowed).

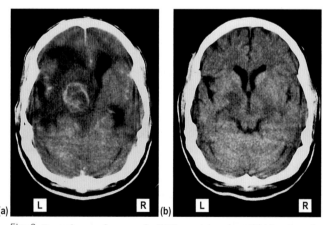

Fig. 2 **Toxoplasma abscesses in AIDS: pre (a) and post (b) treatment.**

Table 1 **Summary of the neurological complications in AIDS**				
Level of nervous system	**Infections**	**Tumours**	**HIV associated**	**Complications of treatment**
Brain	Toxoplasmosis CMV encephalitis PML Cryptococcal meningitis	Primary CNS lymphoma	HIV encephalopathy	Drug-induced confusional states
Spinal cord	CMV myelitis HSV myelitis HZ myelitis		Vacuolar myelopathy	
Cauda equina	CMV polyradiculopathy	Lymphoma		
Peripheral nerve	CMV		Vasculitis*	Nucleoside analogues
Muscle			Myopathy*	Zidovudine

CMV, cytomegalovirus; PML, progressive multifocal leucoencephalopathy; HSV, herpes simplex virus; HZ, herpes zoster
* Relationship with HIV unproven

(oriental liver fluke) are common causes of seizures in different parts of the world. Cerebral malaria is a common cause of coma and death in parts of Africa. All these conditions are seen in people who have travelled in tropical countries, so a travel history is an important clue in the diagnosis of these conditions.

The immunocompromised host
Immunocompromised patients most commonly have:

- iatrogenic cause for immune suppression, such as chemotherapy
- severe general illness such as diabetes or lymphoma
- a specific immune deficiency such as AIDS.

The first two of these are associated with an increased risk of infection from bacteria and fungal infections.

This can involve organisms that are not usually pathogenic. Infection can be difficult to diagnose as there may not be the normal immune response and related clinical features. So in an immunocompromised patient with meningitis there may be a fever and malaise but without symptoms and signs of meningeal inflammation, headache and neck stiffness.

There are some types of infections that occur especially in certain patient groups, for example listeria meningitis in alcoholics, fungal infection in profoundly neutropenic patients. A wide range of neurological problems occurs in human immunodeficiency virus (HIV) infection and AIDS.

HIV infections and AIDS
Neurological complications can occur at any stage of HIV infection. At seroconversion, Guillain–Barré syndrome and facial weakness have been documented. During the asymptomatic phase of HIV infection, chronic demyelinating neuropathies may occur.

Most neurological problems in HIV infection occur as the patient develops significant immunosuppression. Opportunistic infections, tumours, specific neurological problems associated with HIV and neurological complications of the treatment of HIV infection then occur. Different levels of the nervous system are affected and are summarized in Table 1.

Toxoplasmosis
This presents with a focal neurological deficit, headache or seizures, usually developing over a few weeks (Fig. 2). Brain scanning reveals single or multiple ring-enhancing masses with oedema. As this is the most likely diagnosis in this setting, a trial of anti-toxoplasma treatment is given. Further investigation is considered if this fails. The most common differential diagnosis is primary CNS lymphoma. This can be treated with radiotherapy but the response and prognosis is poor.

Progressive multifocal leucoencephalopathy (PML)
This is an infection with JC virus, a human papilloma virus. This presents with progressive focal neurological deficits particularly affecting the occipitoparietal region. MRI demonstrates non-enhancing lesions without mass effect limited to the white matter. There are no specific treatments currently available.

Cryptococcal meningitis
This presents with headache, often with non-specific malaise, and later confusion and multiple cranial nerve palsies. CSF examination usually confirms the diagnosis with india ink staining and antigen detection. This is treated with antifungals, amphotericin B, flucytosine and fluconazole.

Cytomegalovirus
This can affect the nervous system at several levels in AIDS. It can produce an encephalitis, a myelitis, a lumbosacral polyradiculopathy and multifocal neuropathy. Ganciclovir and foscarnet are active against CMV; however, CMV encephalitis carries a poor prognosis even with treatment. Some response is seen in the other conditions.

HIV encephalopathy
This is a subacute dementing process associated with motor slowing. The patient is initially apathetic and later develops behavioural abnormalities with marked memory problems. Reflexes are brisk and there may be prominent frontal withdrawal signs. There is no specific diagnostic test, though cerebral atrophy is commonly observed on CT or MRI of the brain. The neuropathological findings are of multinucleate giant cells with myelin pallor and gliosis. The process is thought to be a direct result of HIV infection though the mechanism is uncertain. There is some suggestion that the antiretroviral agents may slow the progression.

Vacuolar myelopathy
This is a specific clinicopathological entity of uncertain aetiology, though a role for HIV seems likely. Patients develop a spastic paraparesis with prominent posterior column sensory loss.

Peripheral neuropathies
These are common in AIDS. Some distal symmetrical neuropathies are due to agents such as didanosine and zalcitabine. In others the aetiology is unknown. Mononeuritis multiplex associated with vasculitis can occur.

Infections of the nervous system II

- Epidural abscess is a rare cause of radicular pain and fever. This is a medical emergency.
- Syphilis is rare but can produce a wide range of neurological problems.
- The immunocompromised host can develop a wide range of unusual infections.
- HIV is associated with infections at every level of the CNS.

Peripheral neuropathies I: clinical approach and investigations

Peripheral neuropathies are very variable, both in their clinical manifestations and in their aetiology (Table 1). These three sections give an overview of peripheral nerve disease, with the third concentrating on the common isolated peripheral nerve lesions.

Pathology

Peripheral nerves can be affected in three ways (Fig. 1). These mechanisms of injury are not mutually exclusive and in some conditions there are contributions from all three mechanisms:

- axonal degeneration
- demyelination
- vascular nerve damage.

Axonal degeneration

The axon degenerates as a result of many different toxic, metabolic, nutritional and physical (such as cold or trauma) insults and in genetic conditions. The longest axons are most severely affected. These changes result in distal weakness, wasting or sensory loss depending on the involvement of motor and sensory fibres. If the neurone remains intact and the pathological process is reversed, there is scope for regeneration. If the neurone is lost, there is no scope for regeneration.

Demyelination

In this process the myelin is lost but the axon is preserved. The demyelination prevents conduction and produces weakness but not wasting. Repair of demyelination, remyelination, can be quick. Many demyelinating neuropathies also have some associated axonal degeneration. Demyelination can occur in inflammatory diseases, when it tends to be patchy, and in inherited or metabolic neuropathies, when it tends to be uniform.

Vascular nerve damage

The blood supply to peripheral nerves can be disrupted, producing infarcts of peripheral nerves. This then produces isolated axonal degeneration in the axons distal to the site of infarct. This usually occurs with vasculitic illness.

Clinical features

Peripheral neuropathies can be sensory or motor, though usually there is a combination with one predominant. The clinical features depend on the underlying pathological process and the speed of onset. Axonal neuropathies result in wasting of muscles with loss of distal tendon reflexes. Demyelinating neuropathies are not associated with muscle wasting, but usually there is areflexia. In some types of neuropathy the autonomic nervous system can also be affected.

There are four patterns of clinical presentation of peripheral nerve disease (Fig. 2).

- *Distal symmetrical neuropathy.* This is the most common presentation of axonal neuropathies. There is distal sensory and motor dysfunction, affecting the legs more than the arms; sensory changes in the hands are noted when sensory changes in the legs get to the knees.
- *Multifocal neuropathies.* There is an asymmetrical involvement, without involving specifically named nerves. This is usually the presentation of demyelinating or vasculitic neuropathies.
- *Mononeuropathies.* The involvement of an individual named nerve. The most commonly affected nerves are described on page 106.
- *Mononeuritis multiplex.* The involvement of multiple named nerves. This is relatively uncommon and is highly suggestive of a vasculitis.

The speed of onset can be divided into acute, less than 4 weeks, subacute, developing over 1–6 months, and chronic, developing over 6 months. This is useful in the diagnosis of aetiology.

Diagnosis and differential diagnosis

The diagnosis of a peripheral neuropathy falls into two parts.

Is it a peripheral neuropathy?

In most patients this is straightforward, presenting with one of the clinical

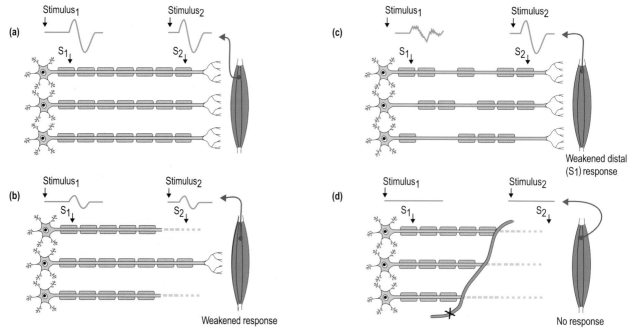

Fig. 1 **Effects on peripheral nerve conduction of common neuropathies. (a)** Normal; **(b)** axonal degeneration; **(c)** demyelination; **(d)** vascular lesion.

syndromes described above. There are a few difficult situations:

■ *Patients with an acute onset weakness of arms and legs.* The differential diagnosis here is between an acute neuropathy, usually Guillain–Barré syndrome, a cervical spinal cord or brain stem lesion, myasthenia gravis and an acute myopathy. Reflex changes, sensory findings and ancillary investigations including nerve conduction studies may be needed to clarify this. NB: The most common and dangerous erroneous differential diagnosis given in patients with acute neuropathies is hysteria.

■ *Patients with weakness and wasting in the limbs without sensory signs.* The differential diagnosis lies between a predominantly motor neuropathy and anterior horn cell disease, such as amyotrophic lateral sclerosis and a myopathy. Neurophysiology may be needed to clarify matters.

What type of peripheral neuropathy is it?
This is a good example of different levels of diagnosis. For example, the clinical diagnosis could be of a chronic distal symmetrical sensorimotor neuropathy. Neurophysiology establishes this to be an axonal neuropathy, and further investigations find this to be a distal symmetrical axonal sensorimotor neuropathy – *caused* by diabetes.

The time course and pattern of clinical presentation along with the neurophysiological disturbance give an indication of likely aetiology, which needs to be confirmed by further investigations. This is summarized in Table 1.

Investigations
The investigations will be directed by the clinical presentation. Nerve conduction studies are essential in understanding the pattern of the neuropathy. Ancillary investigations are directed at establishing associations with the syndrome or finding the aetiology.

In a patient with an acute demyelinating neuropathy, finding an acellular CSF with raised protein is further corroboration of the diagnosis of Guillain–Barré syndrome.

A patient with an axonal distal sensorimotor neuropathy without a clinical indicator of aetiology will need a screen of investigations to look for systemic and deficiency states (Table 2).

The diagnosis of certain inherited neuropathies can now be made by finding the appropriate genetic abnormality using molecular genetics (see below). In other patients in whom there is apparently no family history of neuropathy, a diagnosis can be made by examining the patient's relatives and finding other affected members.

A patient with possible vasculitic neuropathy may need a nerve biopsy if the diagnosis cannot be reached by other means. Nerve biopsy may also be helpful in patients with sarcoidosis, amyloidosis or a disabling neuropathy where the diagnosis has not been made despite extensive investigations.

Formal autonomic function tests may be helpful. Autonomic involvement is prominent in diabetic and amyloid neuropathies, rare inherited neuropathies and Guillain–Barré syndrome.

Table 1 Relationship of presentation of neuropathy to aetiology

	Neurophysiology	Acute	Subacute	Chronic
Distal symmetrical	Axonal	Toxins Porphyria	Systemic disease Deficiency states Toxins Cancer associated Amyloid	As subacute HMSN type 2
	Demyelinating	GBS Diphtheria	CIDP	HMSN type 1 CIDP
Multifocal and mononeuritis multiplex	Axonal	Vasculitis	Diabetes Sarcoidosis	Leprosy
	Demyelinating	GBS	CIDP	CIDP

HMSN, hereditary motor-sensory neuropathy; GBS, Guillain–Barré syndrome; CIDP, chronic inflammatory demyelinating polyradiculoneuropathy

Table 2 Factors associated with neuropathy

Systemic diseases associated with neuropathy
■ Diabetes mellitus
■ Cancer
■ Connective tissue diseases
■ Sarcoidosis
■ AIDS
■ Uraemia
■ Hypothyroidism
■ Critical illness polyneuropathy

Deficiency states associated with neuropathy
■ Thiamine deficiency (B1)
■ Pellagra (niacin deficiency)
■ Pyridoxine deficiency (B6)
■ Pernicious anaemia (B12 deficiency)
■ Folate deficiency
■ Vitamin E deficiency

Toxins associated with neuropathies: selected examples

■ Ethanol	*Drugs*
Industrial	■ Amiodarone
■ Arsenic	■ Cisplatinum
■ Ethylene oxide	■ Dapsone
■ Lead	■ Gold
■ Mercury	■ Isoniazid
■ Organophosphates	■ Metronidazole
■ Thalium	■ Thalidomide
	■ Vincristine

Peripheral neuropathies I: clinical approach and investigations

■ Peripheral nerve damage is either axonal, demyelination or vascular, or a combination of these.

■ Neuropathies can present with distal symmetrical loss, asymmetrical loss, mononeuropathies and, rarely, mononeuritis multiplex.

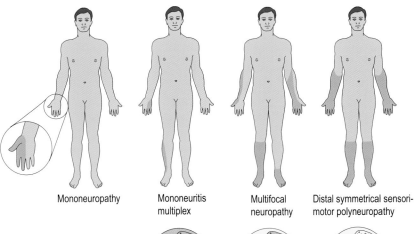

Mononeuropathy Mononeuritis multiplex Multifocal neuropathy Distal symmetrical sensori-motor polyneuropathy

Fig. 2 **Clinical patterns of peripheral nerve involvement in vasculitic neuropathies.**

Peripheral neuropathies II: clinical syndromes

Demyelinating neuropathies

Guillain–Barré syndrome

Guillain–Barré syndrome (GBS) is a monophasic, predominantly motor polyradiculopathy. It develops over days to 4 weeks and can affect limbs and cranial nerves. It can vary in severity from mild weakness to complete paralysis requiring ventilatory support in 10–20% of patients. There are mild sensory symptoms and signs. At onset, reflexes may be present with significant weakness but then soon disappear. The autonomic nervous system is variably affected, producing cardiac arrhythmias and hypo- or hypertension. Recovery begins spontaneously after a few weeks.

GBS affects all ages and occurs in 2 per 100 000 per year. About 70% of patients have a history of antecedent infection: best established are *Campylobacter jejuni*, cytomegalovirus and Epstein–Barr virus.

Diagnosis is primarily clinical with support from neurophysiological studies and a finding of acellular CSF with raised protein. There are some patients whose neurophysiological findings indicate an axonal degeneration, the 'acute axonal' form of GBS, which more commonly follows *Campylobacter* infection.

Management consists of support and specific measures to shorten the illness. It is essential to monitor patients closely with regular measurements of vital capacity (VC) and looking for evidence of autonomic dysfunction. Patients with a VC below 1 litre require ventilation. Close attention to pressure areas, prophylaxis against venous thrombosis, and chest and limb physiotherapy are important in these vulnerable patients.

Neuralgic pain can be treated with pain-modulating agents. Communication aids will be needed in paralysed patients. Helping the patient to understand their predicament and providing psychological support is important.

Two treatments have been found to shorten the course of disease. Plasma exchange and intravenous immunoglobulin will both shorten the illness to a similar degree. Both are more effective the sooner they are given (< 2 weeks). They should be given to patients who cannot walk and are chair- or bed-bound.

The mortality rate is about 5%. Twenty per cent of patients have a continuing motor deficit at 1 year and 3% have a recurrence. The axonal form has a slower and less complete recovery.

The Miller Fisher variant is a rare association of areflexia, ophthalmoplegia and ataxia, and is associated with a specific antiganglioside antibody GQ1b.

Chronic inflammatory demyelinating polyradiculopathy

This is a chronic form of GBS and is considerably rarer. There are two forms: progressive and relapsing. It is responsive to steroids as well as plasma exchange and immunoglobulins. It may be associated with monoclonal gammopathy of uncertain significance.

Axonal neuropathies

Diabetic neuropathies

Diabetes mellitus is the most common cause of neuropathies in the western world. About 15% of patients with diabetes have symptomatic neuropathies, the proportion increasing with duration of disease. Subclinical abnormalities in neurophysiological studies are almost universal after 10 years of diabetes. There are several patterns of peripheral neuropathy in diabetes.

Distal symmetrical neuropathy accounts for 75% of diabetic neuropathies; it occurs more commonly in diabetics with poor glycaemic control and its frequency can be reduced (but not abolished) by tight control. This is predominantly sensory, with parallel autonomic involvement. Some patients have painful paraesthesiae; others simply have numbness. The sensory loss combined with poor circulation can lead to foot ulcers and, on occasion, neuropathic arthropathies (Charcot's

joints). Treatment is improved glycaemic control and symptomatic support.

Asymmetrical proximal neuropathy has a whole range of synonyms, including diabetic amyotrophy or lumbosacral radiculoplexopathy. This presents with asymmetrical painful proximal weakness of the proximal muscles in the legs. It usually occurs in patients with non-insulin-dependent diabetes who have poor glycaemic control and have lost weight. Most patients improve once started on insulin with improved control.

Autonomic neuropathy can occur in association with sensory neuropathy or in relative isolation. The whole range of autonomic failure occurs with postural hypotension, a resting tachycardia, delayed gastric emptying with nausea and vomiting, intermittent diarrhoea and constipation, loss of bladder tone with retention and overflow, impotence and disordered sweating. Treatment is symptomatic (p. 114).

Mononeuropathies and radiculopathies. Isolated peripheral nerve lesions, particularly carpal tunnel, are more common in diabetics. Isolated thoracic radiculopathies also occur and can mimic intra-abdominal disease.

Other systemic diseases

Distal symmetrical axonal neuropathies are seen in a range of other systemic illnesses (Table 1), including hypothyroidism, uraemia, rheumatoid arthritis and systemic lupus erythematosus. The connective tissue diseases can also cause vasculitic neuropathies.

Nutritional deficiencies. Patients with nutritional deficiencies (Table 2, p. 103) often have more than one vitamin deficiency. This can be associated with other problems such as alcoholism, in which the major factor is nutritional deficiency. The clinical presentation is of a painful, predominantly sensory distal symmetrical axonal neuropathy. Treatment is with appropriate vitamins. Vitamin B12 deficiency is more complicated because there is often an associated myelopathy (subacute combined degeneration of the cord). In the full syndrome there is a progressive paraparesis, with loss of proprioception, prominent distal paraesthesiae and associated dementia. Vitamin B12 measurement and the demonstration of antiparietal cell

Table 1	**Types of peripheral neuropathy**
Systemic	
Metabolic	Diabetes, etc.
Toxic	Neurotoxins, ETOH, etc.
Nutritional	Vitamin B12
Extrinsic	
Entrapment mononeuropathies	
Intrinsic	
Metabolic	Refsum's disease, etc.
Immunological	Demyelinating: Guillain–Barré syndrome, chronic inflammatory demyelinating polyradiculoneuropathy
	Vasculitis
Neoplastic	Monoclonal band
Degenerative	Axonal neuropathies
Infectious	Leprosy
Genetic	Hereditary motor and sensory neuropathy, etc.

antibodies and malabsorption of vitamin B12 give a diagnosis.

Toxic neuropathies. Most toxic neuropathies produce a sensorimotor distal symmetrical peripheral neuropathy. Exceptions include lead, which produces a predominantly motor neuropathy. Other signs may point to a particular toxin, e.g. alopecia in thallium poisoning.

Neuropathies associated with neoplasias. Neoplasia can involve the peripheral nerves directly, by nerve invasion or malignant meningitis, or indirectly as a paraneoplastic phenomenon. Direct involvement of the nerves occurs more commonly in lymphoma. Paraneoplastic neuropathies are usually symmetrical distal sensorimotor axonal neuropathies. They occur in about 1% of cancer patients. The whole range of neuropathies are seen as a paraneoplastic phenomenon, though are much rarer.

Infective neuropathies. Leprosy is estimated to affect 12 million people in the developing world. The pattern of peripheral nerve involvement depends on the type of leprosy. In tuberculoid leprosy, where the host reaction predominates with few organisms (paucibacillary), there is marked nerve thickening and a mononeuritis multiplex presentation. In lepromatous

leprosy, with poor host reaction and high number of organisms (multibacillary), there is superficial sensory neuritis, particularly affecting the cooler parts of the body. Typically there are areas of anaesthetic depigmented skin. Intermediate patterns are seen. Treatment is with dapsone and rifampicin. Steroids may also be required to prevent host-mediated tissue damage. Lyme disease, caused by *Borrelia burgdorferi*, is endemic in parts of the USA. Early involvement can affect the facial nerve, radiculopathies or a lymphocytic meningitis. Later, patients can present with a distal symmetrical neuropathy.

AIDS. Several different patterns of neuropathies are associated with HIV infection and AIDS. These are discussed on page 101.

Inherited neuropathies. These neuropathies present as distal symmetrical neuropathies. They are very insidious in onset and there are usually relatively minor symptoms with much more marked signs. In particular, positive sensory symptoms such as paraesthesiae are unusual. Signs such as pes cavus, indicating that abnormalities were present before fusion of the bony epiphyses, may also be found.

Hereditary motor and sensory neuropathies (HMSN) are the most commonly inherited neuropathies. These were previously referred to as Charcot–Marie–Tooth (CMT) disease. The classification is primarily into the demyelinating form (HMSN type 1) and the axonal form (HMSN type 2). HMSN 1 usually presents before age of 30 years and is associated with peripheral nerve hypertrophy. HMSN 2 can present later and patients are usually less severely affected. In both forms of HMSN there is a preferential atrophy of the peroneal muscles to produce the 'inverted champagne bottle' legs (Fig. 1). The genetic basis for some of these has been elucidated (Table 2). There are some forms of HMSN 1 and all forms of HMSN 2 in which the

genetic basis has not been established. Interestingly, a much rarer condition of hereditary liability to pressure palsies has been found to be due to different mutations in the same gene as HMSN 1a.

Rarer hereditary neuropathies. The genetic basis for most forms of familial amyloid polyneuropathies has been determined. These sensorimotor axonal neuropathies with autonomic involvement result from mutations in transthyretin or gelosolin, which result in deposition of amyloid in several tissues, including peripheral nerve. DNA analysis is now the diagnostic method of choice in these patients.

Vasculitic neuropathies

These usually occur in the setting of systemic vasculitic disease such as Wegener's granulomatosis, polyarteritis nodosa, rheumatoid arthritis or Sjögren's syndrome. The diagnosis is made histologically with serological support. Treatment is of the underlying disorder. The previously poor prognosis has improved with the aggressive immunosuppressive regimens now used. Rarely, vasculitis can be restricted to the peripheral nerve, so-called non-systemic vasculitis. This has a better prognosis.

Neuralgic amyotrophy (also called brachial neuritis)

This is an uncommon idiopathic condition. It often occurs after an infection, particularly a vaccination, and begins with severe neuralgic pain in one arm. This is followed by some weakness and, after a few weeks, the pain eases and the patient notices muscle wasting. Typically it affects muscles of the shoulder girdle, particularly serratus anterior, leading to winging of the scapulae, though any muscles in the arm can be affected. There is usually little sensory loss, involving the lateral aspect of the upper arm. The main differential diagnosis is cervical radiculopathies, which usually affect only one root. There is no specific treatment and strength usually returns in 1–3 years.

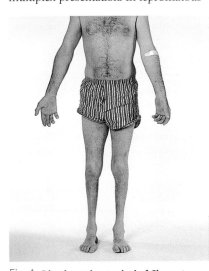

Fig. 1 **Distal wasting typical of Charcot–Marie–Tooth disease.**

Table 2 **Summary of the molecular genetics of hereditary neuropathies**

	Inheritance	Pathology	Chromosome	Gene product
HMSN 1a	AD	Demyelinating	17p	PMP-22
HMSN 1b	AD	Demyelinating	1q	PO
HMSN 1	AD/AR	Demyelinating	?	?
HMSN 2	AD/AR	Axonal	?	?
HLPP	AD	Demyelinating	17p	PMP-22

HMSN, hereditary motor and sensory neuropathy; PMP-22, peripheral myelin protein 22; HLPP, hereditary liability to pressure palsies; AD, autosomal dominant; AR, autosomal recessive

Peripheral neuropathies II: clinical syndromes

- Guillain–Barré syndrome is an important treatable cause of acute generalized neuropathy.
- Diabetes mellitus is the most common cause of axonal neuropathies in the western world.
- A large number of toxins can produce neuropathy.
- Leprosy is a common cause of neuropathy in underdeveloped countries.
- Inherited neuropathies can often be diagnosed using newer genetic techniques.

Common peripheral nerve lesions

Peripheral nerves can be affected in isolation, so-called mononeuropathies. However, only a few peripheral nerves are involved frequently. The commonly involved nerves are usually affected by entrapment at sites of vulnerability. This can be exacerbated by conditions that render the nerves more susceptible, for example diabetes and hereditary liability to pressure palsies. Isolated mononeuropathies can rarely be the onset of mononeuritis multiplex (see above).

The types of nerve injury are given in Table 1. Injuries are usually a combination of neuropraxias with some axonotmesis.

Median nerve

This is the most commonly affected nerve, with the median nerve being compressed at the wrist in the carpal tunnel. The nerve is rarely affected elsewhere. Carpal tunnel syndrome occurs in 10% of women during pregnancy, resolving postpartum. It is associated with rheumatoid arthritis, hypothyroidism, diabetes, acromegaly and myeloma. Most cases are idiopathic.

It commonly presents between 40 and 60 years of age, more often in women. The dominant hand is usually affected first. Initially patients are awoken with tingling and pain in the hand, which they characteristically shake on waking 'like a wet fish'. Later they notice tingling or numbness during the day. They may start dropping things and note some weakness of grip. If severely affected, they may notice wasting of the abductor pollicis brevis (APB) (Fig. 1a).

On examination there may be wasting or weakness of the APB. Sensory changes of varying degrees are found within the median nerve distribution (Fig. 1b). Additional tests include Tinel's test (percussion of the nerve to provoke paraesthesiae in the median nerve distribution) and Phelan's test (dorsiflexing the wrist for 30–60 s). However, there are significant doubts about the sensitivity and specificity of these tests.

Diagnosis is made definitively with nerve conduction studies. The differential diagnosis includes C6 root lesions or more central sensory abnormalities.

Conservative treatment using wrist splints, corticosteroid injections into

Table 1 **Types of nerve injury**		
Type of nerve injury	**Structural changes**	**Rate of recovery**
Neuropraxia	Myelin damage, axon intact	2–12 weeks
Axonotmesis	Loss of axonal continuity, epineurium intact	Regeneration at 1 mm/day from site of lesion
Neurotmesis	Entire nerve trunk separated	No regeneration unless nerve repaired; then 1 mm/day

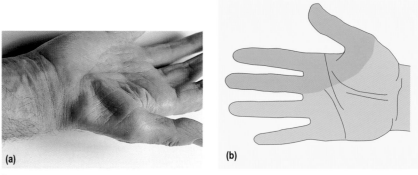

Fig. 1 **Median nerve. (a)** Wasting of abductor pollicis brevis; **(b)** sensory loss of median nerve lesions.

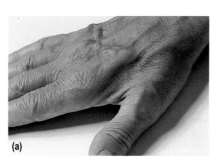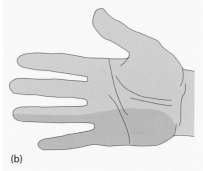

Fig. 2 **Ulnar nerve. (a)** Wasting of interossei; **(b)** sensory loss of ulnar nerve lesions.

the carpal tunnel and diuretics is usually successful in mild cases. More severe cases need surgical decompression of the carpal tunnel at the wrist.

Ulnar nerve

Ulnar nerve lesions usually occur at the elbow, though occasionally they can occur in the hand as the nerve passes the hook of the hamate in Guyon's canal. Bony deformity at the elbow or external pressure are the usual causes.

Numbness and tingling in the little and ring finger and a more diffuse arm pain are the common presentation. The patient may be aware of weakness in the hand. On examination there may be weakness and wasting in the

interossei (Fig. 2a), with weakness of the long flexors of the little and ring fingers. Sensory loss may be demonstrated in the ulnar nerve distribution (Fig. 2b).

Definitive diagnosis depends again on nerve conduction studies. The differential diagnosis of the unilateral wasted hand includes T1 lesions, in which all hand muscles are affected and the sensory loss is in the axilla. If hand wasting is bilateral, the differential diagnosis includes amyotrophic lateral sclerosis (p. 108), more generalized neuropathies (especially HMSN, p. 105) and, very rarely, syringomyelia.

The management depends on severity and aetiology. Following external compression, conservative treatment and

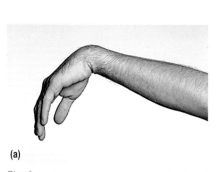

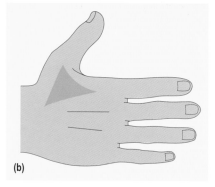

Fig. 3 **Radial nerve. (a)** Finger and wrist drop; **(b)** sensory loss of radial nerve lesions.

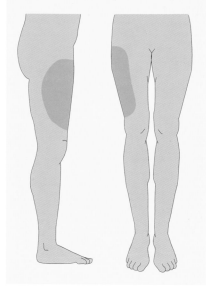

Fig. 5 **Sensory loss of lateral cutaneous nerve of the thigh.**

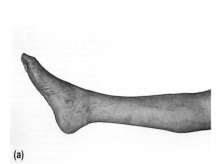

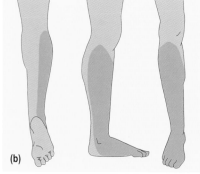

Fig. 4 **Common peroneal nerve. (a)** Foot and toe drop; **(b)** sensory loss of common peroneal nerve lesions.

back pain, and they involve foot inversion.

Treatment depends on aetiology in a similar way to the ulnar nerve. A foot drop splint helps function.

Lateral cutaneous nerve of the thigh (meralgia paraesthetica)

Lesions of this nerve are very common. Patients notice an area of burning or numbness on the outer aspect of the thigh (Fig. 5). A large number of possible causes have been cited with limited evidence, weight change being amongst the most common. This is usually a self-limiting condition and requires no investigation.

Other mononeuropathies

The long thoracic nerve can be affected, producing winging of the scapula. The femoral nerve can be affected, producing weakness and wasting of the quadriceps, with sensory loss on the inner aspect of the thigh.

avoidance of further compression is effective. If the nerve is significantly affected and there is evidence of abnormalities at the elbow, then surgical decompression or transposition can be effective.

Radial nerve

Radial nerve lesions commonly result from compression of the radial nerve against the humerus in the upper arm and usually occur during deep sleep or unconsciousness, for example after an alcoholic binge ('Saturday night palsy'). There is usually a striking weakness in the wrist and finger extensors (Fig. 3). The triceps and brachioradialis are less markedly affected. The triceps reflex is occasionally impaired. There is limited sensory disturbance with a small area of sensory loss at the base of the thumb. Even though the weakness is limited to the extensors of the fingers the patient feels the whole hand is useless. It is important to examine finger abduction and adduction and APB with the hand placed flat (e.g. on a table) and the fingers extended.

The diagnosis can be confirmed neurophysiologically but is usually

clinical. The differential diagnosis includes a C7 radiculopathy and brachial plexus lesions. The sensory abnormality is usually the easiest way to distinguish these.

Most patients improve spontaneously, the speed of recovery depending on the severity of the nerve injury. A lively splint is helpful in improving hand function during recovery.

Common peroneal nerve

The common peroneal nerve is vulnerable as it runs around the fibula head. This can be injured by external pressure (coma, plaster casts, carpet laying, leg crossing), trauma and entrapment in the fibular tunnel. The presentation is of foot drop (Fig. 4a). There may be wasting of tibialis anterior, with weakness of dorsiflexion, toe extension and foot eversion with preservation of foot inversion. The sensory loss is illustrated in Figure 4b.

The differential diagnosis is L5 radiculopathies and more proximal sciatic nerve lesions. These disorders usually have other features to help distinguish them, for example, low

---

Common peripheral nerve lesions

■ Mononeuropathies are common.

■ Mononeuropathies tend to involve nerves at characteristic sites of increased vulnerability.

■ Recovery depends on the type of nerve injury.

Disorders of the motor neurone

The motor neurone, or anterior horn cell, lies in the anterior horn of the spinal cord. Its axon extends to the muscle and is the final common pathway for motor output. Disorders of the motor neurone are uncommon.

Motor neurone disease

The most common disease is motor neurone disease (MND), referred to as amyotrophic lateral sclerosis (ALS) or Lou Gehrig's disease in the USA. The annual incidence is 1 per 100 000 of population. MND usually affects adults aged over 50 years, the risk increasing with increasing age, but occasionally younger adults may be affected. About 5% of cases may be familial and in some of these a genetic abnormality of the enzyme superoxide dismutase (SOD 1, a free radical scavenger) has been identified. The aetiology of the sporadic cases is unknown, but a toxic role has been postulated for the excitatory amino acid neurotransmitter glutamate. Other diseases of the motor neurone are now rare but poliomyelitis was common and its sequelae are still seen.

Pathology

There is degeneration of the motor cortex and anterior horns of the spinal cord with chromatolysis of the motor neurones, which may contain inclusion bodies, and degeneration of the corticospinal tracts and peripheral motor axons.

Clinical features

There are three main patterns of disease (Fig. 1). All are progressive and evolve at different rates. They overlap significantly and in the late stages tend to merge into a diffuse, combined upper motor neurone (UMN) and lower motor neurone (LMN) disorder. The differential diagnosis depends on the pattern of presentation. Sensation must be normal to make the diagnosis. The overall prognosis is poor; death is usually due to respiratory complications from bulbar or respiratory muscle weakness.

Amyotrophic lateral sclerosis

This commonly presents with stiffness and weakness of the hands, muscle cramps and discomfort. In some cases onset may be proximal, resembling a plexopathy or with foot drop, simulating

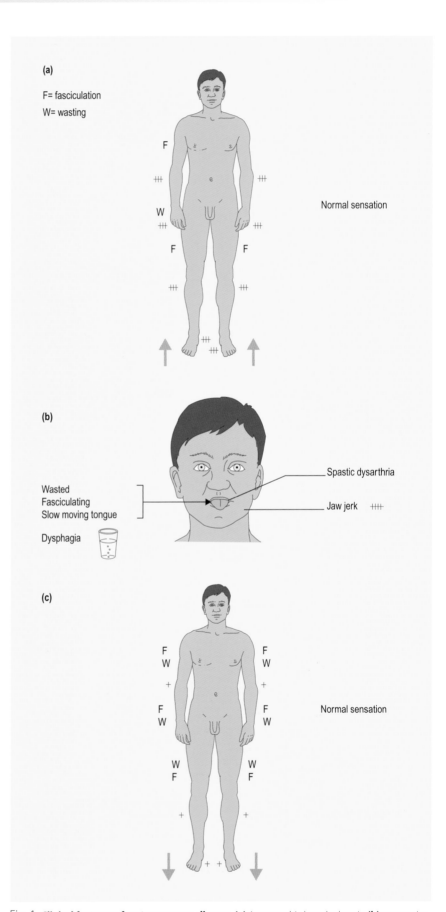

Fig. 1 **Clinical features of motor neurone disease. (a)** Amyotrophic lateral sclerosis; **(b)** progressive bulbar palsy; **(c)** progressive muscular atrophy.

peroneal nerve palsy. Over the following months, more widespread, patchy weakness appears that may affect any muscle, except the extraocular muscles. Weakness becomes more diffuse and spreads to the truncal and bulbar muscles. The hands appear severely wasted and there are often fasciculations in the interossei and sometimes other muscle groups. It may be necessary to observe the patient's trunk and limb muscles for 30 s or more in order to see the fasciculations. Tone is usually normal and weakness is initially patchy. Despite wasting, reflexes are brisk and plantar responses usually become extensor during the disease. The most common differential diagnosis is cervical myeloradiculopathy, sometimes with additional lumbar radiculopathy.

Fifty per cent of patients die within 3 years and 90% by 6 years.

Progressive bulbar palsy

This presents with progressive dysarthria until speech becomes unintelligible. Swallowing becomes difficult and patients spend hours trying to eat each day. They lose weight rapidly and suffer repeated aspiration pneumonia. Emotional lability is common in this form and 10% of patients develop dementia later in the course of the illness. The tongue is usually wasted and fasciculating but moves stiffly, suggesting spasticity. The facial muscles sag and the jaw jerk and facial jerks are brisk. Although 25% of MND presents with this form, most patients later develop limb involvement. The differential diagnosis includes myasthenia gravis, brain stem lesions, cerebrovascular disease, multiple sclerosis and X-linked bulbospinal neuronopathy (see below). Most patients with this form of MND die within 3 years.

Progressive muscular atrophy

This is the rarest form. There is slowly progressive wasting, which is usually symmetrical in both hands. This progresses to more proximal muscles and to the legs over several years. Fasciculations may be present but there are no UMN signs. The differential diagnosis includes other LMN disorders: multifocal motor neuropathy with conduction block, inherited spinal muscular atrophy and post-polio syndrome (see below). Prognosis is best in patients aged under 50 years, with 72% surviving 5 years.

Investigations

There is no single test for MND. Investigations can exclude other causes and support the diagnosis but do not confirm it. Normal nerve conduction studies are used to exclude a neuropathy and electromyography to confirm denervation and show fasciculations in muscles not thought to be affected clinically. MRI may be needed to exclude other causes, depending on the site of clinical involvement: brain for bulbar symptoms and neck for LMN arm features. An MRI brain scan may show corticospinal degeneration.

Treatment

Treatment is supportive and involves most of the paramedical disciplines: physiotherapy (to optimize function, the best use of walking aids, and to advise about positioning); occupational therapy (to optimize the patient's environment); nursing; and speech therapy (to advise about swallowing and provide communication aids). Psychological support for the patient and relatives is important in a difficult, relentlessly progressive disease. Depression is common and can be treated.

Some drug therapy and other medical interventions are useful. Spasticity can be treated with baclofen. Patients with bulbar involvement may benefit from percutaneous insertion of a gastrostomy tube, which is a simple procedure allowing direct enteral feeding to maintain nutrition and reduce the risk of aspiration pneumonia. Some patients with respiratory weakness but otherwise good function may benefit from nocturnal or diurnal respiratory support. This is a delicate, individual decision as patients will continue to deteriorate and the respiratory support may prolong an unsatisfactory quality of life.

Riluzole, a glutamate antagonist, has been shown to improve 18 month survival by 7%, a small but statistically significant benefit.

Polio and post-polio syndrome

Poliomyelitis is due to an RNA virus and usually occurs in childhood. Occasional cases occur in this country after travel abroad or in susceptible adults who change the nappies of babies after they have received oral, live attenuated virus polio vaccine. The disease starts with a mild upper respiratory tract infection and may evolve into meningitis and encephalitis. In some of these cases severe weakness may develop over 24 h affecting any pattern of muscles. Affected muscles become markedly atrophic and do not recover. Subsequent skeletal development is impaired and the typical post-polio limb is flaccid and small. Years later the weakness of the limb may progress. The reason for this is unclear, but probably reflects anterior cell loss due to ageing from a severely depleted population of cells.

Inherited diseases of upper and lower motor neurones

Various rare conditions may include features of UMN and LMN disease. Those most likely to be confused with MND are:

- *Spinal muscular atrophies.* These present with pure LMN disorders. Inheritance is variable and there are three forms: rapidly fatal infantile (Werdnig–Hoffman syndrome), and slowly progressive juvenile (Kugelberg–Welander syndrome) or adult onsets. They are allelic variants of the same gene.
- *Hereditary spastic paraparesis* (usually autosomal dominant). This presents with spasticity of the legs. The arms are stronger, often with compensatory hypertrophy.
- *Adrenoleucodystrophy* (X-linked recessive). This presents with mixed UMN and LMN disease and mild adrenal insufficiency.
- *X-linked bulbospinal neuronopathy.* This presents with bulbar palsy, pronounced action-induced fasciculations, diabetes, gynaecomastia, infertility and mild neuropathy. It is due to a defect of the androgen receptor and has a much better prognosis than MND.

Disorders of the motor neurone

- Motor neurone disease is characterized by progressive upper and lower motor neurone signs with normal sensation.
- There are three main patterns of disease with each different differential diagnosis.
- There is no single diagnostic test for MND.
- Treatment is mainly supportive.

Disorders of the neuromuscular junction

Disorders of the neuromuscular junction (NMJ) are uncommon. The most common is myasthenia gravis (MG), with an annual incidence of 1 per 100 000 and a prevalence of 8–15 per 100 000. There is a bimodal age of onset, affecting young adults, especially females aged 15–30 years, and predominantly males aged 50–70 years. It is important to diagnose MG as it is a dangerous illness that is very amenable to treatment. Other rare disorders of the NMJ are shown in Table 1.

Table 1 Other rare disorders of the neuromuscular junction

Disorder	Mode of action	Comments
Neonatal MG (born to mothers with MG)	Autoimmune, as MG	Hypotonia starts by third day and persists until antibodies leave the baby's system, 2–12 weeks
Congenital myasthenia	Non-autoimmune	MG-type eye and facial weakness, responds poorly to treatment
Botulism (canned food is the usual source)	Botulinum toxin blocks acetylcholine release	Typically acute onset with muscarinic features, e.g. tachycardia and pupil dilatation, as well as weakness. Recently been seen in i.v. drug users
Organophosphate (insecticide) poisoning	Irreversible inhibition of cholinesterase	Presents with cholinergic crisis and confusion. Treatment: atropine for muscarinic effects, ventilatory support, pralidoxime 'releases' cholinesterase
Pseudocholinesterase deficiency	Unable to break down suxamethonium	Prolonged postoperative paralysis due to persisting NMJ block, supportive therapy only required
Snake venom	Alpha-bungarotoxin binds acetylcholine receptor	Long-lasting weakness as binding is irreversible

MG, myasthenia gravis; NMJ, neuromuscular junction

Myasthenia gravis

Pathophysiology

MG is an organ-specific autoimmune disease, with antibodies directed against the acetylcholine receptor. These antibodies compete with acetylcholine released by the nerve terminal, interfering with neuromuscular transmission (Fig. 1). Thymic hyperplasia occurs in 65% of patients, most commonly in young adults. Thymic tumours occur in 15% of patients, usually older men, and 25% of these tumours are malignant, with local invasion; the tumours need treatment in their own right. Antibodies to striated muscle are found in nearly 50% of later-onset patients and 84% of those with thymic tumours. The thymus appears to be important in the pathogenesis of the disease, but its exact role is unclear. Rarely, MG may be due to the drug penicillamine.

Symptoms and signs (Fig. 2)

The cardinal symptom of MG is *variable* muscle weakness. Usually it is possible to elicit a history of *fatiguability*; the more a muscle is used, the weaker it becomes. The distribution of muscle weakness is different from most other conditions: eye movements, eyelids, facial, neck, bulbar and proximal arm muscles, with relative sparing of the lower limbs. Respiratory muscles are commonly affected. Fifty per cent of patients present with ptosis or diplopia and these muscles are affected eventually in over 90%. Typically, diplopia and ptosis develop through the day but have gone the next morning after a night's rest.

The duration of mild symptoms may be months or, rarely, years before the patient comes to medical attention or there may be a sudden *myasthenic crisis*, with bulbar or respiratory failure, precipitated by intercurrent infection or drugs.

In 15% of patients the symptoms remain restricted to the eyes (ocular myasthenia) and in 85% they become generalized, 85% of these within the first year. Acute fulminating myasthenia with respiratory crises is seen more commonly in older patients with thymoma.

In MG, muscle appearance, tone, reflexes and sensation are normal. In mild cases, power may be normal until the muscles are fatigued (Box 1). More commonly there is clear weakness. Typically the defective eye movements of myasthenia do not correspond to any single nerve lesion but MG may mimic any pattern of deficit, including internuclear ophthalmoplegia.

Box 1

Clinical tests for fatiguability

- *Eyes*: maintain upgaze for 30 s and watch for eyelids and eyes to drift down.
- *Bulbar*: observe speech for dysarthria developing in prolonged conversation, ask the patient to count.
- *Arms*: compare shoulder abduction on two sides. Rest one arm and get the patient to abduct the other 20 times, like a chicken flapping its wing, then recompare abduction.

Differential diagnosis

The differential diagnosis includes:

- other causes of ptosis and abnormal eye movements, especially chronic progressive external ophthalmoplegia, midbrain lesions and Guillain–Barré syndrome (Miller Fisher syndrome)
- other causes of bulbar failure: brain stem lesions and motor neurone disease
- other neuromuscular junction disorders (see below).

Investigations

Investigations are directed at confirming the diagnosis and identifying associated thymus disease.

Antibodies directed against the acetylcholine receptor are detectable in the serum of 60% of patients with only ocular symptoms and 85–90% of patients with more widespread symptoms. Titres tend to be highest in patients with thymoma but do not correlate with disease severity.

Electromyography (EMG) may show typical changes of decrement on repetitive stimulation and increased jitter on single-fibre EMG.

The *edrophonium test* involves the use of edrophonium, which is a short-acting cholinesterase inhibitor. It increases acetylcholine availability and therefore overcomes NMJ blockade for 2–3 min and may reverse the signs of MG. The test carries two major risks:

- overactivity at cardiac muscarinic receptors, which may cause dangerous bradycardia
- when testing, if MG patients are undertreated or overtreated, it may tip overtreated patients into respiratory failure.

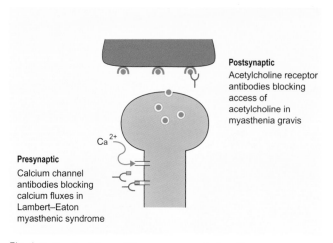

Fig. 1 **Pathophysiology at the neuromuscular junction.**

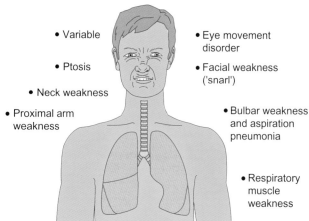

Fig. 2 **Clinical features of myasthenia gravis.**

The tests should only be done where there are resuscitation facilities available. Predosing with atropine reduces the complications. A CT or MRI scan of the thorax can be used for thymoma or thymic hyperplasia.

Treatment

Symptomatic therapy

Cholinesterase inhibitors (pyridostigmine or neostigmine) slow the breakdown of acetylcholine, increasing its availability at the NMJ and overcoming antibody-induced block. Adverse effects are (1) increased muscarinic activity, especially diarrhoea, which may be treated with antimuscarinic drugs such as atropine or propantheline; and (2) *cholinergic crisis*: overtreatment causes increased weakness with prominent muscarinic effects, which may be erroneously diagnosed as the much more common myasthenic crisis (undertreatment). The differentiation may be made by an edrophonium test, with full resuscitation facilities available (see above) and should probably be left to experienced neurologists.

Immune therapy

Immunosuppression to reduce production of the abnormal antibody is required in most cases of generalized myasthenia. Corticosteroids are used, which occasionally produce a paradoxical deterioration in the condition in the first 7–10 days of treatment – patients should be monitored closely. Azathioprine has a steroid-sparing effect but takes months to work.

If the patient is acutely unwell, intravenous immunoglobulin or plasmapheresis may prevent the need for ventilatory support, probably by washing out the abnormal antibodies. It is also effective in apparently antibody-negative patients.

The role of thymectomy in the control of myasthenia remains contentious. Most authorities advocate thymectomy in young patients, increasing the chance of disease remission from 30 to 40% in 3 years. In patients over 40 years old, thymectomy should probably be performed only if thymic enlargement is demonstrated. Thymic tumours need treatment in their own right.

Drugs to avoid

Some drugs interfere with neuromuscular transmission and may precipitate a myasthenic crisis. Sedative drugs may reduce the respiratory drive to critical levels in at-risk patients. Also to be avoided are calcium-channel blockers, beta-blockers, aminoglycoside antibiotics and erythromycin, benzodiazepines and curare-type muscle relaxants. Perioperative care for any intercurrent illness needs to be planned carefully.

Supportive therapy

MG may cause sudden bulbar or respiratory failure. Forced vital capacity (FVC) should be monitored every hour in patients at risk. An FVC below 2 litres is borderline; below 1.5 litres, ventilation may be needed. Bulbar failure may cause aspiration pneumonia and nasogastric feeding may be required temporarily during severe exacerbations.

Prognosis

With modern treatment, most patients can be returned to normal life, but treatment is usually very long term.

Lambert–Eaton myasthenic syndrome (LEMS)

This rare disorder usually affects men. It occurs alone or in association with carcinoma of lung, breast, prostate, stomach or lymphoma. LEMS is due to antibodies to presynaptic voltage-gated calcium channels, which lead to reduced release of acetylcholine from the presynaptic terminal (Fig. 1). There is often a mild coexisting neuropathy.

Patients present with subacute proximal weakness, and sensory and autonomic disturbances, especially a dry mouth. Bulbar and ocular muscles are rarely affected. With effort, strength may improve and the reflexes may increase. EMG shows low-amplitude muscle action potentials and an increment at high stimulation frequencies (in contrast to the decrement of MG). Single-fibre EMG shows increased jitter. Antivoltage-gated calcium channel antibodies can be measured.

Treatment is with guanidine or 3, 4-diaminopyridine. Immunosuppression and plasmapheresis may help some cases.

Disorders of the neuromuscular junction

- MG is a dangerous, but treatable autoimmune disease, associated with thymus disorders.
- Patients present with fatiguable muscle weakness, especially affecting the eyes and bulbar muscles.
- Treatment is with cholinesterase inhibitors and immune suppression.
- Some drugs and intercurrent illness can cause a myasthenic crisis.

Muscle disease

Primary muscle disease is relatively uncommon (prevalence 12 per 100 000) and may be inherited or acquired. This is an area in neurology where the recent rapid developments in molecular genetics are providing new insights into the molecular basis of muscle disease. This is also leading to developments in the classification of muscle disease, for example the channelopathies.

Inherited diseases include:

- *Progressive muscular dystrophies causing progressive weakness.* The patterns of inheritance, age of onset, patterns of muscular involvement and prognoses differ according to type.
- *Metabolic myopathies* may produce progressive deficits, e.g. most mitochondrial myopathies, or intermittent, particularly exertional symptoms, e.g. McArdle's disease.
- *Non-progressive congenital myopathies* present at various ages and may be mild to severe. Examples include central core, myotubular and nemaline myopathies. All are rare.
- *Myotonic syndromes* are characterized by impaired muscle relaxation after contraction, sometimes with muscle weakness.
- *Syndromes of episodic weakness or periodic paralysis* due to disorders of ion channels in the muscle membranes.

Muscular dystrophies

The most common inherited muscle disease is X-linked recessive Duchenne muscular dystrophy (DMD), which affects 1 in 3300 live male births. Thirty per cent of female carriers may be mildly to moderately affected. In DMD there is absence of dystrophin, a protein involved in linking the sarcolemma with actin molecules involved in contraction. This is thought to cause breaks in the membrane during muscle contraction. In Becker muscular dystrophy (BMD), dystrophin is present but abnormal.

Boys with DMD develop weakness of the lower limb girdle by the age of 3–6 years. They adopt the Gower manoeuvre to rise from lying (Fig. 1). Weakness then spreads to other muscle groups in the legs and arms. There may be characteristic rubbery enlargement (pseudohypertrophy) of the calf muscles and 30% have a low IQ. Most are wheelchair-bound by the age of 12 years and die from respiratory complications by the age of 25 years.

Table 1	**Patterns of muscular dystrophies**				
Condition	**Inheritance**	**Age of onset**	**Clinical features**		**Prognosis**
Facioscapulohumeral	Autosomal dominant	10–40	Mild facial weakness with preserved eye movements. Winged scapula and weak biceps, triceps. Preserved deltoid. Legs have minor involvement only		Good
Limb girdle	Autosomal dominant	10–30	Affects limb girdles but spares face. Mild involvement		Good
Emery–Dreifuss	X-linked recessive	4–5	Shoulder girdle and anterior legs. Contractures early and severe		Variable
Oculopharyngeal	Autosomal dominant	30–40	Progressive ptosis, facial weakness and dysphagia. Limbs affected late		Generally good

Investigations include muscle creatine kinase (CK), which is highly elevated, and muscle biopsy, which shows no fibres staining for dystrophin. An ECG is often abnormal. Treatment is supportive, especially prevention of complications, including respiratory infection and contractures. BMD follows a milder course with an onset at age 5–45 years; there is also calf pseudohypertrophy and a highly elevated CK, 20–200 times normal. Other dystrophies are described in Table 1; some have been identified as affecting proteins closely linked with dystrophin.

Metabolic myopathies

These rare disorders may affect carbohydrate or lipid metabolism. The enzyme defects can often be identified on muscle biopsy but these may require specialized studies. Three types of symptom occur:

- Cramps and muscle fatigue, particularly related to exertion: some during exertion, others following. In severe episodes there may be myoglobinuria, which can lead to renal failure. McArdle's disease (myophosphorylase deficiency) and carnitine palmityl transferase deficiency can present this way.
- Generalized, particularly proximal weakness that is slowly progressive. Acid maltase deficiency and mitochondrial myopathies can present this way, the latter with external ocular muscle weakness.
- Symptoms and signs from other organ involvement. This can reflect consequences of the metabolic disturbance in other tissues, for example hepatomegaly in glycogen storage diseases and deafness in mitochondrial diseases or generalized effects such as lactic acidosis in mitochondrial disease.

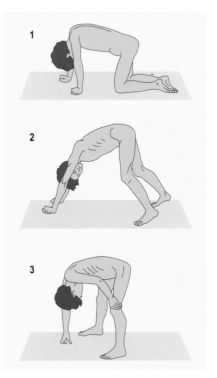

Fig. 1 **Gower's manoeuvre.**

Myotonic syndromes

Myotonic syndromes cause stiffness, limitation of movement and sometimes weakness. Typically, contractions can be provoked by cold and by direct muscle stimulation, e.g. percussion. There is a characteristic EMG pattern of discharges, which, through a loudspeaker, sounds like a dive-bomber. Hypothyroidism may mimic myotonia.

Dystrophia myotonica is the most common cause (prevalence 2 per 100 000). It is an autosomal dominant disorder of a muscle protein kinase, with variable severity and age of onset and a progressive course, whose genetic basis has been elucidated recently. Patients present with muscle cramps triggered by cold, weakness of the hands, or difficulty releasing their grip. There is a characteristic facial appearance with frontal balding, severe temporalis and sternomastoid muscle wasting, bilateral ptosis and facial weakness giving an expressionless, myopathic facies. Limb weakness is worst distally in the hands and feet and there is usually areflexia. The patient cannot suddenly open a clenched fist or release the hand from a handshake. Complications of myotonic dystrophy include cardiac conduction abnormalities and impaired respiratory drive, which may be life-threatening, diabetes mellitus, hypothyroidism, cataracts, male infertility, bowel dysmotility and mental retardation. Myotonia may be improved by phenytoin, procainamide or quinine.

Channelopathies
Some muscle diseases have been found to be due to ion channel abnormalities – 'channelopathies'.

Myotonia congenita occurs in both an autosomal dominant and recessive form. Myotonia is usually symptomatic, patients complain of stiffness, which may interfere with feeding in babies. Stiffness improves with exercise and age. There is associated muscle hypertrophy. Myotonia is usually a prominent sign. A chloride channel defect has been found to be the cause.

Paramyotonia congenita is an autosomal dominant condition caused by a muscle sodium channel defect. Myotonia affects the face and forearms; it is triggered by cold and worsened by repeated exertion (hence *para*myotonia).

Periodic paralysis. The periodic paralyses are rare, usually autosomal dominant conditions in which there may be sudden episodes of generalized weakness and areflexia. They have now been found to be due to ion channel abnormalities. The hyperkalaemic syndromes are due to disorders of the sodium channel and episodes are triggered by exercise and potassium ingestion. They are often associated with myotonia. The hypokalaemic syndromes are due to disorders of calcium channels, are triggered by carbohydrate meals and respond to oral potassium supplements. Acetazolamide is effective in both hypo- and hyperkalaemic periodic paralysis.

Acquired muscle disease
This usually presents with progressive proximal weakness. It is usually secondary to metabolic disturbance (Table 2), inflammatory disease, infection or toxins. Many are treatable.

Common metabolic abnormalities. These often cause typical proximal weakness but CK, electromyography (EMG) and muscle biopsy are

commonly normal. They improve on reversing the metabolic abnormality.

Polymyositis. Polymyositis is the most common inflammatory muscle disease in adults (prevalence 6 per 100 000), especially in women aged 30–60 years. Proximal limb, trunk, neck, pharyngeal and oesophageal muscles may all be involved. The onset is usually subacute or chronic but occasionally acute. Muscles may be painful or tender. CK is usually markedly elevated and EMG often shows myopathic changes with increased spontaneous activity (p. 35). The diagnosis is confirmed by demonstrating inflammatory changes on muscle biopsy. Treatment is with corticosteroids and immunosuppression, most commonly with azathioprine. CK is a marker of disease activity to regulate treatment, which may be long term, and prognosis is good.

Dermatomyositis. This occurs mainly in children, in which similar myositis is combined with a purple 'heliotrope' rash around the eyes and a linear red rash over the knuckles and proximal phalanges: 'Gottron's papules' (Fig. 2). Polymyositis and dermatomyositis may occur in isolation or as part of a more widespread collagen–vascular disease. Sarcoidosis or polyarteritis nodosa may produce a similar clinical picture. There is an increased relative risk of neoplasia in both polymyositis (9%) and dermatomyositis (15%) compared with the general population. Lymphoma and ovarian carcinoma are particularly associated.

Acute myopathy. This may be autoimmune, due to viral or parasitic infections, drugs, trauma, burns and

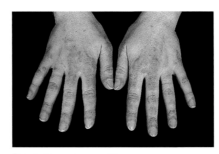

Fig. 2 **Dermatomyositis.**

snake venoms (Table 2). There may be massive muscle damage with myoglobinaemia and myoglobinuria, causing acute renal tubular necrosis. Rhabdomyolisis may also occur after excessive muscle use: prolonged marches, status epilepticus and neuroleptic malignant syndrome (p. 119).

Malignant hyperthermia. This is a pathological sensitivity in 1 in 50 000 halothane anaesthetics. It is thought to be due to an inherited abnormality of the ryanodine receptor, causing acute myonecrosis and systemic complications. An acute myopathy may also occur in very sick patients in the intensive care setting, especially if treated with steroids and neuromuscular blocking agents.

Inclusion body myositis. This is most common in middle-aged men. It is slowly progressive and tends to affect specific muscles in the early stages, e.g. brachioradialis. Characteristic inclusion bodies are seen in the cytoplasm and nuclei of myocytes. The nature of the primary process remains unclear. It responds poorly to immunosuppressive treatment.

Other syndromes of muscle stiffness
Stiff man syndrome. This is an autoimmune condition probably reflecting spinal cord disease. There is axial rigidity, which is worse on exertion. It is associated with autoimmune disease, especially diabetes mellitus and antibodies to glutamate decarboxylase. Treatment is with muscle relaxants and immunosuppression.

Neuromyotonia. The pathogenesis is uncertain, although it presents with features suggesting an autoimmune aetiology. There is a gradual onset with twitching or rippling muscles, then stiffness and an abnormal posture, and these symptoms persist in sleep. There is no percussion myotonia. Antivoltage-gated potassium channel antibodies are found in this condition, resulting in peripheral nerve hyperexcitability.

Table 2 **Causes of acquired muscle disease**	
Metabolic	**Inflammatory**
Renal failure	Polymyositis
Liver failure	Dermatomyositis
Hypocalcaemia	Vasculitis, e.g. polyarteritis nodosa
Hypokalaemia	Acute viral myositis, including HIV
Hypomagnesaemia	Sarcoidosis
Hypothyroidism	**Drugs:** cholesterol-lowering
Hyperthyroidism	'statins', tryptophan, zidovudine
Cushing's syndrome	**Parasites:** cysticercosis, trichinosis,
Addison's disease	toxoplasmosis

Muscle disease

- Muscle disease usually presents with proximal weakness.

- Treatable systemic and inflammatory causes are relatively common.

- Occasionally muscle disease may present with myotonia, episodic weakness and exertional symptoms.

The autonomic nervous system

Anatomy and physiology

The autonomic nervous system controls important functions that are not under voluntary control, i.e. autonomous. The extent of this autonomy varies; initiation of swallowing or micturition is voluntary and subsequent execution is automatic, but there is no voluntary component to gastrointestinal motility. As well as descending control from the CNS, some autonomic structures may function independently, and under humoral control. For example, the heart has an intrinsic pacemaker in the sinoatrial node, which may be modulated by circulating adrenaline and by sympathetic and parasympathetic nerve inputs.

CNS control of autonomic function

CNS structures that are especially important in the control of the autonomic nervous system are in the hypothalamus and the brain stem.

The output from the autonomic nervous system is in two main parts: sympathetic (SNS) and parasympathetic (PSNS). In addition the gut contains a local enteric nervous system, which is largely separate. The predominant actions of the SNS are to facilitate functions required for the 'fight or flight' response and to inhibit other actions. The PSNS tends to have the opposite functions: 'rest and digest'. In addition there are afferent fibres, carrying sensory information regarding the state of the viscera.

Sympathetic nervous system

SNS fibres descend in the brain stem and lateral columns of the spinal cord. They emerge at each spinal level from T1 to L3 to synapse in ganglia, which form a chain close to the spinal column on either side. The preganglionic neurotransmitter is acetylcholine (nicotinic) and the postganglionic neurotransmitter (at effector organs) is noradrenaline (norepinephrine), except at sweat glands (muscarinic acetylcholine).

Parasympathetic nervous system

Preganglionic fibres arise from specific nuclei in the brain stem and base of the spinal cord and pass in discrete nerves to ganglia close to the effector organs. The neurotransmitter is nicotinic acetylcholine in preganglionic and muscarinic in postganglionic neurones. Especially important is the vagus (10th cranial) nerve, which innervates the larynx, heart and abdominal viscera down to the descending colon.

Peripheral autonomic nerves

The peripheral nerves of the autonomic nervous system are small unmyelinated fibres. Afferent autonomic fibres are contained in many peripheral nerves. The spectrum of diseases that affects them overlaps with, but is different from, that affecting unmyelinated fibres in peripheral neuropathies (pp. 102–105)

Causes of autonomic dysfunction

Lesions at all levels of the nervous system may affect autonomic function (Fig. 1) and the site of the lesion determines the pattern of involvement as well as associated deficits. Most autonomic disturbances are acquired but there are some rare inherited causes, e.g. certain inherited neuropathies. Some common neuropathies particularly affect autonomic function, especially those due to diabetes mellitus or alcohol. The autonomic nervous system is also affected by many widely used medications, especially antihypertensive agents.

Primary autonomic failure may occur as a pure syndrome or as part of multisystem atrophy, in association with degeneration in other neurological systems, including the cerebellum, extrapyramidal system and pyramidal tracts. This condition usually presents in middle age and the order in which these neurological systems are affected varies between patients. Commonly, first presentation is with Parkinsonism, which may be difficult to distinguish from idiopathic

Lesion Site	Respiration	Cardiovascular	Urinary	Bowel	Other
1 Frontal	—	—	Incontinence	—	Dementia, ataxia
2 Hypothalamic	Automatic respiration	Postural hypotension	Disturbed salt/water homeostasis	—	Altered hunger, thirst, arousal, sexual function, thermoregulation
3 Brain stem	Altered respiratory pattern and insufficiency	Altered blood pressure and heart rhythm	Retention/ incontinence	Constipation	Dysphagia, cranial nerve abnormalities, tetraparesis
4 Cervical cord	Respiratory insufficiency	Bradycardia/ hypotension	Retention/ incontinence/ dyssynergia	Constipation	Tetraparesis, Horner's syndrome
5 Thoracic cord	Insufficiency if high thoracic	Hypotension	Retention/ incontinence/ dyssynergia	Constipation	Paraparesis
6 Sacral cord	—	—	Retention	Constipation	Paraparesis
7 Peripheral nerve	Respiratory insufficiency (sometimes)	Orthostatic hypotension Tachy-/bradydysrhythmia	Retention	Constipation or diarrhoea	Distal sensorimotor disturbance
8 Skeletal muscle	Respiratory insufficiency	—	—	—	Dysphagia, proximal weakness

Fig. 1 **Patterns of autonomic disturbance with different lesion sites.**

Table 1	**Common autonomic symptoms, their causes and treatments**		
System	**Common symptoms**	**Cause**	**Treatment**
Cardiovascular	Dizziness and blackouts, sudden death	Orthostatic hypertension, tachy- or bradydysrhythmia	Sleep with head-up tilt, compression stockings, antidysrhythmic drugs or cardiac pacing
Respiratory	Sleep apnoea syndrome, stridor, ventilatory failure	Respiratory weakness, upper airway obstruction or failure of central drive	Nocturnal or diurnal ventilatory support Tracheostomy for stridor
Upper GI tract	Dysphagia Vomiting	Incoordination of swallowing Gastroparesis	Altered diet, percutaneous gastrostomy Metoclopramide or doperidone
Lower GI tract	Constipation Diarrhoea	Reduced motility	Aperients Codeine
Bladder	Retention and/or incontinence	Altered detrusor muscle or sphincter or relation between the two	Intermittent or permanent catheterization. Anticholinergic agents, e.g. oxybutynin
Sexual	Impotence, failed ejaculation, anorgasmia	Altered pelvic autonomic function	Papaverine injections for impotence

Parkinson's disease and may partially respond to levodopa. Subsequently, sphincter disturbance and giddiness secondary to postural hypotension develop, giving a clue to the diagnosis. Central respiratory disturbance, e.g. acute stridor, may occur. The prognosis is for gradual deterioration, with survival 5–10 years.

Clinical manifestations of autonomic disturbance

Autonomic disturbance may affect just one system, e.g. cardiovascular, or it may be more generalized. Clinically important consequences affect respiration, swallowing, cardiovascular, bowel, bladder and sexual function (Table 1). Rarely, failure of sweating can result in dangerous hyperpyrexia. There are three main categories of autonomic dysfunction:

- Highest level lesions cause a failure of voluntary modulation of autonomic function, leaving the automatic component intact. For example, locked-in syndrome from a high brain stem lesion causes a failure of voluntary modulation of respiration.
- Lesions of centres integrating autonomic activity, mainly in hypothalamus and brain stem, lead to abnormal patterns of

spontaneous activity, e.g. Cheyne–Stokes respiration or hiccoughs in brain stem lesions. This often coexists with:

- Lesions between the regulating centre and the effector organ, involving especially spinal cord, peripheral nerve, muscle or peripheral neurotransmitters, cause failure of the peripheral organ, e.g. primary ventilatory failure.

In organs with both SNS and PSNS input, the net effect will depend on the balance of pathology affecting the two systems. For example Guillain–Barré syndrome may cause tachydysrhythmia (unopposed SNS) or bradydysrhythmia (unopposed PSNS). The bladder relies on coordination of SNS and PSNS and spinal cord malfunction in multiple sclerosis particularly causes attempted emptying against a closed sphincter, as well as retention or incontinence. This 'dyssynergia' causes urinary urgency, frequency and incomplete voiding.

Investigation of autonomic failure

The first step is confirmation of autonomic dysfunction. Simple clinical tests are described in Table 2. More sophisticated autonomic responses can be measured in a specialized laboratory. These may be supplemented by tests for cause in Table 3, neuroimaging for CNS disease and nerve conduction studies for peripheral disease.

Treatment and prognosis

Treatments for different symptoms of autonomic disturbance are outlined in Table 1. Treatment may also be addressed to the cause, e.g. diabetes mellitus. There is no specific treatment for primary autonomic failure or multisystem atrophy.

Table 3	**Causes of autonomic failure**	
	Central	**Peripheral**
Acute	Stroke	Guillain–Barré syndrome
	Tumour	Drugs: antihypertensive agents, organophosphates
	Drugs: neuroleptics, cocaine, amphetamines, 'ecstasy'	Acute porphyria
	Spinal trauma	Botulism
Chronic	Spinal or brain stem disease, tumour, multiple sclerosis, HIV, syphilis	Neuropathies: diabetes mellitus, alcohol, porphyria, HIV
	Multisystem atrophy	Chagas' disease
	Drugs: antihypertensives, neuroleptics, levodopa, antidepressants	Familial dysautonomia
		Drugs: antihypertensives, adrenergic and cholinergic

Table 2	**Clinical tests of autonomic failure**
What to do	**What it means**
Heart rate response to standing up from supine. Measure ratio of longest R–R interval (30th beat) to shortest R–R interval (15th beat)	Normal >1.21 Tests SNS and PSNS
Fall in systolic blood pressure 1 min after standing from supine	Normal <10 mmHg Abnormal >30 mmHg Tests mostly SNS
Heart variation on deep breathing	Normal >15 bpm Tests mostly PSNS
Valsalva heartbeat ratio. Patient blows out into manometer, maintaining 40 mmHg pressure for 15 s. Ratio of longest R–R interval after the manoeuvre to shortest during it	Normal >1.21 Tests SNS and PSNS
Pupil response to 1/1000 adrenaline (epinephrine) drops	Normal – no response SNS denervation – dilatation
Pupil response to 2.5% methacholine drops	Normal – no response PSNS denervation – constriction
Nocturnal and diurnal pulse oximetry	Measures automatic respiration
Diaphragmatic screening	Measures diaphragm function
Heat trunk for 90 s with electric lamp and measure sweating and hand blood flow	Measures sympathetic outflow to skin

The autonomic nervous system

- CNS structures important in autonomic function are in the hypothalamus, brain stem and spinal cord.

- The two major arms of the autonomic nervous system are anatomically, physiologically and pharmacologically distinct.

- Simple clinical tests can be used to assess autonomic function.

- Autonomic nervous system disturbance may cause potentially fatal cardiac and respiratory complications.

Functional disorders

There are many neurological patients with neurological symptoms and signs that are not due to underlying neurological abnormalities but reflect a psychological problem. In others there is an elaboration of a neurological abnormality so that the signs elicited extend beyond the distribution of the neurological lesion or are out of proportion with the neurological lesion.

There is considerable debate about the diagnoses, classification and terminology used in this area of neurology. Terms commonly used are non-organic, functional, psychogenic or hysterical, though alternatives such as somatiform disorders or abnormal illness behaviour have recently been proposed. These terms have been used in different ways by different neurologists.

Recently, the term somatization has been preferred. Somatization has been defined as 'the expression of distress in the idiom of bodily complaints'. This is an umbrella term which includes diagnoses (such as hysteria), with the notion of an unconscious trigger for the symptoms, and patients with anxiety or depression with unexplained somatic symptoms.

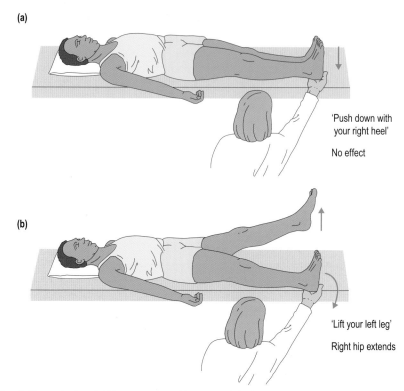

(a)
'Push down with your right heel'
No effect

(b)
'Lift your left leg'
Right hip extends

Fig. 1 **Hoover's sign. (a)** The patient is unable to extend the hip and to press the heel into the bed on request; **(b)** the hip is extended involuntarily when the opposite leg is lifted off the bed.

These disorders, however named, are very important, being a significant factor in up to 20% of neurological outpatients and up to 40% of neurological admissions. There are a large number of different physical manifestations. However, there are several typical clinical syndromes, and they tend to affect patients with some particular features.

Clinical approach

The clinical approach must first determine if there is an underlying organic disease, assess its contribution to the clinical presentation and try to make a positive psychiatric diagnosis. This has been aided by the newer investigative and imaging techniques. How this is done will depend on the clinical presentation. There is always a concern that there is an underlying neurological condition hidden beneath the elaboration.

However, there are some 'classical' features. These include an effect of 'belle indifférence', where the patient seemingly is unconcerned about the disability, and a collapsing weakness, where the power just suddenly gives. These are not specific findings; the latter is also a feature of conditions such as myasthenia gravis and the early stages of Guillain–Barré syndrome (when hysteria is the most commonly given erroneous differential diagnosis).

Non-organic syndromes occur more commonly in women, and usually in younger patients. It is a diagnosis that is made only with great caution in older patients. There is often a history of other physical symptoms and there may be a history of deliberate self-harm or drug overdose.

The management of patients with somatization disorders is difficult once the diagnosis is established. Associated psychiatric illnesses such as anxiety and depression need to be identified and treated. Psychological interventions, including cognitive therapy to try to reattribute the physical symptoms, have been beneficial in some cases. Physiotherapy can be useful in helping a patient to overcome a non-organic paralysis.

In some patients there is a conscious fabrication of a neurological deficit. This is malingering. There are usually more clear-cut financial or other benefits to the patient.

The most common syndromes seen are discussed below.

Non-epileptic attacks or pseudoseizures

Non-epileptic attacks or pseudoseizures are episodes that appear superficially to be seizures. They may be continuous and mimic status epilepticus; indeed, 50% of patients admitted to intensive care units with status epilepticus have been found to have pseudoseizures. In many patients the attacks can readily be distinguished from epileptic seizures; they often include semi-purposeful thrashing ('it took five men to keep me down'); patients remain pink throughout and may flush, but do not become cyanosed; respiration is normal; they do not bite their tongues; incontinence is rare; and recovery is usually quick. There are some patients where it is more difficult to be certain. To establish the diagnosis an EEG during the attack needs to demonstrated to be normal. The attacks tend to occur more often when medical and nursing staff are at hand and obtaining an EEG during an attack is usually more readily achieved than in epileptic seizures.

Measurement of prolactin following a seizure can also be useful, as this is elevated after an epileptic attack.

It is uncertain how many patients with pseudoseizures also have epileptic seizures.

It is important to consider this diagnosis to avoid potential iatrogenic injury to the patient, who may be considered for intubation and ventilation when there is no response to anticonvulsants, and from the adverse effects of multiple anticonvulsants.

Paralysis

In patients with non-organic weakness there is usually an inconsistency in the power of the limb on formal testing and when the patient uses it. Examples include patients who can swing their legs up only on the bed when getting onto it but cannot lift the legs against gravity on formal testing; or patients who can stand with legs slightly flexed at the knees supporting their own weight but who cannot walk. There is usually a characteristic collapsing weakness. There are several manoeuvres that can bring this out, such as Hoover's sign (Fig. 1), or the movement found when testing coordination, which is not obtained on testing power.

Sensory loss

Most patients with organic sensory loss have an incomplete loss, which affects some modalities more than others and accords with a recognizable pattern (p. 60). In patients with non-organic loss the loss is often complete, affecting all modalities and in a distribution that does not conform to an anatomical sensory distribution. There are often inconsistencies on repeat testing. There is usually a discrepancy in the functional loss associated with the sensory loss, for example an arm apparently without joint position sense can still touch the nose with eyes shut or reliably touches the same spot just to one side of the nose.

Sensory loss is often elaborated, so that a mild organic loss is extended in distribution and severity.

Visual loss

This can occur in a wide range of different patterns and in each there is a range of differential diagnoses that need careful consideration. Signs that prove useful are the finding of a 'tube' field loss that does not broaden as it gets further from the eye (Fig. 2).

Physiologically induced sensations and physical symptoms of anxiety

Other types of symptom that fall within somatization are physiologically induced bodily sensations and the physical symptoms of anxiety.

The symptoms associated with hyperventilation account for 2% of neurological outpatients. These symptoms are dizziness or lightheadedness, tingling in the hands, feet and around the mouth, some visual disturbance and sometimes loss of consciousness. Breath-holding time is reduced and forced hyperventilation reproduces the symptoms. Treatment with retraining of breathing by physiotherapists is usually successful.

Anxiety is commonly associated with hyperventilation and many of the physical symptoms attributed to anxiety could be mediated by this mechanism. In addition, patients may be aware of a tremor; sometimes they describe 'a shaking inside'. Recognition of the condition and treatment with anxiolytics is usually successful.

Chronic fatigue syndrome

This syndrome of uncertain aetiology is subject to considerable controversy. The presentation is with disabling fatigue that has lasted for over 6 months where no other medical cause has been found. Symptoms usually include sore throats, low grade fever, joint and muscle pains, headache, poor concentration and sleep disturbance. Many patients have features of depression. It is more common in women.

The aetiology of CFS is much disputed. No organic, especially infective, cause has been found. There are many features in common with other somatization disorders such as fibromyalgia, irritable bowel, etc.

Treatments that have been shown to be effective in clinical trials include tricyclic antidepressants, graded exercises and cognitive behavioural therapy.

Fibromyalgia

In these patients there is a prominent muscle aching, often with fatigue, arthralgia, malaise, sleep disturbance and headaches. There are no definite abnormalities on examination, though some muscles are tender. The reproducibility of these so-called 'trigger points' is contentious. This condition, like CFS, probably represents a somatization disorder. Treatment is as for CFS.

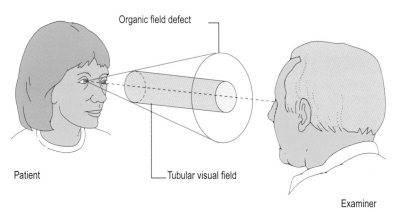

Fig. 2 **Tube visual field is a constant size regardless of distance from the eye.**

> *Functional disorders*
>
> - A significant proportion of patients in neurological clinics or on neurological wards have symptoms or signs that cannot be explained by organic disease.
>
> - Investigation is aimed at excluding underlying neurological disease.
>
> - Characteristic syndromes include pseudoseizures, weakness, and sensory and visual loss.
>
> - Treatment is difficult; cognitive therapy may help.

Neurology and psychiatry

A primary psychiatric diagnosis is present in 13–27% of new neurology outpatients and evidence of psychiatric morbidity in up to 48%.

Introduction

A psychiatric dimension is common in neurological consultations. Neurological and psychiatric illness may be related in several ways:

- Neurological diseases may have psychiatric complications.
- Neurological diseases may present with psychiatric symptoms.
- Psychiatric illness may present with neurological symptoms. Examples are depression presenting as pseudodementia (p. 55) and non-organic neurological illness (p. 116).
- The treatments for psychiatric illnesses can cause neurological complications and vice versa. Drugs of abuse also have neurological and psychiatric complications.
- Psychiatric factors may be important in triggering physical diseases, especially those to which the individual has a predisposition, e.g. epileptic seizures or migraine.

Psychiatric complications of neurological disease

Psychiatric complications of neurological disease may be reactive – a response to the handicap of the disease – or a primary manifestation of the disease itself. In some cases, both mechanisms may be active.

Anxiety

Anxiety is a common occurrence in neurology outpatients, found in 25–35%.

Depression

Depression is a common complication, and occurs especially frequently in certain diseases: Parkinson's disease 50%, Alzheimer's disease 30%, multiple sclerosis 25%, epilepsy 38%, stroke 25% and following head injury 25%. Depression leads to suicide in 6% of patients with Huntington's disease and in epilepsy the suicide risk is 5–25 times that of the general population.

Obsessive–compulsive disorder

This is also seen in movement, especially Parkinson's disease and Huntington's disease.

Euphoria

Euphoria, much vaunted, occurs in only 3% of patients with multiple sclerosis. Emotional lability may also be seen as part of pseudobulbar palsy, usually in multiple sclerosis, cerebrovascular disease or motor neurone disease. Pathological laughter or crying (the act without the underlying emotion) may also occur and usually relates to thalamic or brain stem disease.

Delusions

Delusions and other psychotic symptoms are seen in patients with Alzheimer's disease, vascular dementia, focal epilepsy, multiple sclerosis, treated Parkinson's disease and post-traumatic brain injury.

Complications of epilepsy

Epilepsy is associated with three patterns of psychotic disorder, best defined by the timing of psychotic symptoms in relation to epileptic seizures. They usually occur in patients with focal epilepsy syndromes and with known epilepsy, but occasionally may be a first presentation:

- **Postictal psychosis:** florid psychotic symptoms follow on from a flurry of severe seizures with a consistent time interval, usually 1–7 days. The episode is usually self-limiting within a week, but may require antipsychotic treatment during that time.
- **Ictal psychosis:** psychotic symptoms occur during the epileptic activity itself, usually as a manifestation of non-convulsive status epilepticus, and there is evidence of altered awareness. Patients may be agitated and hit out, but directed aggression is exceptionally rare. In both these situations, the best treatment of psychosis is to prevent seizures with antiepileptic therapy.
- **Interictal psychosis:** timing bears no relationship to identifiable epileptic seizures. Occurs more often in those with structural lesions (23%) than in mesial temporal sclerosis (5%) and is occasionally caused by antiepileptic drug therapy.

Neurological diseases presenting with psychiatric manifestations

The diagnosis of a primary psychiatric illness requires that the symptoms occur in normal consciousness. The presence of altered consciousness or periods of drowsiness suggest a neurological cause (pp. 50, 52). There may, however, be no obvious clouding of consciousness in the early stages and other factors may be helpful in making the diagnosis (Table 1).

Anxiety is seen in metabolic encephalopathies, including hypoxia, thyrotoxicosis, delirium tremens and other drug-induced states. This may progress to a frank psychotic state.

Frontal lobe disorders often present with psychiatric effects. The aetiology is usually a tumour, infarction, trauma, hydrocephalus, encephalitis or focal dementia. There may be release of primitive reflexes: pout, grasp and palmar–mental reflexes. If the lesion extends more posteriorly, there may be more easily identified focal signs: hemiparesis and non-fluent

Table 1 **Comparison of organic brain syndromes and psychiatric disease**		
Symptom	Organic disease	Psychiatric disease
Clouding of consciousness	Common	Rare
Seizures	Common	Rare
Memory	Impaired	Often preserved
Visual hallucinations	Commonly without auditory hallucinations	Rare without auditory hallucinations
Tactile hallucinations	Commonly without auditory hallucinations	Rare without auditory hallucinations
Focal neurological signs	Sometimes	Rare
Disturbed sleep	Reversal of sleep cycle	Insomnia
Paranoia	Common	Common
Feelings of control	Rare	Sometimes
Headache	Sometimes	Sometimes

dysphasia in the dominant hemisphere. There are three recognizable syndromes:

- Disinhibition, with insomnia, hypomanic features and sometimes hypersexuality, is seen in orbitofrontal lesions.
- Apathy, with paucity of speech and motor activity is seen in mesial frontal lesions, especially bilateral infarction of the anterior cerebral artery. Bilateral medial thalamic lesions may produce the same syndrome. There may be urinary incontinence without warning and a gait disorder.
- Impairment of executive function is seen in lateral convexity lesions. These patients find it difficult to maintain attention or to transfer attention from one task to the next. Despite adequate memory function, these patients perform poorly in everyday life.

Auditory hallucinations are common in psychiatric disease and may be accompanied by hallucinations in other modalities, but in organic disease these commonly occur without auditory hallucinations. Visual hallucinations most commonly occur in acute confusional states, where they are often complex (pink elephants in delirium tremens). They may also occur with lesions at any level of the visual system from the eyes to the association cortex, when they may be flashes of light or complex images and may be restricted to an abnormal visual field. Brief, stereotyped images may represent partial seizures but are also seen by normal individuals when falling off to sleep (hypnagogic hallucinations) and, rarely, in brain stem lesions (peduncular hallucinosis). Cortical Lewy body disease causes dementia with visual hallucinations in up to 85% of cases and Parkinson's disease causes nightmares and similar hallucinations when treated with high doses of levodopa. Olfactory, gustatory and somatosensory (crawling ants on the skin) hallucinations also occur in acute organic brain syndromes and in epilepsy (p. 74).

Neurological and psychotropic medication
Drugs used in the treatment of psychiatric illness often have neurological side-effects and vice versa. Withdrawal of the culprit may not be possible; Table 2 lists some alternative strategies.

Antipsychotic and anti-Parkinsonian medication
Drugs used in the treatment of Parkinson's disease are dopaminergic agonists, whereas those used in the treatment of psychosis are predominantly dopaminergic antagonists. Whilst there are several different types of dopamine receptors, allowing some selectivity of action, major side-effects of neuroleptic drugs are movement disorders, which may be acute (oculogyric crisis, neuroleptic malignant syndrome) or chronic (tardive movement disorders), whereas the anti-Parkinsonian drugs cause confusions, hallucinations and psychosis.

Neuroleptic malignant syndrome
Neuroleptic malignant syndrome (NMS) is a life-threatening complication of neuroleptic drugs. The characteristic features are muscle rigidity of an extrapyramidal type, altered consciousness and autonomic disturbance, especially hyperpyrexia, which usually develop acutely. It occurs in up to 1% of individuals receiving neuroleptic medication and may occur at any stage during treatment. The differential diagnosis includes amphetamine or MDMA (ecstasy) abuse, encephalitis, Wilson's disease and primary catatonic schizophrenic psychosis, which are much rarer. NMS may be associated with an elevation of the creatine kinase from muscle damage but there are no diagnostic tests.

The diagnosis is made by exclusion of other causes in the appropriate context of neuroleptic therapy. Treatment is supportive with fluid replacement. Some use intravenous dantrolene sodium or bromocriptine to reduce rigidity. Major complications are renal failure secondary to dehydration, and myoglobinaemia and secondary infection. If the patient can be supported satisfactorily for 10–14 days, there are usually no sequelae and neuroleptics have been restarted in some individuals without recurrence.

Neuropsychiatric complications of drugs of abuse
Drug dependence is a psychiatric disorder, with organic components, physical dependence and tolerance, psychological components and psychological dependence. Most drugs are associated with both neurological and psychiatric complications (Table 3).

Table 2 **Problems with medications used in neurology and psychiatry**			
Drug	**Use**	**Adverse effect**	**Solution**
Dopaminergic agonist	Parkinsonism	Psychosis and hallucination	Quetiapine Donepezil
Dopaminergic antagonist	Psychosis, vomiting, vestibular sedative	Neuroleptic malignant syndrome	See text
Dopaminergic antagonist	Psychosis, vomiting, vestibular sedative	Parkinsonism and other movement disorders	Procyclidine
Anticonvulsant	Epilepsy	Sedation, sometimes depression and psychosis	Antidepressant Antipsychotic
Antidepressant	Depression	Seizures	Antiepileptic

Table 3 **Neuropsychiatric effects of drugs of abuse**		
Drug	**Neurological complications**	**Psychiatric complications**
Alcohol	Intoxication stupor and coma, Wernicke's encephalopathy, Korsakoff syndrome, seizures, delirium tremens, myopathy, neuropathy, cerebellar syndrome	Acute and chronic auditory hallucinosis, personality disintegration, morbid jealousy
Amphetamine	Organic hallucinosis, NMS-type syndrome, cerebral vasculitis	Chronic psychosis
MDMA (ecstasy)	Organic hallucinosis, NMS-type syndrome, destruction of serotonergic fibres	Not yet established
Cocaine	Organic hallucinosis, stroke (common), subarachnoid and cerebral haemorrhage	Depression, mania, phobic disorders, anxiety disorders
Lysergic acid (LSD)	Organic hallucinosis	Chronic psychosis, hallucinatory flashbacks
NMS, neuroleptic malignant syndrome		

Neurology and psychiatry

- In acute psychiatric disorders, drowsiness is a cardinal sign of a physical cause.
- Neurological causes of acute psychiatric symptoms are similar to those for confusion. Neurological causes of acute psychiatric symptoms are similar to those for dementia.
- Treatments for neurological conditions often have psychiatric adverse effects and vice versa.

Rehabilitation

Introduction

Neurological disease may result in chronic neurological deficit, and this accounts for a substantial burden of morbidity in the community. Some disabling diseases are particularly likely to affect young individuals, for example trauma, multiple sclerosis and cerebral palsy. The disability may be stable and long term or slowly progressive in these patients. Severe physical disability affects 420 000 people between the ages of 16 and 59 years in the UK, which is 0.75% of the total population.

Neurological rehabilitation is aimed at optimizing the level of function of the patient within his or her usual environment. This includes maximizing physical ability, preventing deterioration due to secondary disease, optimizing the patient's environment, facilitating psychological adaptation to disability and encouraging social integration (Fig. 1). All these facets need to be assessed in providing the most appropriate support. Most of the burden of caring for the disabled falls on their families and the rehabilitation process involves training relatives and providing them with practical, emotional and psychological support.

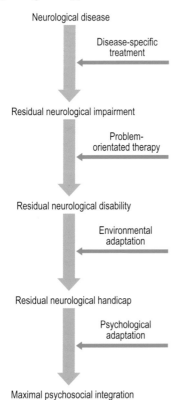

Fig. 1 **Reduction of handicaps by different interventions.** These strategies are used concurrently rather than sequentially.

Impairment, disability and handicap

Neurological impairment, disability and handicap are key concepts in rehabilitation. Neurological *impairment* is a disturbance of the nervous system that results in an abnormality of function. It may occur at any level of the nervous system causing:

- intellectual or emotional impairment
- sensory or motor impairments.

Impairment causes *disability* if there is difficulty performing tasks that are normal for a human being. Disability causes *handicap* if the patient is unable to continue performing his or her normal role as a result of disability. For example, an attack of multiple sclerosis may cause leg weakness. This causes a disability if the patient can only walk short distances. If the patient is a postman, this causes a handicap, as he cannot perform his job, but if his occupation is sedentary, it may not result in the same level of handicap.

Recovery in the nervous system

Neurological recovery

Neurological regeneration may occur after damage, especially in the peripheral nerves. The type of disease is important in this regard; there is usually full recovery after classical demyelinating Guillain–Barré syndrome, but more frequently incomplete recovery after the rarer axonal variant. In the central nervous system there is less scope for regeneration, but recovery may still occur. Two main factors contribute:

- The initial pathological process may subside, e.g. reduction of inflammation in multiple sclerosis.
- Plasticity effects. The central nervous system has less scope for recovery than the peripheral nervous system.

Predictors of neurological recovery

The nature of the disease and its treatment is the first important

Table 1 **Common medical complications of neurological deficit**

Complication	Prevention
Pressure sores	Regular turning
Contractures	Passive movement of joints through the whole range
Thrombosis	Subcutaneous heparin, enhance mobility
Ventilatory failure	Ventilatory support
Pneumonia	Respiratory exercises, protect airway, especially with feeding

predictor. Demyelination is usually followed by more recovery than infarction, because axons are preserved. Severe brain trauma typically affects multiple sites and recovery may be slow. If there is a progressive disease, e.g. tumour, then recovery will be determined by the success of treatment.

The extent of the damage is a key predictor. The greater the extent of the damage, the more incomplete the recovery, because there is less capacity for neuronal plasticity effects.

The age of the patient is also a predictor. Plasticity of the nervous system is greatest in children and declines rapidly with age. Damage to the language centres before the age of 6 years may result in transfer of language to the non-dominant hemisphere, but this is rare at older ages.

Recovery from disability and reduction of handicap

A patient may be able to perform a function even with a residual neurological impairment. For example, the disability of a patient with a foot drop may be treated with a foot splint. He or she may still be handicapped if unable to drive children to school, but this handicap can be treated with a hand-operated car. Alteration of the interaction between the patient and the environment allows the patient to perform tasks important in life, preventing handicap.

Aims of rehabilitation

The aims of rehabilitation are to encourage the facets of recovery described above:

- prevent complications
- promote intrinsic recovery
- teach adaptive strategies
- facilitate function in the patient's normal environment.

Prevention of complications

Neurological diseases cause deficits, which may predispose to numerous complications. These complications may in themselves be life-threatening or cause a deterioration of the underlying neurological condition. This impairs intrinsic recovery and impedes rehabilitation. Much of the acute management of the neurologically ill patient is in prevention and treatment of these complications (Table 1).

Promotion of intrinsic recovery

This is primarily the treatment of the underlying cause of the deterioration, e.g. intravenous steroids speeding recovery from a relapse of multiple sclerosis. Although an active area of research, no therapies have been proven to enhance recovery of the damaged nervous system.

Teaching adaptive strategies

This enables the patient to function despite any residual neurological impairment. Residual handicap can be addressed by assessing the patient's needs in the usual environment and designing further strategies and aids to minimize handicap.

Facilitate function in a normal environment

The patient may be unable to achieve premorbid level of function. Family members may need to take additional roles and community-based services may be needed after discharge from hospital. The patient and carers will need help in psychological adaptation to their new roles.

Problem-orientated team approach

In contrast to the disease-orientated medical model, the rehabilitation approach is problem orientated. The approach is by a team, which addresses different facets of the patient's problems. Rehabilitation is primarily undertaken

Table 2 Physical problems amenable to medical or surgical therapy

Problem	Common cause	Complication	Some treatments available
Spasticity	Upper motor neurone lesions	Painful leg spasms	Baclofen, dantrolene, botulinum toxin, selective surgical lesions of tendons, nerves or roots
Dysphagia	Brain stem lesions, motor neurone disease, myasthenia gravis, myopathy	Aspiration pneumonia, malnutrition	Alteration of diet, postural swallowing techniques, oesophageal dilatation, nasogastric or percutaneous gastrostomy tube feeding
Urinary retention and incontinence	Spinal cord disease, cauda equina lesions, autonomic neuropathy, frontal lobe disease (incontinence)	Overflow incontinence, recurrent infection, renal impairment	Self-intermittent catheterization, recurrent infection, renal indwelling catheter, urinary diversion
Constipation and diarrhoea/incontinence	Spinal cord disease, neuropathies, Parkinson's disease (constipation)	Diarrhoea – skin breakdown	Standard laxatives for constipation, codeine-based and anticholinergic drugs for diarrhoea

by specialist therapists (Fig. 2). The role of the doctor is to integrate this activity, and treat certain physical problems that may be amenable to medical or surgical therapy (Table 2). There are four stages in this process:

1. *Assess* the patient and identify problem areas. Assessment requires a basic physical examination and interpretation of the patient's impairments in the context of daily life, so obtaining a measure of disability and handicap. Disability can occur in various categories of activity (Table 3). The Barthel index provides a useful measure in spheres essential to every individual: 'activities of daily living'.

2. *Set goals* to try and achieve improvements in function. These should be realistic as overambitious

Table 3 Categories of disability

Behavioural
Communication
Personal care
Locomotor
Body disposition (domestic, postural, body movement)
Dexterity
Situational (dependence, endurance, environmental)
Skills, e.g. occupational
Other activities, e.g. hobbies

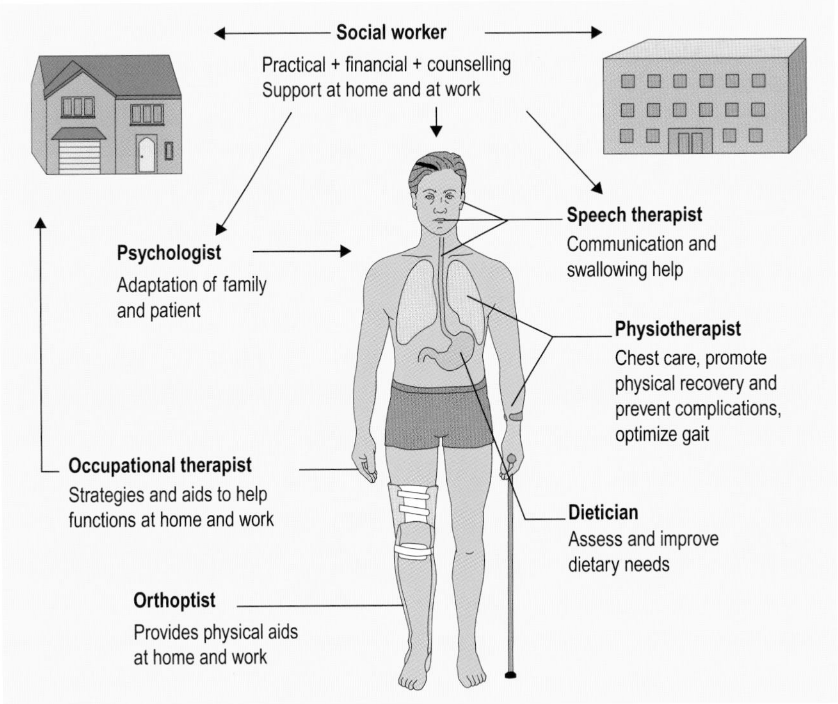

goals may not be achievable and may demoralize patients and staff. For a patient with a multiple sclerosis relapse, the initial goal may be to be able to stand.

3. *Try to achieve these goals* working with specialist therapists (Fig. 2).

4. *Reassess and set new goals* once these goals are achieved. Once the multiple sclerosis patient can stand, the aim may be to take a few steps with help. If the goal is not achieved, an alternative strategy may be needed: for example, if a patient is unable to strengthen the hands enough to use ordinary cutlery, then modified cutlery may allow normal eating.

When the patient is nearing maximum recovery, he or she needs to visit home and workplace with a physiotherapist and occupational therapist to assess specific needs in the usual environment.

Social worker
Practical + financial + counselling
Support at home and at work

Psychologist
Adaptation of family and patient

Speech therapist
Communication and swallowing help

Physiotherapist
Chest care, promote physical recovery and prevent complications, optimize gait

Occupational therapist
Strategies and aids to help functions at home and work

Dietician
Assess and improve dietary needs

Orthoptist
Provides physical aids at home and work

Fig. 2 **Team approach to rehabilitation.**

Neurological rehabilitation

- Neurological impairment, disability and handicap are key concepts in neurorehabilitation.
- Rehabilitation involves assessing and optimizing function in all spheres of the patient's usual environment.
- Rehabilitation uses a problem-orientated, team approach to achieve realistic goals.
- Rehabilitation involves the patient's carers and community services.

Case histories

Cases

Neurology cannot really be learnt from a book. Once you have the tools to make sense of neurological presentations and a framework of understanding of the range of neurological conditions, you are in the position to learn neurology from clinical practice – patient by patient as you help solve their clinical problems.

To get you on your way here are some clinical cases, with examples of many common or important neurological conditions. The questions for all are the same – reflecting clinical practice rather than any kind of exam practice – 'what is your diagnosis?' and 'what would you do next?' Some are accompanied by results of investigations, which, as in real life, may not be relevant. Brief answers are given on page 125 with reference to the relevant section of the book.

Case 1

A 48-year-old woman complains of numbness in both hands. She first noticed this 18 months ago, but initially it was intermittent and most often at night or when she was driving. For the last 3 months it has been continuous and she has had trouble with fine movements – such as doing buttons up.

Examination is normal apart from mild weakness of abductor pollicis brevis in both hands and a subjective alteration to pinprick in the thumb, index and middle fingers.

Case 2

A 35-year-old man is brought to Accident and Emergency with a headache that has become increasingly severe over the preceding 6 h. The paramedics reported he had had a seizure in the ambulance. He is febrile and unwell. He has a stiff neck and is confused with no focal neurological signs.

Case 3

A 24-year-old woman has a 6 week history of intermittent double vision. She notices images can be displaced either side by side or on top of one another. She has otherwise felt well.

On examination she has a mild right-sided ptosis which fatigues, and a variable double vision looking up with vertically displaced images, with the outer image in the right eye. The remainder of the examination is normal.

Case 4

You are asked to see an 18-year-old man urgently. He had two generalized seizures without any warning 2 months ago, attended hospital and was started on carbamazepine. Since then he has had increasingly frequent generalized seizures despite increasing doses of carbamazepine. He tells you that he has also had some blank spells, when he has missed some time. You ask him if he has any sudden jerks of his limbs, and he says he has and has had for many years, though recently he has been getting many more.

Examination is normal apart from the bite mark on the side of his tongue from a seizure he had earlier in the day.

Case 5

A 68-year-old woman complains of dizziness. She has had episodes of feeling dizzy, with a sensation of rotation lasting a minute or so, which then leaves her feeling wobbly for 10–15 min. She finds it occurs on looking up or rolling over in bed.

Conventional neurological examination is normal. On getting her to lie back flat with her head to the right you notice torsional vertigo to the right which comes on after 5 s, and lasts about 10 s, when she tells you she feels dizzy, before fading.

Case 6

A 68-year-old man presented with a 4 week history of progressive right-sided weakness. His family had noticed that this had been associated with some problems with his speech, as he sometimes seemed to find it difficult to find the right words, and a general slowness in thinking. He had been in a minor road traffic accident 2 months ago. He had been put on aspirin 3 years ago for mild angina.

On examination his speech was non-fluent and he had a mild right hemiparesis with brisker reflexes on the right and an extensor right plantar response. Sensory examination was normal.

Case 7

A 54-year-old man presented with a 4 day history of difficulty walking. He had been decorating 5 days before when he developed a pain between his shoulder blades with some numbness in his little fingers. Since then he had increasing numbness in his hands and gradually deteriorating walking with increasing leg weakness. He had developed urinary urgency. When he coughed he felt his symptoms were worse.

On examination his cranial nerves were normal. He had mild weakness of finger extension and elbow extension with moderate weakness affecting both legs, particularly hip flexion, knee flexion and foot dorsiflexion. Tone was increased in his legs. The biceps reflexes were absent, with reflex spread to finger flexion. Knee and ankle reflexes were brisk with bilaterally extensor plantars. Vibration sense was lost to the sternum, proprioception impaired at the toes, with a level to pinprick at T4 on the chest with loss on the medial forearm and hand to the middle finger.

Case 8

A 33-year-old man presents with a 3 day progressive history of weakness and sensory loss. He had just got over a cold when he began to get numbness in both feet which spread up his legs and to his hands and arms over the next few days, with an increasing heaviness and weakness. He had not been able to get out of bed this morning because of weakness.

On examination he was afebrile. Cranial nerves were normal. He had generalized weakness with all arm muscles grade 4 and legs 3. He was areflexic. Plantars were unresponsive. Vibration sense was lost to the anterior superior iliac spines, proprioception was normal and there was pinprick and temperature loss to knees.

Case 9

A 44-year-old woman presents complaining of headaches. These had begun 3 years ago with a pain around the top of her head. This was constant, though on some days the pain became more severe. She was taking co-codamol, 2 tablets 4 times a day, which helped a little. Previously she had more discrete headaches that lasted 6–8 h and were preceded by flashing lights, which occurred perhaps once a month, though she had not had one for maybe 18 months.

Neurological examination was normal, with normal retinal venous pulsation on fundoscopy.

Case 10

An 18-year-old girl is referred after she had a blackout in a nightclub. She recalls being in the nightclub and feeling unwell and sweaty. She made her way to the exit and got outside. She next recalls coming to on the floor with her friends around her, but knew exactly where she was. She had been incontinent. She tried to get up but briefly blacked out again.

Her friends report that she said she felt awful as she went outside. She then fell to the ground where she twitched slightly for about 20 s before coming to and making good sense. They tried to sit her up and she went out again for a few seconds. It was too dark to see her colour. She had never had any other episodes and examination was normal.

Case 11

A 68-year-old man reports that the day before presentation he had lost the use of his right arm and speech for about 10 min. It had come on suddenly and gradually improved. He otherwise had felt well. He had never had similar problems before. He had mild hypertension, for which he took atenolol, but was otherwise well.

Neurological examination was normal. He was in sinus rhythm, BP 155/90, normal cardiac examination with no carotid bruits.

Case 12

A 55-year-old man presents with an increasing weakness in his right hand. This has come on gradually over the last 6–8 months, particularly interfering with using the key in the door and writing. He feels his grip is weaker. He has noted some numbness in his little finger. He is otherwise well.

On examination he has wasting of the right first dorsal interosseous with weakness in that muscle and in right abductor digiti minimi and the long flexors of the little and ring fingers. Other muscles are normal. Reflexes are normal. There is a loss of pinprick sensation over the little finger and medial half of the ring finger on the right.

Case 13

A 33-year-old woman presents with a 1 week history of dizziness and 3 day history of double vision. She had noticed her left side felt clumsy over the last couple of days. She recalls having an episode when she lost vision in her right eye for a few weeks 5 years ago.

On examination she has an impairment of left eye adduction with normal right eye abduction on looking to the right, with some nystagmus in the right eye. She has a pale right optic disc with normal acuity and field. Power in her limbs is normal with normal reflexes. Sensation is normal. Her gait is ataxic and she has ataxia in the left arm and leg.

Case 14

A 75-year-old man reports a 12 month history of increasing difficulty using his left hand. He had noted he had more difficulty doing up buttons. He had noticed that his automatic winding watch had stopped winding, which he realized was because his arm had stopped swinging when he walked. His left shoulder felt stiff.

On examination he was well. His facial expression was normal, as was examination of his cranial nerves. His gait was slightly stooped and his left arm was slightly flexed and did not swing. Tone was increased in his left arm with cogwheeling. Power was full with symmetrical reflexes. There was mild slowing in fast repeating movements in his left hand and slightly in his left foot. Sensation was normal.

Case 15

A 68-year-old woman reported a 6 month history of increasing difficulty with her speech, which was becoming progressively slurred, and 1 month of difficulty swallowing. She had some cramps in her hands and thighs. She had lost a little weight, though was not sure how much.

On examination she was thin; examination of the eyes and eye movements were normal. Her speech was slow and slurred. Her tongue was wasted and fasciculating; tongue movements were very slow. There were fasciculations in all muscles in the shoulder girdle and in both quadriceps; however, power in both

arms and legs was normal. All her tendon reflexes were brisk with bilaterally upgoing plantars. Sensory examination was normal.

Case 16

A 37-year-old man presents to Accident and Emergency with a headache. This had come on suddenly 12 h before while he was jogging. He had to stop and sit down and then called his wife to take him home. He had been in bed since and vomited once. The headache was persisting. He had occasional mild headaches in the past but nothing like this.

Neurological examination was normal but his neck was a little stiff. A CT brain scan was reported as normal.

Case 17

A 48-year-old man presents with a history of progressive difficulty walking over the last 4 months. He has noticed his right leg is stiff and there is slight clumsiness of his right hand. His wife comments he sometimes seems to mix his words up and say the wrong word. On three occasions in the last 2 weeks his right leg has jerked repeatedly for about 5 min and then has felt even weaker, so he cannot walk for a further half hour.

On examination there is a supinator catch in the right arm and increased tone in the right leg. Reflexes are increased in the right leg with an extensor plantar response. Sensation is normal. He circumducts his right leg slightly as he walks and the ankle is slightly plantarflexed.

Case 18

A 38-year-old woman presents with sudden onset of weakness, nausea and double vision. She tells you that 10 days ago she injured her neck playing squash and that for the last 5 days she has had pain in the left side of her neck.

On examination the left pupil is smaller than the right and there is a partial left ptosis. The left eye fails to abduct on looking to the right, though other eye movements are normal. The right arm and leg are slightly weak with reduced sensation to pinprick. There is finger–nose incoordination of the left arm and heel–shin incoordination of the left leg. Reflexes are brisk on the right with an extensor plantar response. She is unable to walk.

Case 19

A 57-year-old man presents with a sudden onset of mild left-sided weakness with no other symptoms. He has a history of rheumatic fever in childhood but no other medical problems.

On examination he is in atrial fibrillation and is normotensive. His neurological examination reveals slight drooping of the left side of his mouth. His left arm and leg are slightly weak with increased tone and brisk reflexes. The plantar response is uncertain.

Case 20

A 65-year-old man is brought to you by his wife who says he is becoming forgetful. He retired from work 4 years ago because he was starting to make mistakes and his memory has declined since then. He remembers the names of only three of his five grandchildren. His wife says at times he has become more aggressive and different from his usual self and has accused her of stealing things from him. He recently got lost when they were out shopping together in town.

His physical examination is normal but he remembers only one of three objects at 1 min and fails to draw intersecting pentagons. He cannot remember the date or month. He scores 23/30 on mini-mental state examination.

Case 21

A 58-year-old woman is referred from the medical wards. Her family describe an illness starting 3 months earlier with memory disturbance and she has deteriorated rapidly. Six weeks ago her walking started to become unsteady and they brought her to hospital; tests including her CT brain scan and general blood tests are normal.

On examination you find that there are asynchronous spontaneous jerks of her limbs, which seem to be triggered by loud noises. She has difficulty cooperating with the examination and seems drowsy. She does not speak and her family tell you they are not sure if she recognizes them. A full examination is difficult but there are no obvious cranial nerve signs, no wasting and tone is normal. Reflexes are brisk but with flexor plantar responses.

Case 22

A 73-year-old woman complains of headache of 3 weeks' duration. The pain is made worse by chewing and she has found that her scalp is tender when she combs her hair. She has been off colour and lost 2 kg in the same period.

Her neurological examination is normal.

Case 23

A 28-year-old woman presents with stereotyped sensations that have been occurring for 1 year. They tend to cluster in the week before her period. She feels a strange feeling rising from her stomach and a sensation that everything is very familiar. On one occasion the feeling was so intense that she had to pull over for 3 min before she could continue driving home. Her husband has seen one and said she looked pale, appeared to be chewing something and did not answer him during the attack. She took a few minutes to recover and had no recollection of the episode.

She is previously well and her examination is normal.

Case 24

A 33-year-old man presents with headache for 4 weeks and a right-sided lower motor neurone facial weakness for 3 days. He has had night sweats for the last 2 weeks and has lost 5 kg in weight. On the day of admission he had developed deafness in his left ear.

He is mildly confused and has a temperature of 37.7°. His neck is slightly stiff but there are no other signs. His CT scan shows mild ventricular dilatation.

Answers

Case 1: Carpal tunnel syndrome
(p. 106)
The history of numbness in the hands waking the patient from sleep is classical for carpal tunnel syndrome. As the median nerve compression progresses the symptoms intrude into the day and a fixed deficit in median nerve distribution may emerge. Nerve conduction studies usually confirm the diagnosis and treatment is with decompression at the wrist.

Case 2: Acute bacterial meningitis
(p. 98)
The fever points to infection and the neck stiffness suggest meningitis. The time course is typical for acute bacterial meningitis, which may be complicated by seizures. Seizures are more common in encephalitis but the evolution is usually slightly slower in onset and there is less neck stiffness. He should be treated with antibiotics prior to having a scan and lumbar puncture.

Case 3: Myasthenia gravis
(p. 110)
The variability in the history, fatiguability, and a pattern of diplopia not fitting with any specific cranial nerve, make the diagnosis highly likely to be myasthenia gravis. Diagnostic tests are acetylcholine receptor antibodies, neurophysiology and edrophonium test. Treatment is with pyridostigmine and immunosuppression.

Case 4: Juvenile myoclonic epilepsy (p. 74)
The history of myoclonic jerks for many years before a tonic-clonic seizure is typical and many patients also have absences. This form of epilepsy is often made worse by carbamazepine and the most effective treatment is usually sodium valproate.

Case 5: Benign paroxysmal positional vertigo (BPPV)
(p. 47)
This is the typical history for BPPV and the manoeuvre described is Hallpike's test, which confirms the diagnosis. Treatment is the Epley's manoeuvre.

Case 6: Subdural haematoma (SDH) (pp. 67 and 78)
The history and signs point to a progressive left hemisphere lesion. With a head injury preceding the onset, the first diagnosis is SDH. These are more common in patients on warfarin or aspirin. Alternative diagnosis is a tumour unrelated to the injury.

Case 7: Cervical cord compression
(pp. 80–83)
He has lower limb spasticity due to bilateral upper motor neurone dysfunction pointing to a spinal lesion. The highest abnormal sign is the absent biceps reflexes, implying a lower motor neurone abnormality at the level of the biceps motor roots and therefore a motor level at C6. Worsening with cough suggests the cause is compressive; spondylosis or tumour. He should have emergency MRI of cervical spine and neurosurgical referral.

Case 8: Guillain–Barré syndrome
(p. 104)
The patient has generalized weakness and loss of reflexes pointing to a diffuse lower motor neurone disturbance, and a sensory disturbance consistent with a neuropathy. The subacute course and preceding infection are typical of GBS. Nerve conduction abnormalities and elevated protein level in the cerebrospinal fluid are common but may take time to develop; treatment is with i.v. immunoglobulin or plasmapheresis on the basis of the clinical picture.

Case 9: Migraine and analgesic misuse headache (p. 43)
The earlier history of discrete headaches is typical of migraine. This has changed to a more continuous headache only partially treated by analgesia, typical of analgesic misuse headaches. Common culprits are codeine, caffeine, paracetamol and triptans. No investigation required. Treatment is to withdraw analgesia and consider migraine prophylaxis.

Case 10: Syncope (p. 44)
People who faint often try first to get out into fresh air. The history of passing out again when she tried to get up is also typical. Most faints are associated with some limb twitching and this does not mean they have had a seizure. Most cases in healthy young individuals require no investigation but recurrent or atypical episodes may merit ECG, 24 h ECG, tilt testing or echocardiography.

Case 11: Left carotid territory transient ischaemic attack (TIA)
(pp. 70–71)
The tempo points to a TIA and the speech disturbance puts it into carotid artery territory. He should have Doppler carotid arteries and receive aspirin. He is mildly hypertensive and other vascular risk factors should also be addressed and treated.

Case 12: Ulnar neuropathy
(pp. 106–107)
The distribution of weakness and numbness are typical of ulnar neuropathy. Investigation is with nerve conduction studies, which usually show conduction delay across the elbow, due to compression. Conservative treatment is sometimes effective but surgical decompression or transposition may be required.

Case 13: Multiple sclerosis
(pp. 19 and 84–87)
The earlier history and signs in her right eye are typical of previous optic neuritis. The new signs are of a left internuclear ophthalmoplegia and ataxia which both indicate a lesion in the brain stem. Thus, she has lesions disseminated in time (now and some years ago) and place (the optic nerve and brain stem) making a clinical diagnosis of MS. Investigations are MRI brain, sometimes lumbar puncture and visual evoked potentials and blood tests to exclude rare mimics of MS, where indicated.

Case 14: Parkinson's disease
(pp. 88–91)
Reduced armswing is a typical early symptom of PD. Stiffness may lead the condition to be mistaken for a rheumatological disorder. The other symptoms and signs are also typical. One-third of patients have no tremor at presentation. There are no diagnostic investigations, but a careful history and examination may help to

excluded other, rarer Parkinsonian syndromes.

Case 15: Motor neurone disease (amyotrophic lateral sclerosis, ALS) (pp. 108-109)

Widespread fasciculations and wasting point to a diffuse lower motor neurone disturbance including bulbar muscles. The brisk reflexes and upgoing plantars indicate an upper motor neurone lesion. She has no sensory signs. Thus, she demonstrates mixed upper and lower motor neurone involvement in multiple regions, typical of ALS. The progressive course is typical. Nerve conduction studies and EMG will provide support for the diagnosis and exclude mimics.

Case 16: Subarachnoid haemorrhage (SAH) (pp. 72–73)

Any sudden onset headache, especially during exertion, is SAH until proven otherwise. The duration is rather long for benign exertional headaches, which have also usually occurred several times by presentation. A CT scan is normal in about 10% of SAH and a lumbar puncture with spectrophotometry for haemoglobin breakdown products is needed to exclude the diagnosis.

Case 17: Left hemisphere tumour (p. 94)

The symptoms and signs point to an upper motor neurone lesion and with the associated speech disturbance this is likely to be in the left cerebral hemisphere. The progressive time course makes a tumour the most likely cause. The jerking episodes are focal seizures followed by 'Todd's paresis'. Investigation with CT or MRI is indicated and a screen for primary tumours, including chest X-ray, ultrasound or CT abdomen, blood count, renal and liver function. Rarer causes include cerebral abscess or chronic subdural haematoma. He should be treated with an antiepileptic drug such as carbamazepine. If a tumour is found then corticosteroids may be indicated prior to surgery/biopsy.

Case 18: Left vertebral artery dissection (pp. 64–69)

The physical signs include a left Horner's syndrome and left 6th nerve palsy. These are in the brain stem above the decussation of the descending pathways, explaining the right hemiparesis and sensory loss, and involvement of the ipsilateral cerebellar pathways explains the ipsilateral ataxia. The acute onset is typical of a stroke. The history of neck trauma and pain suggests dissection of the left vertebral artery. Arterial dissection is the commonest identifiable cause of stroke in young adults, and pain over the vessel preceding infarction is typical. Investigation is with specially tailored MRI. Optimal treatment is not established: either aspirin or anticoagulation.

Case 19: Cardioembolic stroke (pp. 64–69)

The signs are of a right hemiparesis and the sudden onset points to a vascular cause. In a patient with atrial fibrillation, embolism of a cardiac thrombus is likely but the history of previous rheumatic fever also raises the rarer possibility of infective endocarditis. He should have CT scan, Doppler carotids and echocardiogram, with ESR, CRP and blood cultures if there is any suggestion of infection. If there is no alternative cause, he should receive long-term warfarin.

Case 20: Alzheimer's disease (pp. 54–55)

He has a slowly progressive memory disturbance affecting episodic and visuospatial memory (bihemispheric disturbance) with alteration of personality and no physical problem; the typical picture of AD. Investigation is with CT/MRI, renal and liver function, thyroid function, blood count, ESR and syphilis serology.

Case 21: Sporadic Creutzfeldt–Jakob disease (CJD) (pp. 55 and 99)

This is the typical history of sporadic CJD with rapidly progressive dementia, ataxia and startle-sensitive myoclonic jerks. MRI brain may show increased signal in the basal ganglia or thalamus and EEG may show characteristic periodic complexes. There is no absolute antemortem diagnostic test and no specific treatment. Management is supportive.

Case 22: Giant cell arteritis (GCA or temporal arteritis) (p. 40)

GCA is the most important diagnosis to consider in elderly patients with recent onset headaches. The clinical features of this case are classical but are not always present. Over 90% have either a raised ESR or CRP in the blood and a temporal artery biopsy is usually diagnostic. Treatment with high-dose corticosteroids should be instituted as soon as the diagnosis is suspected and a biopsy should be undertaken within a few days.

Case 23: Focal epilepsy (pp. 74–79)

These are typical focal seizures of temporal lobe origin. MRI brain and EEG are required but may be normal and, as she has had multiple episodes, she needs antiepileptic treatment; carbamazepine would be the most commonly used drug. She should be advised not to drive and to inform the DVLA and her insurance company and advised regarding avoiding situations that would put her or others at risk if she were to have a seizure. She should be informed about the risk of carbamazepine interacting with the oral contraceptive and warned regarding teratogenicity.

Case 24: Tuberculous meningitis (TBM) (pp. 38 and 97)

Headache and neck stiffness with fever suggest an infective meningeal process. Infarction of facial and vestibulocochlear nerves and mild hydrocephalus on CT scan are due to inflammation of the basal meninges. The subacute onset, with symptoms coming over weeks, with weight loss and multiple cranial nerve lesions are typical of TBM. The next test is cerebrospinal fluid analysis by lumbar puncture, if considered safe from CT scan appearances, or by cisternal puncture if not. Treatment is 1 year of antituberculous therapy guided by organism sensitivities. Underlying HIV needs to be considered.

Appendix

Glasgow Coma Scale

Introduction

The Glasgow Coma Scale is a simple yet reliable scoring system for measuring a patient's level of consciousness. It is widely used and it is important to be very familiar with it. It is best to record the three elements of the score separately as well as the total (e.g. Eyes 3, Verbal 2, Motor 3: Total 8/15). Remember 3 is the lowest possible score!

	Score
Eyes open	
Spontaneously	4
To verbal stimuli	3
To pain	2
Never	1
Best verbal response	
Orientated and converses	5
Disorientated and converses	4
Inappropriate words	3
Incomprehensible words	2
No response	1
Best motor response	
Obeys commands	6
Localizes pain	5
Flexion – withdrawal to pain	4
Abnormal flexion (decorticate rigidity)	3
Abnormal extension (decerebrate rigidity)	2
No response	1
Total	

Index